T0342492

Controversies in Pediatric Neurosurgery

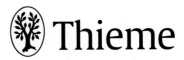

Controversies in Pediatric Neurosurgery

Thieme

Controversies in Pediatric Neurosurgery

George I. Jallo, MD
Associate Professor
Division of Neurosurgery, Pediatrics, and Oncology
Clinical Director
Division of Pediatric Neurosurgery
Director
Neurosurgery Residency Program
The Johns Hopkins Hospital
Baltimore, Maryland

Karl F. Kothbauer, MD
Chief
Division of Neurosurgery, Department of Surgery
General and Pediatric Neurosurgery
Lucerne Cantonal Hospital
Lucerne, Switzerland

Gustavo Pradilla, MD
Resident
Department of Neurosurgery
The Johns Hopkins Hospital
Baltimore, Maryland

Thieme
New York • Stuttgart

Thieme Medical Publishers, Inc.
333 Seventh Ave.
New York, NY 10001

Editorial Director: Michael Wachinger
Executive Editor: Kay Conerly
Editorial Assistant: Dominik Pucek
International Production Director: Andreas Schabert
Production Editor: Richard Rothschild
Vice President, International Sales and Marketing: Cornelia Schulze
Chief Financial Officer: James W. Mitos
President: Brian D. Scanlan
Compositor: Thomson Digital
Printer: Gopsons Papers Ltd.

Library of Congress Cataloging-in-Publication Data

Controversies in pediatric neurosurgery / [edited by] George I. Jallo, Karl F. Kothbauer, Gustavo Pradilla.
      p. ; cm.
   Includes bibliographical references and index.
   ISBN 978-1-60406-074-4 (alk. paper)
   1. Nervous system—Surgery. 2. Children—Surgery. I. Jallo, George I. II. Kothbauer, Karl F. III. Pradilla, Gustavo.
   [DNLM: 1. Neurosurgical Procedures—methods. 2. Child. 3. Infant. 4. Nervous System Diseases—surgery. WL 368 C7647 2010]
   RD593.C598 2010
   617.4'80083—dc22

                                    2009043169

Copyright © 2010 by Thieme Medical Publishers, Inc. This book, including all parts thereof, is legally protected by copyright. Any use, exploitation, or commercialization outside the narrow limits set by copyright legislation without the publisher's consent is illegal and liable to prosecution. This applies in particular to photostat reproduction, copying, mimeographing or duplication of any kind, translating, preparation of microfilms, and electronic data processing and storage.

Important note: Medical knowledge is ever-changing. As new research and clinical experience broaden our knowledge, changes in treatment and drug therapy may be required. The authors and editors of the material herein have consulted sources believed to be reliable in their efforts to provide information that is complete and in accord with the standards accepted at the time of publication. However, in view of the possibility of human error by the authors, editors, or publisher of the work herein or changes in medical knowledge, neither the authors, editors, nor publisher, nor any other party who has been involved in the preparation of this work, warrants that the information contained herein is in every respect accurate or complete, and they are not responsible for any errors or omissions or for the results obtained from use of such information. Readers are encouraged to confirm the information contained herein with other sources. For example, readers are advised to check the product information sheet included in the package of each drug they plan to administer to be certain that the information contained in this publication is accurate and that changes have not been made in the recommended dose or in the contraindications for administration. This recommendation is of particular importance in connection with new or infrequently used drugs.

Some of the product names, patents, and registered designs referred to in this book are in fact registered trademarks or proprietary names even though specific reference to this fact is not always made in the text. Therefore, the appearance of a name without designation as proprietary is not to be construed as a representation by the publisher that it is in the public domain.

Printed in India

5 4 3 2 1

ISBN 978-1-60406-074-4

We thank our families, Michelle, Ingrid, Florian, and Diana, for their patience and support of this endeavor, which made busy schedules busier and long workdays longer. This would not be possible without you.

We also dedicate this book to our mentor, Dr. Fred Epstein, who taught us that if controversy did not exist, then no advances would be made.

Contents

Foreword

Should I be asked what *Controversies in Pediatric Neurosurgery* conveys to the reader, my answer would be a sense of freedom. Aside from independently deriving different ways to approach a given pathologic condition, this sensation of freedom is also generated by the editors' willingness to deny a predetermined conclusion or appropriate answer for each given controversy. Consequently, most of the information is provided in a sort of colloquial way among friends aimed at achieving a unified purpose, rather than a debate of opposing absolutes and incompatible truths. Additionally, the "Lessons Learned" by the editors at the end of each chapter tend to mediate the positions of the contributing authors and likewise individuate the essential points of discussion. Obviously, the intention is to offer the reader a convergent view, rather than to accentuate the dubious.

Generally, one of the main limits and risks a multiauthored volume may suffer from is a quality of unevenness among the various chapters. In many of these cases, editors propend to offer a somewhat rigid scheme for their contributors to adhere to in order to make their book as uniform as possible. This book is unique in that it is evident that the authors enjoyed the opportunity to employ their own style when delivering their message or sharing their personal experience. The lack of a dogmatic attitude by both the editors and the authors amounts to a very readable book with a surprisingly agile architecture apt for conveying and updating information effectively.

The readability of this book is further enhanced by the authors' and editors' shared understanding that an attitude of assured knowledge must be renounced when addressing these controversies, avoiding contraposition, and emphasizing the reasons for the multifaceted approaches often required to treat pediatric neurosurgical conditions. Occasionally, as in the excellent contribution by Albright in Chapter 19, it is expressly declared that the will to avoid considering controversial therapeutic approaches must be challenged in the interest of delivering the best possible care.

The editors have chosen 20 controversial subjects that cover the spectrum of pediatric neurosurgery, including disorders of cerebrospinal fluid dynamics, congenital cranial and spinal malformations, tumors, vascular congenital and acquired disorders, intracranial infections, and intractable epilepsy. These topics certainly belong to those areas of pediatric neurosurgery where treatments still bring doubt and discussion. However, after reading this book, one may wonder whether the essential core of pediatric neurosurgery, or even the entire discipline, should be thought of as controversial, as physiopathogenetic interpretation remains obscure. A controversial spirit could argue that other similarly debated pediatric neurosurgical subjects were not covered. However, considering the excellence of this work as it stands, even such a critic would be compelled to admit that the field might demand a second volume by the same editors, covering the remaining nosographic entities of pediatric neurosurgery whose pathogenesis, not to mention treatment, is quite debatable.

Over the years, controversy has arisen over the advantages and disadvantages of pursuing the specialty of pediatric neurosurgery in comparison with that of general neurosurgery. Almost always, this debate is solicited by general neurosurgeons and might have comprised the first chapter of the book, but luckily we were spared such a fruitless discussion. Indeed, pediatric neurosurgeons appear to have a firm appreciation for the element of controversy inherent in their discipline and do not feel a need to seek some kind of legitimization of purpose. The controversies in pediatric neurosurgery, such as those dealt with in this interesting book, demonstrate unequivocally how open the field is to young and curious minds eager to further develop the specialty. In this respect, the editors should be praised for having chosen to challenge themselves by facing unsolved problems with a flexible discernment, rather than conforming to the status quo by working in a field where the knowledge is already well established, its principles fully accepted.

Concezio Di Rocco
Rome

Preface

"Knowledge is a process of piling up facts; wisdom lies in their simplification."

—*Martin H. Fischer*

Considerable numbers of conditions in pediatric neurosurgery are approached in various ways throughout the world. These different treatment modalities are greatly dependent upon surgical training and experience, location in the world, and available resources. Due to the relatively small numbers of cases and the lack of studies providing hard evidence, considerable debate exists regarding the "correct" way of treating such conditions. The diverse algorithms that pediatric neurosurgeons use to approach patients with Chiari I malformations and tethered cords are perennial subjects of such debate. How aggressive the surgical resection of craniopharyngiomas and ependymomas ought to be is another. We have attempted to address these controversies by inviting opinion leaders in their respective fields to provide their points of view based on the best evidence and the most extensive experience to date. The authors were entirely free to express their viewpoint, while the editors summarized their points in the "Lessons Learned" sections following each subject of controversy, sometimes taking sides, sometimes just framing the open questions, as they remain open.

This book is intended to expose readers to the various strategies available and to assist practitioners in their discussions with patients and their families in an unbiased manner. The book is divided into two sections, intracranial and intraspinal disease processes. We hope that this textbook will serve as a reference with its diverse opinions and approaches for all pediatric neurosurgical diseases. Furthermore, we hope that the "controversies" addressed here will allow us to expand our knowledge and understanding of these conditions.

We are grateful to all contributors for their efforts. Our thanks extend to the editorial team of Kay Conerly, Dominik Pucek, Ivy Ip, and Emma Lassiter at Thieme Medical Publishers for their patience and dedication to the project.

Contributors

Rick Abbott, MD
Professor
Department of Neurosurgery
Division of Clinical Neurosurgery
Children's Hospital at Montefiore
Montefiore Medical Center
New York, New York

A. Leland Albright, MD
Professor
Department of Neurosurgery and Pediatrics
University of Wisconsin School of Medicine
    and Public Health
University of Wisconsin Health Center
Madison, Wisconsin

Richard C. E. Anderson, MD
Assistant Professor
Department of Neurosurgery and Pediatric Neurosurgery
Columbia University Medical Center
New York, New York
Director
Division of Pediatric Neurosurgery
St. Joseph's Children's Hospital
Paterson, New Jersey

Frank J. Attenello, MS
Department of Neurosurgery
The Johns Hopkins University School of Medicine
Baltimore, Maryland

Anthony M. Avellino, MD, MBA, FACS
Professor
Department of Neurological Surgery
Director
University of Washington School of Medicine
    Neurosciences Institute
Harborview Medical Center
Seattle, Washington

Constance M. Barone, MD, FAAP, FACS
Clinical Professor
Department of Neurosurgery
University of Texas Health Science Center at San Antonio
San Antonio, Texas

Ethan A. Benardete, MD, PhD
Assistant Professor
Department of Neurosurgery
SUNY Downstate Medical Center
New York, New York

Su Gülsün Berrak, MD
Associate Professor
Department of Pediatrics
Division of Pediatric Oncology
Marmara University Medical Center
Istanbul, Turkey

Donald J. Blaskiewicz, MD
Department of Neurological Surgery
SUNY Upstate Medical Center
Syracuse, New York

Paolo Bolognese, MD
The Chiari Institute
Harvey Cushing Institutes of Neuroscience
North Shore–Long Island Jewish Health System
Great Neck, New York

Frederick A. Boop, MD
Associate Professor
Department of Neurosurgery
University of Tennessee College of Medicine
Chief
Division of Pediatric Neurosurgery
Le Bonheur Children's Medical Center
Memphis, Tennessee

Ingrid M. Burger, MD, PhD
Radiology Resident
Department of Radiology
University of California–San Francisco
San Francisco, California

Benjamin S. Carson, MD
Professor
Departments of Neurosurgery, Oncology, Plastic Surgery, and Pediatrics
The Johns Hopkins University School of Medicine
Director
Division of Pediatric Neurosurgery
Co-Director
The Johns Hopkins Craniofacial Center
Department of Neurosurgery
The Johns Hopkins Hospital
Baltimore, Maryland

Oğuz Çataltepe, MD
Associate Professor
Departments of Neurosurgery and Pediatrics
University of Massachusetts Medical School
Division of Neurosurgery
UMass Memorial Medical Center
Worcester, Massachusetts

Sid Chandela, MD
Department of Neurosurgery
Albert Einstein College of Medicine
New York, New York

D. Douglas Cochrane, MD, FRCS(C)
Division of Neurosurgery
BC Children's Hospital
Vancouver, Canada

Alan R. Cohen, MD, FACS, FAAP
Reinberger Professor, Chief
Department of Pediatric Neurosurgery
Surgeon-in-Chief
Department of Neurological Surgery
Rainbow Babies and Children's Hospital
Cleveland, Ohio

Shlomi Constantini, MD
Director
Department of Pediatric Neurosurgery
Dana Children's Hospital
Tel Aviv Medical Center
Tel Aviv, Israel

Moise Danielpour, MD
Director
Department of Pediatric Neurosurgery
    and Residency Training
Cedars-Sinai Medical Center
Los Angeles, California

S. Dobson, MD, FRCP(C)
Departments of Surgery and Pediatrics
University of British Columbia
BC Children's Hospital
Vancouver, Canada

Sudesh J. Ebenezer, MD, EdM
Neurosurgeon
Department of Neurosurgery
Providence Health & Services
Olympia, Washington

Richard G. Ellenbogen, MD
Department of Neurological Surgery
University of Washington School of Medicine
Harborview Medical Center
Seattle, Washington

Robert E. Elliott, MD
Resident
Department of Neurosurgery
NYU Medical Center
New York, New York

Philippe Gailloud, MD
Division of Interventional Neuroradiology
The Johns Hopkins Hospital
Baltimore, Maryland

Saadi Ghatan, MD
Columbia University College of Physicians and Surgeons
Children's Hospital of New York
New York, New York

Ronald T. Grondin. MD, MSc, FRCSC
Shillito Neurosurgery Fellow
Department of Neurosurgery
Harvard Medical School
Children's Hospital
Boston, Massachusetts

Nalin Gupta, MD
Assistant Professor
Department of Neurological Surgery
University of California–San Francisco
San Francisco, California

Gregory G. Heuer, MD, PhD
Department of Neurosurgery
University of Pennsylvania
Philadelphia, Pennsylvania

George I. Jallo, MD
Associate Professor
Division of Neurosurgery, Pediatrics, and Oncology
Clinical Director
Division of Pediatric Neurosurgery
Director
Neurosurgery Residency Program
The Johns Hopkins Hospital
Baltimore, Maryland

John A. Jane Jr., MD
Associate Professor
Department of Neurosurgery and Pediatrics
Department of Neurosurgery
University of Virginia Health System
Charlottesville, Virginia

David F. Jimenez, MD, FACS
Professor and Chairman
Department of Neurosurgery
University of Texas Health Science Center–San Antonio
San Antonio, Texas

Nadia Khan, MD
Clinical Instructor, Cerebrovascular Surgery
Department of Neurosurgery
Stanford University Medical Center
Stanford Hospital and Clinics
Stanford, California

Erin N. Kiehna, MD
Neurosurgery Resident
Department of Neurosurgery
University of Virginia Health System
Charlottesville, Virginia

Karl F. Kothbauer, MD
Chief
Division of Neurosurgery, Department of Surgery
General and Pediatric Neurosurgery
Lucerne Cantonal Hospital
Lucerne, Switzerland

Mark D. Krieger, MD
Department of Neurological Surgery
Keck School of Medicine
University of Southern California
Division of Pediatric Neurosurgery
Children's Hospital of Los Angeles
Los Angeles, California

David J. Langer, MD
Assistant Professor
Department of Neurosurgery
Albert Einstein College of Medicine
Director of Cerebrovascular Surgery
Roosevelt Hospital Medical Center
New York, New York

Christopher E. Mandigo, MD
Department of Neurosurgery
Columbia University Medical Center
Neurological Institute
New York, New York

J. Gordon McComb, MD
Department of Neurological Surgery
Keck School of Medicine
University of Southern California
Division of Neurosurgery
Children's Hospital of Los Angeles
Los Angeles, California

Matthew J. McGirt, MD
Division of Neurosurgery
The Johns Hopkins Hospital
Baltimore, Maryland

Thomas E. Merchant, DO, PhD
Chief
Division of Radiation Oncology
St. Jude Children's Research Hospital
Memphis, Tennessee

Thomas H. Milhorat, MD
The Chiari Institute
Harvey Cushing Institutes of Neuroscience
North Shore–Long Island Jewish Health System
Great Neck, New York

Jonathan P. Miller, MD
Director
Department of Functional and Restorative Neurosurgery
Assistant Professor
Department of Neurological Surgery
Case Western Reserve University School of Medicine
University Hospitals of Cleveland
Cleveland, Ohio

W. Jerry Oakes, MD
Section of Pediatric Neurosurgery
Division of Neurosurgery
Children's Hospital
Birmingham, Alabama

M. Memet Özek, MD
Professor
Department of Neurosurgery
Division of Pediatric Neurosurgery
Marmara University Medical Center
Istanbul, Turkey

Monica S. Pearl, MD
Fellow
Division of Interventional Neuroradiology
The Johns Hopkins Hospital
Baltimore, Maryland

David W. Pincus, MD, PhD
Associate Professor
Department of Neurosurgery and Pediatrics
University of Florida Medical School
Gainesville, Florida

Gustavo Pradilla, MD
Resident
Department of Neurosurgery
The Johns Hopkins Hospital
Baltimore, Maryland

Mark R. Proctor, MD
Assistant Professor
Department of Neurosurgery
Harvard Medical School
Division of Neurosurgery
Children's Hospital
Boston, Massachusetts

Jeffrey A. Pugh, MD, MSc, FRCSC
Assistant Professor
Department of Surgery
University of Alberta Faculty of Medicine
Division of Neurological Surgery and Pediatric Surgery
University of Alberta Hospital and Stollery Children's
    Hospital
Mackenzie Health Sciences Centre
Edmonton, Canada

Harold L. Rekate, MD
Chairman
Department of Pediatric Neurosciences
Barrow Neurological Institute
St. Joseph's Hospital and Medical Center
Phoenix, Arizona

Sandrine de Ribaupierre, MD
Assistant Professor
University of Western Ontario Schulich School of Medicine
Division of Neurosurgery
London Health Sciences Centre
Victoria Hospital
London, Canada

Bénédict Rilliet, MD
Service of Neurosurgery
Centre Hospitalier Universitaire Vaudois
Lausanne, Switzerland

James N. Rogers, MD
Professor
Department of Anesthesiology
University of Texas Health Science Center at San Antonio
San Antonio, Texas

Chan Roonprapunt, MD, PhD
Assistant Professor
Department of Neurosurgery
Albert Einstein College of Medicine
Roosevelt and Beth Israel Medical Centers
New York, New York

Jonathan Roth, MD
Department of Pediatric Neurosurgery
Dana Children's Hospital
Tel Aviv Medical Center
Tel Aviv, Israel

David I. Sandberg, MD
Associate Professor
Department of Neurological Surgery
University of Miami School of Medicine
Division of Clinical Neurological Surgery and Pediatrics
Miami Children's Hospital
Miami, Florida

Daniel M. Sciubba, MD
Assistant Professor
Department of Neurosurgery
The Johns Hopkins University School of Medicine
Division of Neurosurgery
The Johns Hopkins Hospital
Baltimore, Maryland

R. Michael Scott, MD
Neurosurgeon-in-Chief
Children's Hospital
Boston, Massachusetts

Spyros Sgouros, MD
Professor
Department of Neurosurgery
Attikon University Hospital
Athens, Greece

Ali Shirzadi, MD
Resident Physician
Department of Neurosurgery
Cedars-Sinai Medical Center
Los Angeles, California

Oliver Simmons, MD
Division of Pediatric Plastic Surgery
The Johns Hopkins Hospital
Baltimore, Maryland

Edward R. Smith, MD
Assistant Professor
Harvard Medical School
Assistant in Neurosurgery
Division of Neurosurgery
Children's Hospital
Boston, Massachusetts

Paul Steinbok, MD
Professor
University of British Columbia
Head
Division of Pediatric Neurosurgery
BC Children's Hospital
Vancouver, Canada

Phillip B. Storm, MD
Division of Neurosurgery
Children's Hospital of Philadelphia
Philadelphia, Pennsylvania

Charles Teo, MD, MBBS, FRACS
Director
Centre for Minimally Invasive Neurosurgery
Prince of Wales Private Hospital
Sydney, Australia

Ulrich W. Thomale, MD
Selbständiger Arbeitsbereich Pädiatrische Neurochirurgie
Charité, Campus Virchow Klinikum
Berlin, Germany

Dominic N. P. Thompson, FRCS
Department of Neurosurgery
Great Ormond Street Hospital for Children NHS Trust
London, England

R. Shane Tubbs, PhD
Section of Pediatric Neurosurgery
Division of Neurosurgery
Children's Hospital
Birmingham, Alabama

Olivier Vernet, MD
Service of Neurosurgery
Centre Hospitalier Universitaire Vaudois
Lausanne, Switzerland

John C. Wellons III, MD
Associate Professor
Department of Neurosurgery and Pediatrics
University of Alabama at Birmingham
Section of Pediatric Neurosurgery
Division of Neurosurgery
Children's Hospital
Birmingham, Alabama

Jeffrey H. Wisoff, MD
Associate Professor
Department of Neurosurgery and Pediatrics
Division of Pediatric Neurosurgery
NYU Medical Center
New York, New York

David A. Yam, MD
Resident Physician
Department of Neurosurgery
University of Tennessee
Le Bonheur Children's Medical Center
Memphis, Tennessee

Yasuhiro Yonekawa, MD
Professor Emeritus
University of Zurich
Neurosurgeon
Klinik im Park
Zurich, Switzerland

Gabriel Zada, MD
Department of Neurological Surgery
Keck School of Medicine
University of Southern California
Division of Neurosurgery
Children's Hospital Los Angeles
Los Angeles, California

Controversies in Pediatric Neurosurgery

Controversies in Pediatric Neurosurgery

I Intracranial

1 Arachnoid Cysts

♦ Cystoperitoneal Shunting

Gabriel Zada and Mark D. Krieger

Arachnoid cysts are developmental anomalies occurring between layers of the arachnoid membrane that are frequently encountered in pediatric patients. Often they are discovered incidentally and remain clinically silent. In a minority of cases, however, arachnoid cysts can cause symptoms via mass effect on surrounding structures, spontaneous rupture or hemorrhage, or obstruction of cerebrospinal fluid (CSF) outflow pathways. They have been associated with a wide spectrum of clinical presentations in pediatric patients, including headaches, macrocephaly, hydrocephalus, seizures, and motor/developmental delays.[1–6]

Patient evaluation is a key factor in the management of arachnoid cysts, as a majority of these lesions can be managed conservatively with sequential imaging. In the past, the optimal initial management of symptomatic arachnoid cysts requiring surgical intervention has been debated. Although several options for treating arachnoid cysts have been used in the past, by far the two most frequently used modalities have been CSF shunting procedures, such as cystoperitoneal shunting, and craniotomy with fenestration of the cyst membrane.[5] Either shunting or fenestration can be employed as a primary procedure, and each approach carries with it its own set of risks and benefits. Both procedures clearly have a useful role in the management of arachnoid cysts, and the optimal management of pediatric patients is likely more contingent on knowing when to use the correct procedure. Fenestration offers the clear benefit of potentially rendering patients shunt independent for life, yet it is unsuccessful in a certain proportion of cases. Cystoperitoneal shunting is usually relied on as a definitive backup measure when fenestration is unsuccessful or as a primary treatment for arachnoid cysts when there is clear evidence of coexisting hydrocephalus.

Benefits of Cystoperitoneal Shunt Procedures

Shunt procedures have been used as a treatment for arachnoid cysts for decades. Although cystoperitoneal shunts remain the most commonly performed diversion procedure for treating arachnoid cysts, other shunt procedures, such as ventriculoperitoneal, cystoventriculoperitoneal, cystocisternal, and cystoventricular shunts, have been used by some surgeons.[7–9] CSF fluid shunting procedures offer several advantages over open craniotomy with fenestration for the treatment of arachnoid cysts. Foremost, the overall success rate of cystoperitoneal shunt procedures in decreasing the size of arachnoid cysts and reducing mass effect on surrounding structures is higher than in major reported series of craniotomy and fenestration.[1,4,10,11] Nevertheless, fenestration procedures are frequently attempted by many centers because a major emphasis is placed on shunt avoidance, if possible.

It has been theorized that cystoperitoneal shunts address the underlying problem relating to arachnoid cysts and a potential underlying mechanism for their expansion, namely impaired CSF flow dynamics. Furthermore, shunt procedures are frequently required following attempted craniotomy with fenestration, whether in the form of a cystoperitoneal shunt, ventriculoperitoneal shunt, or subdural-peritoneal shunt[3,12] (**Fig. 1.1**). The rate of shunt dependence following craniotomy with fenestration has been reported as 43 to 80% in larger series.[2,9,10,13] A study by Ciricillo et al reported that 12 of 15 children (80%) treated initially with fenestration were shunt dependent following surgery.[10] A previous study from our institution reported an overall postfenestration shunt dependence rate of 55%.[9]

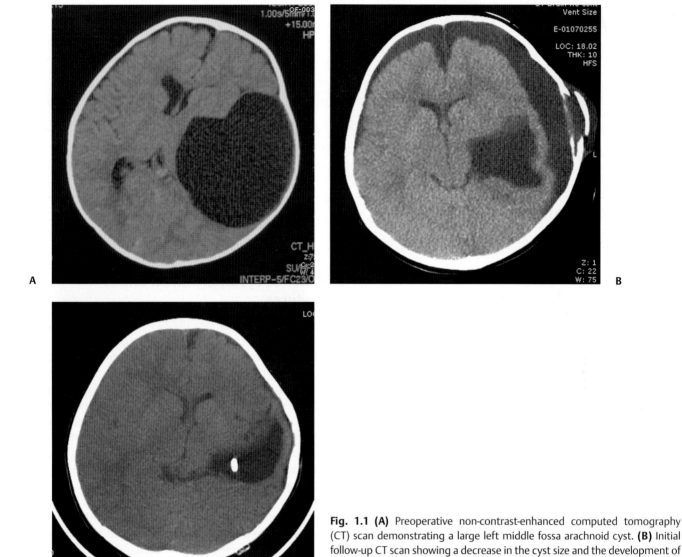

Fig. 1.1 (A) Preoperative non-contrast-enhanced computed tomography (CT) scan demonstrating a large left middle fossa arachnoid cyst. **(B)** Initial follow-up CT scan showing a decrease in the cyst size and the development of subdural hygromas. **(C)** Follow-up CT scan obtained after placement of a cystoperitoneal shunt revealing improvements in the cyst size and hygromas.

The requirement for shunting following fenestration depends significantly on the presence or absence of hydrocephalus.[2,9,13] Most authors are in agreement that patients with hydrocephalus and an arachnoid cyst will require a shunt procedure[1,2,9,10,13,14] (**Fig. 1.2**). Along the same lines, infants with arachnoid cysts presenting with macrocephaly, without underlying hydrocephalus, are also significantly more likely to be shunt dependent following a fenestration procedure.[13] A more recent study from our institution assessed the rate of postcraniotomy shunt dependence for patients younger than 2 years of age with arachnoid cysts, when grouped by clinical presentation. The proportion of postfenestration shunt dependency according to patients' clinical presentation was 83% in patients with hydrocephalus,

57% in patients with macrocephaly, and 7% in patients presenting with all other symptoms (p = .0039, two-tailed Fisher's exact test).[13] These findings suggest that patients presenting with arachnoid cysts and macrocephaly without ventriculomegaly (in addition to patients with hydrocephalus) have an underlying aberrancy with CSF flow and absorption, perhaps resulting in a forme fruste state of hydrocephalus. Of note, some authors have reported that an even more influential factor than the type of surgical intervention used in determining the success rate of treatment is the location of the cyst.[10,15]

Some surgeons have indicated that a major goal in the treatment of arachnoid cysts is establishing equilibration of intracystal pressure with intraventricular pressure. For this

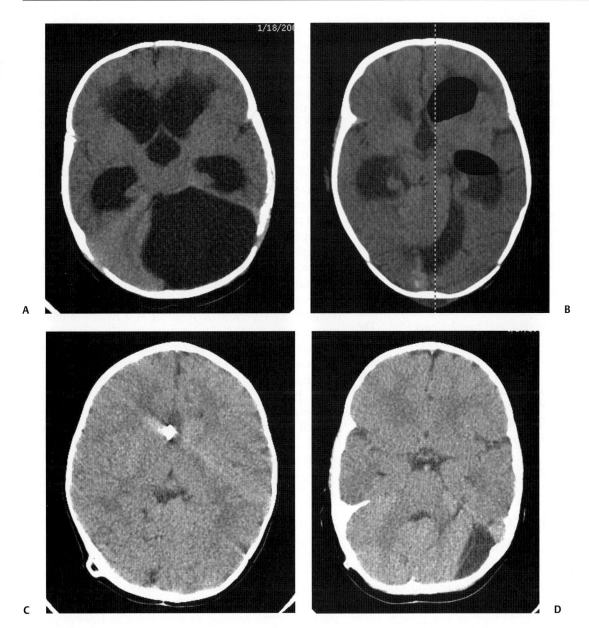

Fig. 1.2 (A) Initial non-contrast-enhanced CT scan exhibiting a posterior fossa cyst and hydrocephalus. **(B)** Postoperative CT scan obtained after fenestration showing improvement in the cyst size as well as ventriculomegaly. **(C,D)** Follow-up CT scans revealing the patient's status following placement of a ventriculoperitoneal shunt.

reason, some reports have stated that cystoperitoneal shunts do not adequately restore physiologic intracranial pressure but instead result in overdrainage of the cyst compartment.[16] This dynamic, of course, depends in part on the valve system that is employed in the cystoperitoneal shunt system. One concern that has been raised with the use of shunt systems is rapid overdrainage of arachnoid cysts, potentially resulting in extra-axial hematomas.[17,18] Similarly, many authors have reported that complete obliteration of a cyst is not required to achieve improvement in patients' symptoms, but that a small decrease in cyst size is usually sufficient in doing so.[8] In recent years, programmable shunt valves have been increasingly used with excellent surgical results, potentially due to the regulated, gradual reduction offered by these systems.[17,19–21] Some authors have advocated cystoventriculoperitoneal diversion procedures in an effort to equilibrate the intracystal and intraventricular pressures.[4,14] Others have been less supportive of this technique, given the more complex Y-shaped connection requirement and the need for additional catheter insertion.[2,8] In an effort to restore the communication between all intracranial CSF spaces, some surgeons have advocated the use of cystoventricular shunt systems with acceptable surgical results in patients without hydrocephalus.[7,8]

Risks of Cystoperitoneal Shunt Procedures

In addition to often being the more definitive procedure for the management of arachnoid cysts, cystoperitoneal shunt procedures are associated with a relatively low risk profile.[4,10,22–24] The risks of cystoperitoneal shunt insertion or revision are generally reported as being lower than for craniotomy with fenestration.[4,10,11,25] Shunt insertion for arachnoid cysts is generally a less invasive procedure than craniotomy with fenestration, although endoscopic fenestration and the use of adjunct neuronavigation have certainly provided minimally invasive fenestration of cysts in recent years.[15,26,27] Open craniotomy for cyst fenestration has been associated with a higher risk profile and has been reported to cause postoperative complications, including hemiparesis, cranial nerve palsies, hypothalamic injury, increased seizure frequency, and postoperative hematomas.[2,3,10,12,28,29]

Shunt procedures, however, carry with them the lifelong burden of shunt dependence and associated potential risks, such as infection, malfunction, and overdrainage.[1,4,10,23] The rate of subsequent revision for cystoperitoneal or associated shunts has been reported as 10 to 50%.[1,2,4,9–11] Undoubtedly, a minority of patients will require multiple shunt revisions. In one large series of 77 patients treated with cystoperitoneal shunts, 8 patients (10%) experienced a total of 12 shunt malfunctions over a mean follow-up time of 7.7 years.[1] The mean time to shunt malfunction following shunt operation was 4.8 years.

It has been noted that successful cystoperitoneal shunting can lead to opposition and eventual scarring of the arachnoid membranes, resulting in obliteration of the cyst.[1,10] In these cases, subsequent shunt malfunction may not result in reexpansion of the cyst or recurrence of symptoms. Arai et al noted that the degree of long-term shunt dependency was related to the size of the cyst, with larger cysts being more likely to present with shunt malfunction and intracranial hypertension.[1] Furthermore, they reported successful removal of cystoperitoneal shunts without cyst recurrence in 12 cases, with a mean follow-up time of 3.3 years.

In conclusion, patients with symptomatic arachnoid cysts can be treated with a variety of surgical interventions. Each patient must be assessed on an individual basis in regard to the requirement for surgery and the optimal first-line intervention. Key factors in this decision-making process include the location and size of the cyst, the proximity to adjacent cisternal spaces, and the presence or absence of hydrocephalus. Cystoperitoneal shunting is a relatively low-risk and effective method of treating arachnoid cysts, especially in cases of unsuccessful fenestration and in patients with hydrocephalus. Given the major emphasis placed on shunt avoidance at our institution, fenestration remains a preferred primary treatment in patients with symptomatic cysts, especially in those without hydrocephalus and macrocephaly. Nevertheless, cystoperitoneal shunting remains a useful, often definitive procedure in the management of pediatric arachnoid cysts.

♦ Open or Endoscopic Fenestration

Jeffrey A. Pugh and John C. Wellons III

Arachnoid cysts are the most common nontraumatic intracranial lesions, with a reported frequency as high as 1 in 1000. First recognized in 1831, they can present with headaches, seizures, accelerated head growth, or associated hydrocephalus; however, given the relatively higher frequency in autopsy studies, most are asymptomatic.[30] As such, the natural history of arachnoid cysts is poorly understood, with reports in the literature of both spontaneous resolution and progressive enlargement.[31–33] Furthermore, the pathophysiology of arachnoid cysts is not well understood. Most theories center on a gradual accumulation of CSF into a congenitally abnormal compartment via a "ball-valve" effect. Oftentimes, areas thought to be arachnoid cysts may in actuality be regions of periventricular encephalomalacia following perinatal infarction and may respond to standard CSF diversion (i.e., ventriculoperitoneal shunting or endoscopic third ventriculostomy). Alternatively, loculated fluid collections resulting from intraventricular adhesions, more common in children with hydrocephalus

due to intraventricular hemorrhage of prematurity or meningitis, may also occur. This discussion will center on arachnoid cysts believed to be congenital; however, many of the same surgical principles may be extrapolated for secondary pathology.

Galassi et al classified arachnoid cysts of the middle cranial fossa based on imaging characteristics and clinical response to surgical management.[34] Type I cysts communicate with the subarachnoid cisterns, are often incidental findings, and frequently do not require treatment. Type II cysts may or may not communicate with adjacent cisterns and are more likely to require treatment. Type III cysts do not communicate with the subarachnoid space, cause local mass effect, are more often symptomatic, and require surgical management.[34] Di Rocco et al monitored local intracranial pressure (ICP) in patients with middle fossa arachnoid cysts and found constantly elevated pressure in patients with type III cysts in contrast to normal pressure in patients with type I cysts. In patients with type II cysts, recording elevated ICP assisted in surgical decision making in their series.[35]

Intraventricular, suprasellar, quadrigeminal plate, and posterior fossa arachnoid cysts present additional surgical challenges due to location and proximity to delicate neurovascular structures. Additionally, cysts in these locations are more likely to present with associated hydrocephalus and as such were commonly managed by ventriculoperitoneal shunting. The wide variability in clinical presentation of arachnoid cysts further complicates a systematic approach to best management.

Early studies evaluating the best treatment for arachnoid cysts demonstrated that ventriculoperitoneal or cystoperitoneal shunting was associated with fewer serious complications and best overall outcome.[36-40] Harsh et al reviewed their experience managing intracranial arachnoid cysts in 16 pediatric patients.[36] Five of nine patients treated by craniotomy and cyst fenestration into the basal cisterns demonstrated recurrence, in contrast to successful reduction in cyst size and clinical improvement in all seven patients treated by cystoperitoneal shunting primarily and all four patients who underwent secondary cystoperitoneal shunting after failed fenestration. Ciricillo et al reported similarly poor success rates for primary cyst fenestration.[37] Only 3 of 15 patients experienced long-term benefit from cyst fenestration. In seven patients with middle fossa arachnoid cysts treated by cyst shunting, all experienced clinical improvement, and none required revision, whereas 6 of 14 patients with cysts in other locations required shunt revision for cyst recurrence.

In some patients the presence of an arachnoid cyst may be an indication of a more widespread imbalance in CSF physiology. Patients with progressive macrocephaly and/or hydrocephalus in association with a middle fossa arachnoid cyst are probably the best candidates for ventricular or cyst shunting.[41] Raffel and McComb and later Fewel et al demonstrated that patients presenting without hydrocephalus do better with cyst fenestration alone compared with those patients with hydrocephalus.[42,43] Two thirds of patients with hydrocephalus required prior or subsequent cystoperitoneal or ventriculoperitoneal shunting. Zada et al later reported on their experience with cyst fenestration in patients younger than 2 years of age.[44] They found that five out of six (83%) patients with hydrocephalus were shunt dependent and that 57% of patients with nonspecific macrocephaly required a subsequent shunt. This is in contrast to successful fenestration as the only treatment in 14 of 15 patients without hydrocephalus or macrocephaly. An important note is that 55% of shunts placed during this study required revision during a median follow-up of 33 months, demonstrating the complicated CSF flow dynamics in these patients.[44]

Although shunting procedures have demonstrated improved outcome, CSF shunt systems continue to have early risks of overdrainage and foreign body infection, as well as long-term risks of shunt malfunction and cyst recurrence. Unfortunately, advances in shunt technology, including programmable valves, have not made a significant impact in the rate of these complications. In contrast, improvements in microsurgical techniques, neuroimaging, and neuroendoscopy have markedly decreased the complications associated with surgical management of arachnoid cysts and offer patients the opportunity for shunt freedom.[45-54]

In the past cyst location was an important factor in directing surgeons toward fenestration versus shunting. Middle fossa arachnoid cysts frequently underwent open surgical excision and marsupialization with additional fenestration of the deep wall into the basal cisterns. Thus, either a major intracranial or a cystoperitoneal shunt procedure was performed. As such the early advantage as far as complication rate and morbidity were concerned understandably favored shunting procedures. As more minimally invasive procedures were developed, the complication rates for surgical management became more alike. To avoid the long-term complications associated with shunting, open and now endoscopic surgical fenestration has become the favored approach.

One criticism of cyst wall excision and marsupialization, particularly of large middle fossa arachnoid cysts, is the risk of subdural hygroma or hematoma formation.[55] In the absence of adequate fenestration into the basal cisterns, cyst fluid accumulates in the subdural space, which communicates poorly with any sites for CSF absorption. Kang et al demonstrated that excision of the cyst wall and fenestration into the basal cisterns was more successful than shunting (79% vs 66%); however, in their study, neither of two patients who had cyst wall excision without fenestration improved.[56] In an attempt to reduce the risk of subdural fluid collections, Elhammady et al performed transcortical endoscopic fenestration of middle fossa arachnoid cysts into the basal cisterns.[57] In their small series, two of three patients with direct access to the arachnoid cyst developed significant subdural fluid collections in comparison to one of three patients undergoing transcortical fenestration who developed a small fluid collection that resolved spontaneously. Minimally invasive approaches through keyhole craniotomies with the aim to minimize disruption of the superficial cyst wall and maximize the fenestration into the basal cisterns have proven to be more successful.[48,58-61] Levy et al demonstrated a decrease in cyst size in 82% of patients using standard microsurgical instruments via a microcraniotomy to obtain wide fenestration of the basal cisterns.[61] Godano et al employed the neuroendoscope to improve visualization of the deep cyst membrane while working with standard microsurgical instruments alongside the endoscope, demonstrating complete resolution of symptoms in 11 of 12 patients.[48]

As endoscopic equipment and techniques evolve, minimally invasive management of the arachnoid cysts will continue to be performed with greater success and fewer complications. Greenfield and Souweidane have reported successful endoscopic cyst fenestration in 32 of 33 patients.[49] The one failure in their series responded to a second endoscopic fenestration, demonstrating that in appropriately selected patients, cyst fenestration can safely and effectively treat arachnoid cysts without the need for shunting.

Prepontine or suprasellar cysts were probably underappreciated as a cause of hydrocephalus before widespread use of magnetic resonance imaging (MRI).[62] Once these cysts became recognized, treatment still centered on management of the hydrocephalus because surgical excision or fenestration of these cysts was technically challenging and associated with significant morbidity.[63] With advancements in neuroendoscopy, suprasellar cysts have become more accessible.[64–66] Gangemi et al summarized the results of 176 patients with suprasellar arachnoid cysts from their review of the literature.[67] They reported that 90% of patients were successfully treated by endoscopic cyst fenestration into the third ventricle and prepontine cistern compared with 81% success by other surgical interventions (cyst resection, shunting, or percutaneous ventriculocystostomy). We approach the endoscopic management of suprasellar arachnoid cysts as having three surgical steps: fenestration into the roof of the cyst, fenestration through the floor of the cyst into the prepontine cistern, and coagulation shrinkage of the cyst wall until the anatomy of the third ventricle is restored and the cerebral aqueduct can be visualized. Di Rocco et al reported on the resolution of clinical symptoms in 12 patients undergoing endoscopic ventriculocystostomy, with or without third ventriculostomy, despite radiographic improvement in only 9 out of 12.[47] Wang et al successfully treated six patients with dual fenestration and confirmed active CSF flow and patency of all fenestrations with MRI.[62] These reports demonstrate the safety of endoscopic cyst fenestration but do not address the long-term success or rather the potential for cyst recurrence. Cyst recurrence and obstruction of the cerebral aqueduct are the main reasons for failure of simple endoscopic cyst fenestration. Coagulation shrinkage of the cyst wall, though opening up CSF pathways, is criticized for the risk of thermal injury to the hypothalamus. Sood et al reported on one child who developed precocious puberty following cyst wall coagulation in eight patients.[68] The remaining seven patients did not demonstrate any hypothalamic dysfunction following this procedure.

Arachnoid cysts in the posterior fossa and the quadrigeminal cistern frequently present with hydrocephalus due to compression of the cerebral aqueduct, cerebellum, and fourth ventricular outflow. Cysts in these locations are perhaps the most difficult to manage through a microsurgical approach. Advances in neuroendoscopic techniques have made cyst fenestration safer. Quadrigeminal plate or pineal region cysts can be approached via the posterior wall of the third ventricle, fenestrating the cyst into the ventricular system and performing an endoscopic third ventriculostomy at the same time. Alternatively, an occipital bur hole approach over the superior cerebellar surface provides minimally invasive access to these cysts. Similarly, retrocerebellar cysts and cerebellopontine angle (CPA) arachnoid cysts can be approached through minimally invasive occipital or retrosigmoid bur holes. The neuroendoscope provides superior illumination of the deep surface of such cysts, enabling fenestration into the basal cisterns. Direct cyst fenestration has been shown to reduce cyst size, restoring native CSF circulation pathways and relieving hydrocephalus without the need for cyst or ventricular shunts.[69–73]

Conclusion

Improvements in neuroimaging, microsurgical techniques, image-guided surgery, and neuroendoscopy have all contributed to lowering the complication rate of arachnoid cyst excision, marsupialization, and fenestration, as well as improving the efficacy of treating these cysts. However, the best management of intracranial arachnoid cysts remains uncertain. Given the well-recognized complications of shunts (specifically, overdrainage, malfunction, and infection), our preference is to find solutions that enable patients to be shunt independent. The pathophysiology of arachnoid cysts is not well understood and is likely not uniform across cysts of different locations, size, and presenting symptoms. Certainly, it is possible, even likely, that middle fossa arachnoid cysts presenting with hydrocephalus or macrocephaly have an underlying derangement of CSF dynamics. For these patients, shunt independence is particularly challenging to accomplish. However, a minimally invasive endoscopic cyst fenestration is very appropriate as the first approach to manage these patients in the hope that they may enjoy shunt freedom. If this fails to alleviate symptoms, a cystoperitoneal or ventriculoperitoneal shunt can be placed secondarily. Patients with middle fossa arachnoid cysts presenting with headaches, seizures, or focal neurologic deficits are well served by cyst fenestration, with the majority experiencing symptom relief without the need for shunting. Hydrocephalus associated with arachnoid cysts in other locations has been shown to be very effectively treated by cyst fenestration and third ventriculostomy. These patients are well managed by restoring natural CSF pathways and eliminating the need for shunts. As technological advances continue to enable more and more minimally invasive surgical approaches with improved visualization and better microsurgical and endoscopic instruments, the management of patients with intracranial arachnoid cysts will continue to improve and enable more patients to benefit from symptom resolution and shunt independence.

◆ Lessons Learned

Arachnoid cysts are a superb example of how much our decision preferences are influenced by certain preformed concepts.

Most of us have a strong preference to avoid shunts, as we are all experiencing the downsides of shunting with those patients who continue to come back with the next shunt malfunction.

Therefore, the treatment of arachnoid cysts without shunts of several types is greatly preferred. Indeed the open, endoscopic, or endoscope-assisted fenestration of arachnoid cysts of various locations has improved with time.

Nonetheless, as Zada and Krieger have nicely outlined, the shunting of arachnoid cysts is actually more effective than fenestration. Both articles outline the important pretreatment aspects: the most important one is to identify those patients who are likely to experience complications from or failure of shunting. These are patients with concomitant hydrocephalus and infants with macrocephaly and a cyst. Treating these patients with fenestration alone is probably justified only when an adequate treatment of hydrocephalus with endoscopic third ventriculostomy is possible. If not, it may be better to just go for a shunt right away.

References

1. Arai H, Sato K, Wachi A, Okuda O, Takeda N. Arachnoid cysts of the middle cranial fossa: experience with 77 patients who were treated with cystoperitoneal shunting. Neurosurgery 1996;39(6):1108–1112, discussion 1112–1113

2. Fewel ME, Levy ML, McComb JG. Surgical treatment of 95 children with 102 intracranial arachnoid cysts. Pediatr Neurosurg 1996;25(4):165–173

3. Galassi E, Gaist G, Giuliani G, Pozzati E. Arachnoid cysts of the middle cranial fossa: experience with 77 cases treated surgically. Acta Neurochir Suppl (Wien) 1988;42:201–204

4. Harsh GR IV, Edwards MS, Wilson CB. Intracranial arachnoid cysts in children. J Neurosurg 1986;64(6):835–842

5. Oberbauer RW, Haase J, Pucher R. Arachnoid cysts in children: a European co-operative study. Childs Nerv Syst 1992;8(5):281–286

6. Rengachary SS, Watanabe I, Brackett CE. Pathogenesis of intracranial arachnoid cysts. Surg Neurol 1978;9(2):139–144

7. D'Angelo V, Gorgoglione L, Catapano G. Treatment of symptomatic intracranial arachnoid cysts by stereotactic cyst-ventricular shunting. Stereotact Funct Neurosurg 1999;72(1):62–69

8. McBride LA, Winston KR, Freeman JE. Cystoventricular shunting of intracranial arachnoid cysts. Pediatr Neurosurg 2003;39(6):323–329

9. Raffel C, McComb JG. To shunt or to fenestrate: which is the best surgical treatment for arachnoid cysts in pediatric patients? Neurosurgery 1988;23(3):338–342

10. Ciricillo SF, Cogen PH, Harsh GR, Edwards MS. Intracranial arachnoid cysts in children: a comparison of the effects of fenestration and shunting. J Neurosurg 1991;74(2):230–235

11. Stein SC. Intracranial developmental cysts in children: treatment by cystoperitoneal shunting. Neurosurgery 1981;8(6):647–650

12. Anderson FM, Segall HD, Caton WL. Use of computerized tomography scanning in supratentorial arachnoid cysts: a report on 20 children and four adults. J Neurosurg 1979;50(3):333–338

13. Zada G, Krieger MD, McNatt SA, Bowen I, McComb JG. Pathogenesis and treatment of intracranial arachnoid cysts in pediatric patients younger than 2 years of age. Neurosurg Focus 2007;22(2):E1

14. Serlo W, von Wendt L, Heikkinen E, Saukkonen AL, Heikkinen E, Nystrom S. Shunting procedures in the management of intracranial cerebrospinal fluid cysts in infancy and childhood. Acta Neurochir (Wien) 1985;76(3–4):111–116

15. Karabatsou K, Hayhurst C, Buxton N, O'Brien DF, Mallucci CL. Endoscopic management of arachnoid cysts: an advancing technique. J Neurosurg 2007;106(6, Suppl):455–462

16. Aoki N, Sakai T, Umezawa Y. Slit ventricle syndrome after cyst-peritoneal shunting for the treatment of intracranial arachnoid cyst. Childs Nerv Syst 1990;6(1):41–43

17. Germanò A, Caruso G, Caffo M, et al. The treatment of large supra-tentorial arachnoid cysts in infants with cyst-peritoneal shunting and Hakim programmable valve. Childs Nerv Syst 2003;19(3):166–173

18. Wester K. Arachnoid cysts in adults: experience with internal shunts to the subdural compartment. Surg Neurol 1996;45(1):15–24

19. Belliard H, Roux FX, Turak B, Nataf F, Devaux B, Cioloca C. [The Codman Medos programmable shunt valve: evaluation of 53 implantations in 50 patients.] Neurochirurgie 1996;42(3):139–145, discussion 145–146

20. Reinprecht A, Czech T, Dietrich W. Clinical experience with a new pressure-adjustable shunt valve. Acta Neurochir (Wien) 1995;134(3–4):119–124

21. Zemack G, Romner B. Seven years of clinical experience with the programmable Codman Hakim valve: a retrospective study of 583 patients. J Neurosurg 2000;92(6):941–948

22. Kaplan BJ, Mickle JP, Parkhurst R. Cystoperitoneal shunting for congenital arachnoid cysts. Childs Brain 1984;11(5):304–311

23. Kim SK, Cho BK, Chung YN, Kim HS, Wang KC. Shunt dependency in shunted arachnoid cyst: a reason to avoid shunting. Pediatr Neurosurg 2002;37(4):178–185

24. Locatelli D, Bonfanti N, Sfogliarini R, Gajno TM, Pezzotta S. Arachnoid cysts: diagnosis and treatment. Childs Nerv Syst 1987;3(2):121–124

25. Sprung C, Mauersberger W. Value of computed tomography for the diagnosis of arachnoid cysts and assessment of surgical treatment. Acta Neurochir Suppl (Wien) 1979;28(2):619–626

26. Elhammady MS, Bhatia S, Ragheb J. Endoscopic fenestration of middle fossa arachnoid cysts: a technical description and case series. Pediatr Neurosurg 2007;43(3):209–215

27. Wang JC, Heier L, Souweidane MM. Advances in the endoscopic management of suprasellar arachnoid cysts in children. J Neurosurg 2004;100(5, Suppl Pediatrics):418–426

28. Aicardi J, Bauman F. Supratentorial extracerebral cysts in infants and children. J Neurol Neurosurg Psychiatry 1975;38(1):57–68

29. Garcia-Bach M, Isamat F, Vila F. Intracranial arachnoid cysts in adults. Acta Neurochir Suppl (Wien) 1988;42:205–209

30. Boop FA, Teo C. Congenital intracranial cysts. In: McLone DG, ed. Pediatric Neurosurgery, Surgery of the Developing Nervous System. 4rth ed. Philadelpia: WB Saunders; 2001:489–498

31. McDonald PJ, Rutka JT. Middle cranial fossa arachnoid cysts that come and go: report of two cases and review of the literature. Pediatr Neurosurg 1997;26(1):48–52

32. Rao G, Anderson RC, Feldstein NA, Brockmeyer DL. Expansion of arachnoid cysts in children: report of two cases and review of the literature. J Neurosurg 2005;102(3, Suppl):314–317

33. Artico M, Cervoni L, Salvati M, Fiorenza F, Caruso R. Supratentorial arachnoid cysts: clinical and therapeutic remarks on 46 cases. Acta Neurochir (Wien) 1995;132(1–3):75–78

34. Galassi E, Gaist G, Giuliani G, Pozzati E. Arachnoid cysts of the middle cranial fossa: experience with 77 cases treated surgically. Acta Neurochir Suppl (Wien) 1988;42:201–204

35. Di Rocco C, Tamburrini G, Caldarelli M, Velardi F, Santini P. Prolonged ICP monitoring in sylvian arachnoid cysts. Surg Neurol 2003; 60(3): 211–218

36. Harsh GR IV, Edwards MS, Wilson CB. Intracranial arachnoid cysts in children. J Neurosurg 1986;64(6):835–842

37. Ciricillo SF, Cogen PH, Harsh GR, Edwards MS. Intracranial arachnoid cysts in children: a comparison of the effects of fenestration and shunting. J Neurosurg 1991;74(2):230–235

38. Pascual-Castroviejo I, Roche MC, Martínez Bermejo A, Arcas J, García Blázquez M. Primary intracranial arachnoidal cysts: a study of 67 childhood cases. Childs Nerv Syst 1991;7(5):257–263

39. Voormolen JH. Arachnoid cysts of the middle cranial fossa: surgical management for headache. Clin Neurol Neurosurg 1992;94(Suppl): S176–S179

40. Jamjoom ZA. Intracranial arachnoid cysts: treatment alternatives and outcome in a series of 25 patients. Ann Saudi Med 1997; 17(3): 288–292

41. Levy ML, Meltzer HS, Hughes S, Aryan HE, Yoo K, Amar AP. Hydrocephalus in children with middle fossa arachnoid cysts. J Neurosurg 2004;101(1, Suppl):25–31

42. Fewel ME, Levy ML, McComb JG. Surgical treatment of 95 children with 102 intracranial arachnoid cysts. Pediatr Neurosurg 1996;25(4): 165–173

43. Raffel C, McComb JG. To shunt or to fenestrate: which is the best surgical treatment for arachnoid cysts in pediatric patients? Neurosurgery 1988;23(3):338–342

44. Zada G, Krieger MD, McNatt SA, Bowen I, McComb JG. Pathogenesis and treatment of intracranial arachnoid cysts in pediatric patients younger than 2 years of age. Neurosurg Focus 2007;22(2):E1

45. Boutarbouch M, El Ouahabi A, Rifi L, Arkha Y, Derraz S, El Khamlichi A. Management of intracranial arachnoid cysts: institutional experience with initial 32 cases and review of the literature. Clin Neurol Neurosurg 2008;110(1):1–7

46. Daneyemez M, Gezen F, Akbörü M, Sirin S, Ocal E. Presentation and management of supratentorial and infratentorial arachnoid cysts: review of 25 cases. J Neurosurg Sci 1999;43(2):115–121, discussion 122–123

47. Di Rocco F, Yoshino M, Oi S. Neuroendoscopic transventricular ventriculocystostomy in treatment for intracranial cysts. J Neurosurg 2005;103(1, Suppl):54–60

48. Godano U, Mascari C, Consales A, Calbucci F. Endoscope-controlled microneurosurgery for the treatment of intracranial fluid cysts. Childs Nerv Syst 2004;20(11–12):839–841

49. Greenfield JP, Souweidane MM. Endoscopic management of intracranial cysts. Neurosurg Focus 2005;19(6):E7

50. Helland CA, Wester K. A population-based study of intracranial arachnoid cysts: clinical and neuroimaging outcomes following surgical cyst decompression in children. J Neurosurg 2006;105(5, Suppl): 385–390

51. Huang Q, Wang D, Guo Y, Zhou X, Wang X, Li X. The diagnosis and neuroendoscopic treatment of noncommunicating intracranial arachnoid cysts. Surg Neurol 2007;68(2):149–154, discussion 154

52. Paladino J, Rotim K, Heinrich Z. Neuroendoscopic fenestration of arachnoid cysts. Minim Invasive Neurosurg 1998;41(3):137–140

53. Schroeder HW, Gaab MR, Niendorf WR. Neuroendoscopic approach to arachnoid cysts. J Neurosurg 1996;85(2):293–298

54. Tamburrini G, D'Angelo L, Paternoster G, Massimi L, Caldarelli M, Di Rocco C. Endoscopic management of intra and paraventricular CSF cysts. Childs Nerv Syst 2007;23(6):645–651

55. Tamburrini G, Caldarelli M, Massimi L, Santini P, Di Rocco C. Subdural hygroma: an unwanted result of sylvian arachnoid cyst marsupialization. Childs Nerv Syst 2003;19(3):159–165

56. Kang JK, Lee KS, Lee IW, et al. Shunt-independent surgical treatment of middle cranial fossa arachnoid cysts in children. Childs Nerv Syst 2000;16(2):111–116

57. Elhammady MS, Bhatia S, Ragheb J. Endoscopic fenestration of middle fossa arachnoid cysts: a technical description and case series. Pediatr Neurosurg 2007;43(3):209–215

58. Ozgur BM, Aryan HE, Levy ML. Microsurgical keyhole middle fossa arachnoid cyst fenestration. J Clin Neurosci 2005;12(7):804–806

59. Hernàndez Leòn O, Pérez Falero RA, Arenas Rodrìguez IF, Lozano Crespo Palacio C. Microsurgical keyhole approach for middle fossa arachnoid cyst fenestration. Neurosurgery 2005;56(5):E1166

60. Chernov MF, Kamikawa S, Yamane F, Hori T. Double-endoscopic approach for management of convexity arachnoid cyst: case report. Surg Neurol 2004;61(5):483–486, discussion 486–487

61. Levy ML, Wang M, Aryan HE, Yoo K, Meltzer H. Microsurgical keyhole approach for middle fossa arachnoid cyst fenestration. Neurosurgery 2003;53(5):1138–1144, discussion 1144–1145

62. Wang JC, Heier L, Souweidane MM. Advances in the endoscopic management of suprasellar arachnoid cysts in children. J Neurosurg 2004;100(5, Suppl Pediatrics):418–426

63. Rappaport ZH. Suprasellar arachnoid cysts: options in operative management. Acta Neurochir (Wien) 1993;122(1–2):71–75

64. Fitzpatrick MO, Barlow P. Endoscopic treatment of prepontine arachnoid cysts. Br J Neurosurg 2001;15(3):234–238

65. Kirollos RW, Javadpour M, May P, Mallucci C. Endoscopic treatment of suprasellar and third ventricle-related arachnoid cysts. Childs Nerv Syst 2001;17(12):713–718

66. Nakamura Y, Mizukawa K, Yamamoto K, Nagashima T. Endoscopic treatment for a huge neonatal prepontine-suprasellar arachnoid cyst: a case report. Pediatr Neurosurg 2001;35(4):220–224

67. Gangemi M, Colella G, Magro F, Maiuri F. Suprasellar arachnoid cysts: endoscopy versus microsurgical cyst excision and shunting. Br J Neurosurg 2007;21(3):276–280

68. Sood S, Schuhmann MU, Cakan N, Ham SD. Endoscopic fenestration and coagulation shrinkage of suprasellar arachnoid cysts: technical note. J Neurosurg 2005;102(1, Suppl):127–133

69. Bahuleyan B, Rao A, Chacko AG, Daniel RT. Supracerebellar arachnoid cyst: a rare cause of acquired Chiari I malformation. J Clin Neurosci 2007;14(9):895–898

70. Erdinçler P, Kaynar MY, Bozkus H, Ciplak N. Posterior fossa arachnoid cysts. Br J Neurosurg 1999;13(1):10–17

71. Gangemi M, Maiuri F, Colella G, Magro F. Endoscopic treatment of quadrigeminal cistern arachnoid cysts. Minim Invasive Neurosurg 2005;48(5):289–292

72. Gangemi M, Maiuri F, Colella G, Sardo L. Endoscopic surgery for large posterior fossa arachnoid cysts. Minim Invasive Neurosurg 2001;44(1):21–24

73. Jallo GI, Woo HH, Meshki C, Epstein FJ, Wisoff JH. Arachnoid cysts of the cerebellopontine angle: diagnosis and surgery. Neurosurgery 1997;40(1):31–37, discussion 37–38

2 Communicating Hydrocephalus

◆ Nonadjustable (Fixed Pressure) Shunt Valves

Spyros Sgouros

The introduction of ventricular shunts in the early 1950s[1] revolutionized the treatment of hydrocephalus and converted it from a terminal disease[2] to a treatable condition with overall good physical and cognitive outcome.[3–8] These early shunts contained a one-way valve, which opened and allowed passage of cerebrospinal fluid (CSF) when the difference of pressure between its input and output reached a preset threshold level. This type of valve is now referred to as pressure-regulated or differential pressure and in its most common implementation, which has been marketed for 4 decades, contains a silicone diaphragm mechanism that bends under pressure and opens circumferentially a narrow passage through which CSF escapes. Other designs also exist with similar pressure characteristics, for example, proximal or distal slit, "spring-ball," "ball-in-cone," "duckbill," cruciform, and diamond slit.[9] In all designs, the deformation characteristics of an elastic material are taken advantage of to create a one-way mechanism that opens whenever the proximal (ventricular) pressure exceeds a preset level. This preset pressure level is intended to simulate normal intracranial pressure (ICP) within the cerebral ventricular system; hence it is set around 10 to12 cm H_2O, the nominal normal ICP. Early on it was appreciated that different patients may respond better clinically if this preset pressure was higher or lower than the average "medium" setting; thus, "high" and "low" pressure valves were designed.

Evolution of Valve Designs

Despite tremendous technological improvements over the last several decades, there has been little change in shunt valve design in essence, if one excludes the improvement in materials, that has had a measurable effect on the long-term mechanical complications of shunts. A major breakthrough came in the 1980s, when the syndrome of shunt overdrainage due to "siphoning" (rapid loss of CSF from the

head) in the erect position was appreciated. Different technological solutions were pursued to overcome this. Two main types of devices were developed: "antisiphon" or "siphon control" devices and "flow control" valves. Antisiphon devices come in different designs; common ones use either a dome to sense atmospheric pressure and apply increased resistance to flow in the erect position (e.g., Delta chamber, Medtronic PS Medical, Goleta, California) or gravity-controlled balls that progressively occlude the CSF passage and increase the resistance to flow (e.g., ShuntAssistant, Christoff Miethke GmbH & Co. KG, Potsdam, Germany; and SiphonGuard, Codman & Shurtleff Inc., Raynham, Massachusetts). Most manufacturers have incorporated differential pressure valves and antisiphon devices in single-case shunts (e.g., Delta valve = differential pressure valve + Delta chamber, Medtronic PS Medical). Flow control valves provide constant flow of CSF over a wide range of pressures. The best example is the Orbis-Sigma OSV II valve (Integra LifeSciences Corp., Plainsboro, New Jersey), which contains a dome connected to a movable ruby pin with variable profile that allows a stable flow of CSF to a wide pressure range, while including an overflow mechanism in case the CSF pressure becomes too high. Recently, the OSV valve was developed in a lower flow setting as well, to suit patients with normal pressure hydrocephalus (NPH) who may be more prone to chronic subdural hematomas following shunting.

Adjustable Valves

In the 1980s, an adjustable valve was produced, the Hakim-Medos programmable valve (now called the Codman Hakim programmable valve, Codman & Shurtleff), which was able to change the opening pressure setting percutaneously with the help of a magnet system. It offered the facility to change the opening pressure in 18 steps of 10 mm H_2O over a wide range, from 30 to 200 mm H_2O. It was an interesting concept, certainly advanced for its time. The Codman Hakim was marketed as a programmable valve, but it is better thought of as adjustable, as the user can change only its opening pressure, not its essential functional characteristics; in other words, it operates on only one program, at different pressure levels. The Codman Hakim is a differential pressure valve, with a ruby ball and seat controlled by a stainless steel spring of adjustable height. Although its market acceptance (by market, we mean neurosurgeons worldwide who implant shunts) was slow, it is still in production today in its original form. Over the past 5 years the concept of changeable opening pressure has gained acceptance. Other adjustable valve designs have appeared as well, and they are gradually gaining market acceptance or market share. Incidentally, the use of financial terms when discussing scientific devices like shunts is appropriate, because the technological evolution that became available for clinical use is directly related to the economic realities that apply to the manufacture and distribution of these devices.[10,11]

Recently, manufacturers have combined adjustable pressure/differential pressure valves with antisiphon devices in a single case. Three notable examples are the Strata valve (Medtronic PS Medical), an adjustable Delta valve (diaphragm differential pressure valve + Delta chamber) with five pressure settings; the Miethke Pro-GAV (Christoff Miethke GmbH & Co. KG, Potsdam, Germany), which combines a ball-in-cone differential pressure valve and a gravity-controlled ball antisiphon device; and the Codman Hakim programmable valve, which has been combined with the SiphonGuard (Codman & Shurtleff) in the same case. These newer devices offer improved laboratory characteristics but have not been available long enough to ascertain their clinical performance.

Flow control valves are not yet available in adjustable models.

Controversies Regarding Shunt Valves

After 5 decades of shunt design evolution, laboratory and clinical studies, and considerable scientific debate at countless meetings, the issues of superiority of shunt valve design remain unresolved. This by implication signifies the difficulties with the development of implantable medical devices, as well as the economies of scale that affect medical devices in comparison with commercial electronic goods, for example, which incorporate infinitely more complicated technology than shunt valves and are sold for a fraction of the price. At the same time, it has been rather striking how polarized neurosurgeons' views are on the choice of shunts, though no conclusive scientific evidence exists, which implies that significant factors in the choice of shunts play to the history of education of

each individual surgeon (most surgeons choose valves that their mentors were using when they were training, in parallel to the known assertion in commerce that most drivers will choose the same make of car when they change, provided they had no major problems with the previous one), and the ability of the industry to penetrate the local environment of neurosurgeons using the usual market techniques (advertisements, personal contacts, social trends, etc.).

Several in vitro studies have examined the hydrodynamic properties of shunt valves, with particular reference to antisiphon action.[12,13] Two major valve-testing facilities exist: in Cambridge, UK, and in Heidelberg, Germany, in the respective Departments of Neurosurgery. Both of these testing facilities have consistently shown that most shunt valves do not counteract effectively the overdrainage phenomenon in the erect position, despite manufacturers' claims.[12,13] The standard differential pressure valves have major susceptibilities to overdrainage, the Codman Hakim programmable valve cannot counteract overdrainage in the erect position even in its higher settings, and the dome-designed antisiphon devices (e.g., Delta chamber, Medtronic PS Medical) are susceptible to subcutaneous pressure.[14] This last problem has been shown to render the devices inactive with time, as they are implanted in the subcutaneous tissue, which encases them in fibrous tissue, and they lose their reference to atmospheric pressure, which deactivates the whole mechanism of increased resistance to CSF flow.

Considerable controversy exists still on whether flow-regulated valves offer a better clinical long-term outcome than pressure regulated devices. Several clinical studies and a randomized clinical trial have not yet proven this conclusively. It seems that, although in the laboratory, flow-regulated valves are better than differential pressure valves in counteracting the siphoning effect and maintaining normal ICP, in actual clinical practice, the overall shunt survival time (the time from implantation to the shunt's first revision due to some complication, commonly obstruction) is not substantially different between the two shunt types, the only difference being the types of complications that affect them.[15-17] Differential pressure valves are associated with a higher proximal obstruction rate, whereas flow control valves are associated with a higher valve obstruction rate. Furthermore, differential pressure valves are associated with a higher incidence of slit ventricles seen on radiology, but only a minority of patients develop the clinical features of the syndrome (**Fig. 2.1**).

Cost comparison studies, performed mainly for the realities of the developing world, have shown no difference in clinical outcome in differential pressure valves costing $60 and $600,[11,18] demonstrating clearly the tremendous differences in performing neurosurgery in developing and developed countries, and by implication the overpricing and

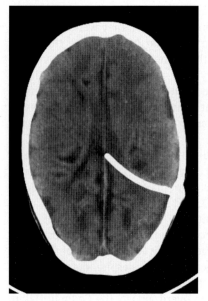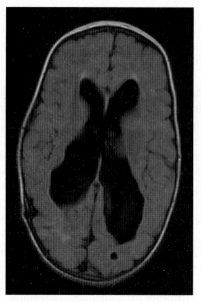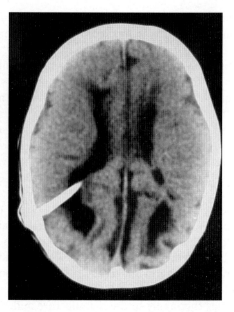

A-C

Fig. 2.1 Computed tomography (CT) scans of children with posthemorrhagic hydrocephalus obtained a few years after shunting. Differences in the size of the ventricles are observed. The smallest ventricles are seen in the child with **(A)** a differential pressure valve, the largest ventricles in the child with **(B)** a flow control valve. **(C)** The child with a valve with an antisiphon device has moderate-size ventricles.

inflationary effect of the medicolegal and commercially driven environment.

For most hydrocephalic children older than 2 years and most adults, a medium-pressure valve with an antisiphon device offers good long-term results. Adult patients are not particularly susceptible to overdrainage, so even valves without antisiphon devices offer good results. Neonates, young infants, and children in the first 2 years of life probably benefit most by a flow control valve, as they are the most likely to develop slit ventricle syndrome. Children with established slit ventricle syndrome can be difficult to manage and often require several valve trials. They are most likely to need change from a differential pressure to flow control valve and can benefit often by adjustable valves if they have developed poor compliance and are very sensitive to small changes of pressure. Young infants with very big ventricles and a small cortical mantle are particularly susceptible to overdrainage, collapse of the cortical parenchyma, and development of subdural hematomas; thus, they should have high resistance valves (high pressure + antisiphon or flow control or adjustable set at high pressure).

Fixed Pressure versus Adjustable Pressure Valves

Another controversy that has arisen in the last few years is whether adjustable pressure valves are superior to fixed pressure valves. This debate has evolved for two main reasons: the shunt manufacturers decided to promote the marketing of adjustable valves as the concept seemed to gain market

acceptance, and NPH has become a more prominent focus in comparison to 10 or 20 years ago, with the view, promoted by shunt manufacturers, not proven by robust clinical trials, that adjustable shunts are more suitable to patients with NPH. Critical assessment of the published evidence does not support the idea of any superiority of adjustable pressure valves.

Before embarking on comparisons between these two types of differential pressure valves, it is important to remember that for at least 3 decades children and adults worldwide have been treated with fixed pressure shunts with very good results. Fixed pressure shunts have a consolidated profile of complications,[19–23] which makes management of patients predictable and, to a large extent, easy. On average, a newly implanted fixed pressure valve, whether differential pressure with or without antisiphon device or a flow-controlled valve, has a 1-year survival rate of 70%, a 5-year survival rate of 55 to 60%, a 10-year survival rate of 20%, and an immediate postimplantation complication rate (including infection) of ~10%.[22] Symptomatic slit ventricle is a clinical problem often difficult to solve, but thankfully it is not that common, seen probably in < 20% of shunted children, and rarely in adults. Millions of children worldwide have benefited from fixed pressure shunts, completed school, completed higher education of some kind, and enjoy a near-normal life. This was not possible before the invention of the differential pressure valve.

Several clinical studies have established the use of adjustable valves in both children and adults.[24–29] All studies declared that adjustable valves have the same rate of complications as fixed pressure valves, not less. A randomized,

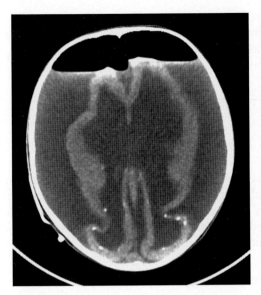
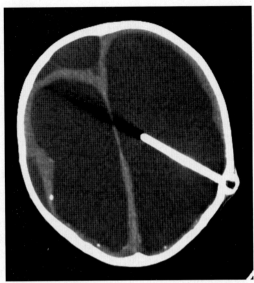

A

B

Fig. 2.2 CT scans of a neonate with hydrocephalus and an abnormally thin cerebral mantle. **(A)** A few days after insertion of a valve with an antisiphon device, large subdural collections developed. **(B)** The original valve was removed, and an adjustable valve was inserted and gradually increased in opening pressure, until the subdural collections were absorbed.

controlled study by Pollack et al between the Codman Hakim programmable valve and fixed pressure valves was not designed to demonstrate if the ability of pressure change confers any clinical advantage; it was only designed to show if the two types of valves had similar complication rates.[25] The main advantage of adjustable valves is the facility to change the opening pressure of the valves without resorting to an operation. Most studies with large patient numbers have demonstrated that 50 to 60% of patients required at least one adjustment of the pressure setting. Nevertheless, in all studies it is clear that there is no well-defined protocol for changing the opening pressure. Some surgeons use adjustable pressure valves in all cases,[27–29] whereas others use them selectively for patients who may require pressure change (e.g., in slit ventricle syndrome).[24] Another shortcoming is the lack of recommendations regarding the startup setting and the criteria for changing the pressure setting. It seems that pressure change has been done at surgeons' discretion or interpretation of the symptoms or because of a lack of improvement on the part of patients. An exception is patients who develop postshunting subdural hematomas who invariably have the valve pressure setting increased. Even in these patients, additional drainage of the subdurals via a burr hole has been required in a significant percentage.[25,26] Although no clear consensus exists, it appears that adjustable valves may be useful in children who suffer from slit ventricle syndrome and have tried other valves and in adults with NPH. They may be useful in other circumstances where incremental change of intraventricular pressure may be beneficial, for example, in neonates with very large ventricles with a thin cerebral mantle, where there is a significant risk of subdural collections

following shunting (**Fig. 2.2**), and in children with large convexity arachnoid cysts where fixed pressure valves in a cystoperitoneal shunt can cause overdrainage.[30]

Invariably, all adjustable pressure valves have a significantly higher cost than standard fixed pressure valves, on the order of 30 to 50%, depending on local pricing policies. Some proponents of the routine use of adjustable valves for all patients and all ages have tried to argue that the excess cost is being offset by the long-term saving that the option of pressure change incurs. That economic argument has not been proven yet. A speculative study has been performed,[10] but it has no real value, as it attempted to calculate the projected economical saving rather than compare prospectively actual cost efficiencies in implanted patients. There is no prospective study that compares the cost of adjustable versus nonadjustable valves, and it would be impossible to carry out such a study, having in mind the problems that patients with hydrocephalus, especially children, have over several years (repeat admissions for possible obstructions, repeat scans for investigations of headaches, doctors' differing attitudes to symptoms, etc.). Certainly, the current evidence in the literature does not justify the routine use of adjustable valves in all patients and all ages.

Conclusion

Fixed pressure shunts have an established profile of success, complication, and long-term failure rates. They have proven their value with time. Many new shunt designs have appeared in the past 20 years, but none have managed to make a dramatic impact on the success, complication, and long-term failure rates. Adjustable pressure shunts may be good for specific types of patients, such as children with symptomatic slit ventricle syndrome or adults with NPH. The routine use of adjustable pressure shunts has not been proven justifiable yet.

♦ Programmable Shunts

Ethan A. Benardete

History

The development of the first valves for CSF diversion shunts occurred in the 1950s. Because ventriculoatrial shunts were common at the time, Matson and Alexander realized that a one-way valve was necessary to prevent reflux of blood from the atrium of the heart into the ventricular system.[31] Several basic valve designs were developed, including ball-in-cone, diaphragm, and slit valves.[32,33]

During the ensuing decades, as ventriculoperitoneal shunts became preferred, a further benefit of shunt valves was recognized, the shunt valve's ability to regulate CSF flow. It is this capability that led to the next innovation in valve technology: adjustable shunt valves. The earliest adjustable designs date to the 1970s and 1980s.[31] Adjustable shunt valves provide a way to change the amount of CSF drainage without the need for further surgery.

CSF Dynamics

In the early 20th century, insightful experiments by Dandy and Blackfan, among others, demonstrated the nature of obstructive and communicating hydrocephalus.[34] As was later observed, all hydrocephalus is obstructive in point of fact, but when the obstruction is at the level of the subarachnoid space or arachnoid granulations, it is commonly referred to as communicating.[35]

The normal in vivo situation is not well mimicked by a CSF shunt. It has been observed that normal CSF flow is pulsatile, whereas the flow in a ventriculoperitoneal shunt tube is largely continuous and subject to gravitational forces as well as ICP.[36] Differential pressure valves then compensate for these forces by providing a fixed opening pressure so that continuous drainage does not occur. Below the opening pressure, CSF flow decreases to negligible amounts, whereas above the opening pressure, the pressure head behind the valve drives the flow.

What determines the right opening pressure for a given patient? The shunted patient is an artificial situation in which slight changes in position may potentially dramatically alter the pressure difference across the valve. Brain physiology must adapt to this foreign situation, but we have no way of telling what the ideal opening pressure may be a priori. Some patients may do well with their initial fixed differential pressure valve. Nonetheless, in a significant proportion of patients, the initial fixed differential pressure valve may cause problems. These problems, which will be considered more fully later, are related to either over- or underdrainage.

Valve Technology

Briefly, we will review the basic facts of shunt valve design. Fixed differential pressure valves come in a variety styles. The original Holter valve uses two tubes with slits to both produce one-way flow and create a fixed resistance, or opening pressure. Valves of a similar nature include the Phoenix valves (Vygon Neuro, Valley Forge, Pennsylvania). Another variation on the slit valve is the miter valve, such as the Mishler valve (Integra).

Other fixed valves use a ball and spring to put resistance across the small opening inside the valve chamber. The Hakim valve (Codman & Shurtleff) is a ball-and-spring type well known for its durability. The GAV and Paedi-GAV (Aesculap Inc., Center Valley, Pennsylvania) combine a ball-and-spring design with an integral antisiphon device, which uses weighted balls to compensate for the effects of patient position. Several other valve designs, for example, the PS Medical valves (Medtronic), use a diaphragm to regulate flow across the valve opening.

Flow control valves represent a different concept in valve design. These valves attempt to hold flow constant across a broad range of pressures. The well-known valves in this category are the Orbis-Sigma valve and the OSV II (Integra). Fluid pressure drives a small conical piston so that, when pressure is higher, the opening for fluid flow is smaller. This allows relatively even flow over a wide range of pressures. The shunt design trial of the 1990s failed to show any benefit to this design over fixed pressure valves in terms of failure rate or patient outcome.[37]

The concept of a noninvasively adjustable valve dates to at least the 1970s.[31] Several adjustable shunt valves are on the market today. The Codman Hakim programmable valve uses a ratchet mechanism to control the resistance of the spring mechanism that controls a ball across the valve opening. The ratchet mechanism is adjustable by an external magnet using an electrically operated programming unit. The standard valve is adjustable from an opening

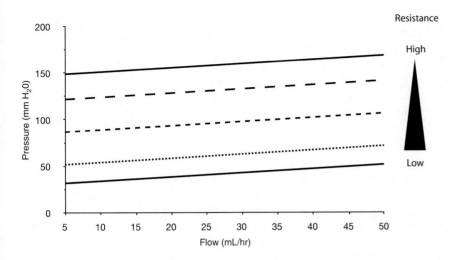

Fig. 2.3 Graphical representation of adjustable shunt valve function. Each line represents the pressure versus flow curve for a given setting of the adjustable valve. As the valve is set to higher opening pressures, less flow occurs at any given pressure.

pressure of 30 to 200 mm H_2O. After programming, the setting of the valve can be checked using a skull radiograph by comparing the position of a movable radiopaque marker with fixed markers on the valve. The valve is also available with a separate antisiphon component. Because this valve and other adjustable valves rely on a magnet to program the opening pressure, rechecking the setting is suggested following magnetic resonance imaging (MRI) scans.

Similarly, the Medtronic PS Medical Strata and Strata II valves use a magnet to noninvasively adjust the tension on a spring, which seats a ball inside a conical opening. Increasing tension on the spring increases valve resistance. The setting of the valve can be obtained without radiographs using a handheld indicator tool, which comes in both a manual and an electronic version. This valve typically comes with an integral antisiphon device; however, the valve is also available without the antisiphon component. The valve is adjustable to five different levels of resistance or "performance" levels, from 0.5 to 2.5.

The Sophy valve, manufactured by Sophysa (Orsay, France) and first introduced in 1985, is the oldest commercially available adjustable valve. It also uses a magnetically movable fulcrum to adjust the tension on a synthetic ruby ball that is seated within the flow pathway. The Polaris valve, which is marketed as MRI-compatible, is an updated version of the Sophy adjustable valve.

Aesculap markets the pro-GAV adjustable valve based on the fixed GAV shunt design (Miethke). This valve is housed in a titanium metal casing unlike the plastic coverings of the other valves. Similar to the others, tension on a ball is adjusted with an external magnet and read with an indicator tool. The design also incorporates an antisiphon device.

In summary, several adjustable shunt valves are available, each with minor variations. There are no clinical studies that evaluate one design over another. Surgeon preference

regarding such subtleties as size, ease of use, availability, and familiarity largely drives the decision over which one of the adjustable valves to use.

Clinical Uses

Ventriculoperitoneal (or ventriculoatrial or ventriculopleural) shunts are conceptually simple devices, and the clinical uses of adjustable shunt valves are straightforward. Adjusting the valve opening pressure lower results in less resistance to flow, and higher CSF flow rates are obtained. Similarly, higher opening pressures result in higher resistances and less flow under similar conditions. When plotted as a pressure versus flow curve, the different valve settings typically give a series of parallel curves (**Fig. 2.3**). Each line in **Fig. 2.3** represents the performance of the valve at a different resistance setting.

This adjustable resistance feature is useful in several clinical situations. Because the correct opening pressure for a given patient is initially unknown, a starting opening pressure must be estimated. A typical dilemma occurs with patients with large ventricles. These types of pediatric patients are not uncommon in centers where treatment for hydrocephalus is delayed. One must weigh the desire to provide high CSF flow to reduce the size of the ventricles against the risk of causing a subdural hematoma by rapid collapse of the ventricles. Numerous publications have documented the utility of having an adjustable shunt valve in this situation. By raising the opening pressure of the valve, an incipient subdural hematoma can be treated noninvasively without the need for valve revision or evacuation of the subdural fluid (**Fig. 2.4**).

A second type of patient in which an adjustable valve can be useful is the patient with slit ventricles. Here shunt overdrainage leads to an abnormally small amount of CSF within the ventricular system. Symptoms include

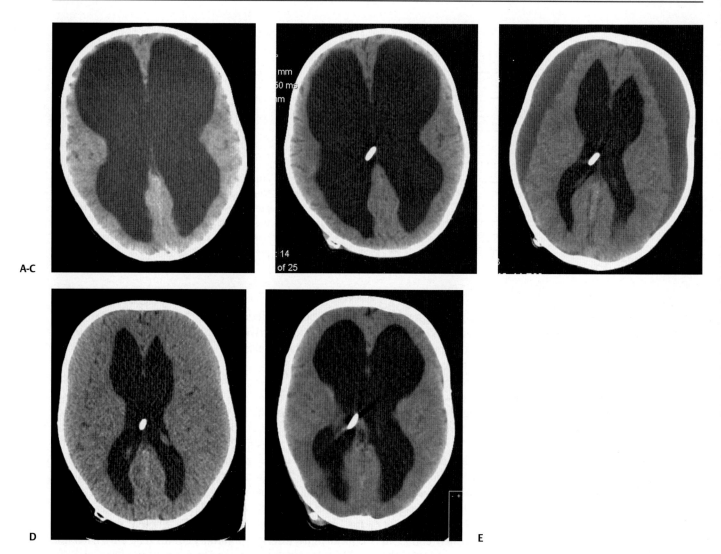

A-C

D

E

Fig. 2.4 Clinical examples of adjustable shunt valve use. **(A)** This patient presented at 16 months of age with severe communicating hydrocephalus and a head circumference of 61 cm. **(B)** The patient underwent placement of a right occipital ventriculoperitoneal shunt with an adjustable shunt valve. **(C)** Over the course of several months, large bilateral subdural hematomas developed. **(D)** The patient's shunt valve was reset to a higher resistance with gradual resolution of the chronic subdural collections. **(E)** Long-term follow-up shows complete resolution of the subdural hematomas. The patient continued to improve neurologically after placement of the shunt.

chronic headaches and frequent shunt malfunctions. Gradual elevation of the opening pressure can allow for reexpansion of the ventricles.[38] This reexpansion may also lead to fewer proximal malfunctions, as the ventricular walls are not coapted. Noninvasive manipulation of the opening pressure makes this procedure much more tolerable.

Occasionally, the neurosurgeon will encounter situations where shunt underdrainage is a problem. In neonates, in particular, underdrainage is often accompanied by accumulation of subgaleal CSF collections. These collections can put the healing incision at risk. After a shunt obstruction has

been ruled out, this situation can sometimes be treated noninvasively by decreasing the opening pressure of the valve.

Clinical Studies and Evidence

Efficacy

Numerous retrospective studies have documented the effectiveness of adjustable shunt valves for various purposes. In 2005 Kestle et al published a prospective multicenter study of the Strata valve documenting its efficacy and safety.[39] The first-year revision rate for these patients was similar to patients with fixed pressure valves. Nevertheless, the adjustable property was found to be useful in a large number of patients. Similar favorable results with other types of adjustable valves have been found by others.[40–42]

Several studies have shown that readjustment of the opening pressure in a patient with large ventricles can arrest the development of subdural fluid collections and allow for their resorption. In 1987 Dietrich et al reported on such a case.[43] Their experience with 74 patients was also summarized in 1990.[44] Similarly, a retrospective study of 75 patients with the Sophy valve reported 10 cases of subdural fluid collections managed by valve adjustment.[45]

Patients with slit ventricle syndrome or shunt overdrainage can also be treated by noninvasive adjustment of the shunt valve. Kondageski et al published a report on 24 patients with shunt overdrainage symptoms who were managed by insertion of a Strata valve and shunt valve adjustment.[46] Although patients with subdural fluid collections were not excluded, inclusion in the study was predicated on clinical symptoms as well as documented low ICP (measured with a fiberoptic ICP probe). A significant reduction in symptoms occurred after insertion of the valve, and insertion of the adjustable valve was also significantly associated with reduction in the need for further surgery.

Further studies have focused on the value of these valves in neonates. In the early postinsertion period, low opening pressure can be set to avoid subgaleal fluid accumulation.[47] After several days, the opening pressure can then be increased to prevent overdrainage-type symptoms.

Adjustable Shunt Complications

Significant concern regarding the susceptibility of adjustable shunt valves to stray magnetic fields has led to several published studies. An in vitro study by Nomura et al showed that cellular phones could theoretically influence the setting, but that valves in the standard frontal or occipital locations are unlikely to be influenced by the magnetic field of cellular phones.[48] An in vitro and in vivo study of the Codman Hakim valve found it to be particularly susceptible to magnetic fields,[49] and further studies have found both the Sophy and Codman Hakim valves at risk.[50,51]

In my experience, inadvertent changing of the shunt valve setting is relatively uncommon. Nevertheless, it is reasonable to recheck the valve setting after MRI imaging and at each follow-up visit or emergency consultation. The major manufacturers of adjustable valves are all developing devices that will be less susceptible to magnetic pulses such as MRI (e.g., Polaris).[52]

Comparison with Fixed Differential Pressure Valves

No prospective, randomized trial of adjustable shunt valves versus fixed differential pressure valves has ever been published. It is unlikely that such a trial would ever be undertaken because of difficulties with enrollment and design. The shunt trial of the 1990s did seem to indicate that no particular shunt valve design was superior to any other.[37] But similar to other trials in neurosurgery, comparisons such as this often fail to demonstrate superiority because of indiscriminant patient selection. There are undoubtedly certain valve designs that work better for certain patients, but without selecting those patients a priori, it is usually impossible to see an effect.

Recent published reports have found in a retrospective analysis that adjustable shunt valves are effective in reducing proximal shunt malfunction and need for shunt revision.[53]

There is little evidence to suggest that adjustable valves from the major manufacturers malfunction more frequently than other valves. In my experience, valve malfunction represents the least likely cause of shunt malfunction.

Cost

Another common argument against adjustable shunt valves is that they cost more that the standard differential pressure valve. However, proponents of adjustable shunt valves argue that the cost of the valve is more than compensated for by avoidance of additional surgery and time in the hospital to "switch over" to a different fixed pressure valve. In addition, if a certain number of slit ventricle syndromes or subdural hematomas were avoided, this might make up for the cost of the valve. One study has addressed these issues and found that the adjustable valves were a cost benefit.[54] Similarly, Arnell et al concluded that a primary programmable valve insertion in pediatric patients was cost-effective.[40]

Conclusion

Treatment of hydrocephalus with the use of ventriculoperitoneal (or other terminus) shunts is a nonoptimal solution to a difficult problem. Shunts do not mimic what we know about the way CSF is absorbed in the normal physiologic situation. However, adjustable shunt valves improve the performance of CSF-diversion shunts in many patients. Numerous reports support the notion that these adjustable valves are effective in noninvasively treating syndromes of both over- and underdrainage. I recommend an adjustable shunt valve as the initial valve in all cases of pediatric communicating hydrocephalus unless interference from magnetic fields (i.e., very frequent MRI scans) is a major concern.

◆ Antibiotic-Impregnated Catheters

Gustavo Pradilla, Daniel M. Sciubba, and George I. Jallo

Hydrocephalus constitutes one of the most prevalent clinical entities requiring neurosurgical treatment. CSF diversion remains the mainstay of therapy.[55] Regardless of the location and system used, patients with implanted shunts frequently present with system failures that result in considerable morbidity and mortality.[56,57] Among shunt-related complications, infections continue to challenge neurosurgical specialists and clinicians alike, despite standardized prophylactic antibiotics and strict sterile techniques.[58] Recent advances in sustained drug delivery technology facilitated the development of antibiotic-coated catheters.[59–62] The purpose of this article is to familiarize the readers with the clinical nuances of hydrocephalus treatment, to describe the pathophysiology of shunt-related infections, to discuss the principles of sustained drug delivery applied to antibiotic-coated catheters, and to present clinical data that evaluate its safety and efficacy.

Hydrocephalus

CSF circulation may be altered by congenital or acquired conditions altering normal transit pathways, resulting in obstructive hydrocephalus, or by either impaired absorption or CSF overproduction. Hydrocephalus can develop at any age. Common causes of hydrocephalus include prematurity (following germinal matrix hemorrhage), congenital central nervous system (CNS) disorders such as myelomeningoceles, Dandy-Walker malformation, arachnoid cysts, posthemorrhagic development following aneurysmal or posttraumatic subarachnoid hemorrhage, postinfectious development after meningitis or meningoencephalitis, and congenital skull deformities such as Crouzon and Pfeiffer syndromes.[63]

The incidence of acquired hydrocephalus is inconsistently reported, but congenital hydrocephalus data suggest that it occurs in ~0.4 to 3.16 of every 1000 live births.[64–67] Until the mid-20th century, patients with hydrocephalus faced progressive and devastating neurologic dysfunction, often resulting in death. Historical accounts attribute the earliest description of hydrocephalus and the first documented attempts of ventricular puncture to Hippocrates (5th century BC); however, it appears that the technique only resulted in drainage of the subdural space.[68–70] Head wrapping, bloodletting, trephination, and other techniques were used unsuccessfully from the 16th to the 18th centuries. In the late 19th and early 20th centuries, experimentation with CSF diversion as a treatment for hydrocephalus was started using venous grafts and artificial cannulas without significant results.[71] Under Harvey

Cushing's leadership, members of the Hunterian Laboratory at Johns Hopkins, including Walter Dandy, greatly contributed to the understanding of CSF physiology. This work allowed Dandy to later develop bilateral choroid plexectomies and third ventriculostomies as the first efficacious surgical treatments for infantile hydrocephalus.[70–72] Endoscopic ventriculostomy and ventriculocysternostomy quickly followed with variable rates of success. CSF diversion to a body cavity was extensively investigated by Matson and colleagues at Boston Children's Hospital.[73] This work focused primarily on ureteral diversion but lost favor to other sites due to significant infection rates and other delayed complications.

Although multiple sites were tested, significant progress in the field was modest until the development of biocompatible materials and unidirectional valves. In the 1950s work by Nulsen and Spitz on ventriculojugular shunts provided a simple valve mechanism[71] that in conjunction with the introduction of silicone shunt tubing by Pudenz set the foundation for the systems used today.[74–76] The first patient treated with a silicone ventriculoatrial shunt died 2 years later from a shunt obstruction, but silicone has remained a preferred material in shunt tubing manufacturing and is currently used to produce the new generation of antibiotic-coated catheters.

Treatment

Patients presenting with acute hydrocephalus secondary to intraventricular hemorrhage (IVH), acute shunt malfunction, or other etiologies require prompt CSF diversion with either temporary drainage or permanent shunting. Temporary alternatives to shunt placement include administration of diuretics, repeated lumbar punctures, lumbar drainage, repeated ventricular punctures, external ventricular drainage, and ventriculosubgaleal shunts.

Medical therapies for hydrocephalus are aimed at decreasing CSF production and involve the administration of diuretics. The most commonly used diuretics, acetazolamide and furosemide, have been used alone and in combination with variable efficacy. Acetazolamide blocks the formation of H^+ and HCO_3. from CO_2 and H_2O, which results in urinary bicarbonate excretion, and furosemide inhibits the Na–K–2Cl symporter in the thick ascending limb of the loop of Henle, both resulting in diuresis. Although their mechanisms of action differ, combination therapy results in a synergistic reduction of CSF production. Clinically, the efficacy of these medications is moderate and temporary. As illustrated in a clinical trial, their use has been associated with increased mortality, increased shunt placement, and higher neurologic disability at 1 year when compared with serial lumbar punctures[77] in pediatric patients with posthemorrhagic hydrocephalus.

Repeated lumbar punctures and continuous lumbar drainage have been previously advocated to prevent hydrocephalus and relief intracranial hypertension in patients with IVH. It was hypothesized that the removal of degrading blood and protein from the CSF decreased the risk of hydrocephalus and reduced the need for permanent ventricular shunting. For premature infants with ultrasound-documented IVH (with or without hydrocephalus), this hypothesis has been tested in randomized trials. Results from these studies were evaluated by a systematic Cochrane foundation review, which showed no reduction in the risk of shunt dependence, disability, multiple disability, or death when early lumbar punctures or ventricular taps were performed.[78,79] This analysis also showed that repeated taps were associated with an increased risk of CNS infection. Because of this, the authors recommend that repeated punctures be reserved for patients with symptomatic intracranial hypertension.

Premature neonates suffering from germinal matrix hemorrhages tend to have multiple comorbidities and very low birth weights. Significant morbidity of repeated ventricular punctures and inability to place permanent ventricular shunts led to the development of ventriculosubgaleal shunts. Willis and colleagues evaluated the efficacy and related complications of this procedure over a 1-year period.[80] Their study showed that ventriculosubgaleal shunts stabilized the clinical and radiographic progression of hydrocephalus in all six premature patients and prevented permanent shunting in one patient (16.6%). Four patients, however, developed shunt infections involving either the ventriculosubgaleal shunt itself (one patient) or the subsequent ventriculoperitoneal shunts (three patients). The overall rate of infection in the study was two thirds (infection rates for primary ventriculoperitoneal shunt placement in the authors' institution at the time of the study was 1%). The results of this study suggested that ventriculosubgaleal shunts were effective for temporary CSF diversion in neonates with posthemorrhagic hydrocephalus, although the observed infection risk was significant. Several other studies have validated the use of ventriculosubgaleal shunts since, with lower infection rates.[80-82]

Permanent CSF diversion can be accomplished by placement of ventricular or lumbar catheters using several techniques, including frameless stereotaxis and neuroendoscopy. Selection of an adequate location for placement of the distal catheter can have a significant role in the longevity and rate of postoperative complications of the shunt. Regardless of the location and technique used, postoperative shunt infections remain the most prevalent complication of CSF diversion.

Shunt Infections

CSF shunt implantations constitute nearly 50% of all surgical procedures performed by pediatric neurosurgeons, with ~30,000 shunt procedures performed annually in the United States alone.[83] Although infection constitutes the most prevalent complication following shunt placement in the pediatric population,[84] the rate of shunt infections varies considerably in the literature and from center to center, ranging from 0.33 to 39.0%.[85,86] Postoperative nosocomial meningitis after shunt placement has been reported in up to 33% of patients in some series; it carries mortality rates as high as 20%.[87] As reported by Dallacasa and others, most infections tend to occur within a few months of surgery, with 91% occurring within 9 months of shunt placement.[88] In general, these "early" infections frequently result from direct inoculation of nonpathogenic skin flora into the shunt components at the time of surgery.

Coagulase-negative staphylococci constitute the most prevalent organisms isolated (45–72%),[89-91] followed by gram-negative bacilli (19–22%).[92] Pathogens normally found in skin flora such as *Propionibacterium* acnes and other gram-positive rods are common especially in adolescents, but environmental and intestinal floras such as *Haemophilus influenzae* and *Enterococcus* are also frequently described.[92-96] Fungal pathogens have been reported with less frequency (2–17%).[84,85] Infections occurring beyond the postoperative period are less likely to result from *Staphylococcus aureus* and are frequently associated with abdominal pseudocysts and other sources of infection.[83]

Although risk factors for shunt infection remain controversial, young age and a history of prematurity have been frequently identified and have been associated with poorly developed immune systems, compromised skin quality with higher bacterial density, and increased incidence of systemic infections and sepsis.[88,97] In patients presenting with postoperative or early shunt infections following shunt placement, bacterial colonization of the hardware during surgery could be an initiating factor. After implantation the response of local and systemic immune mechanisms can be significantly altered by the presence of the shunt, which acts as a foreign body and therefore facilitates bacterial proliferation.[98] Perioperative risk factors were analyzed prospectively by Kulkarni and colleagues, who found that intraoperative exposure of the hardware to breached surgical gloves and postoperative incisional CSF leak were significantly associated with higher infection rates.[93-95,97] In addition, a correlation between lower rates of infection and increased surgeon experience has been found in several studies.[99-101]

Patients with shunted hydrocephalus commonly present with concomitant comorbidities that require abdominal, thoracic, or other types of surgeries in the vicinity of the implanted hardware. Although the incidence of symptomatic shunt infections resulting from intra-abdominal surgeries has been low in retrospective series, shunted patients presenting with fever or abdominal pain following urological or intra-abdominal procedures should be monitored closely for symptoms of shunt infection as well.[102] Similarly, ventriculoperitoneal shunt catheters are at risk for infection from intra-abdominal sources, and given the higher virulence of intestinal flora following CNS penetration, shunt removal from the peritoneal cavity is commonly recommended in these cases.

Open neural tube defects facilitate the penetration of organisms found in epidermal and intestinal flora and constitute an independent risk factor for shunt infection. It has been hypothesized that concomitant repair of the spinal defect with shunt implantation may decrease the incidence of CSF leakage by relieving ICP. The risk of infection, however, could be higher as the CNS could have been colonized prior to the closure of the defect.[103,104]

Diagnosis

Early diagnosis of shunt infections in patients with non-specific signs and symptoms remains challenging, as reliable predictive factors are lacking. Common signs and symptoms include fever, irritability, meningismus, and seizures.[88] The presence of fever and seizures appears to be more frequently associated with shunt infections and may help the clinician differentiate infection from mechanical shunt malfunction.[88,105]

Fevers may be low grade and intermittent, with mild generalized symptoms, unless more virulent organisms, such as gram-negative bacteria, are involved. The presence of seizures in this patient group is multifactorial and may be related to the higher incidence of seizure disorders in patients with hydrocephalus as compared with the general population, or due to the frequent episodes of high fevers with shunt infection,[105] which decreases seizure threshold. Although shunt infections may present simultaneously with shunt malfunctions, they may develop in the presence of a functioning shunt. Headaches are clinically unspecific in this patient population and may develop as a result of the infection or due to a concomitant shunt malfunction. Incisional erythema, warmth, and pain along the shunt tract can be seen but are not required criteria for diagnosis. In patients with intraperitoneal distal catheters, abdominal pain may result from peritonitis[106] or arise from CSF pseudocysts (loculated peritoneal collections).[107,108]

In patients presenting with clinical suspicion of shunt infection, spinal fluid sampling can confirm the diagnosis. The method of choice for CSF sampling depends on several factors, such as shunt configuration, age, spinal anatomy, and condition of the skin at the sampling site. Selection of lumbar puncture over shunt tap is therefore based on clinical analysis in a case-by-case manner. The incidence of infection following a shunt tap has not been adequately studied, but in published series it ranges from negligible to 32%.[109-112]

Laboratory Studies

Peripheral leukocytosis and serological markers, including C-reactive protein (CRP) and erythrocyte sedimentation rate (ESR), can be useful markers of acute infection and therapeutic response. Microbiological CSF analysis can orient the diagnosis in conjunction with high clinical suspicion. Confirmation of diagnosis, however, must not delay prompt antimicrobial therapy and surgical intervention. Biochemical and cytological profiles are helpful markers of CNS infection, with hypoglycorrhachia, elevated protein concentration, and polymorphonuclear infiltration strongly suggesting active infection. As reported by Lan and colleagues, CSF neutrophil counts $> 100/mm^3$ have a 96% specificity and a 0.55 positive predictive value for shunt infection.[105]

Gram staining can provide further insight and facilitates characterization of the pathogens involved. As reported by Tung et al,[113] patients with CSF eosinophilia have a higher risk of developing shunt malfunction and shunt infections; however, based on the findings of Lan and colleagues, eosinophilia is significantly more prevalent in patients with malfunction when compared with those with infection.[105] Causative pathogens can be identified in up to 85.7% of cases.[114] Antibodies against *Staphylococcus epidermidis* can be useful in detecting chronic ventriculoatrial shunt infections.[115]

Treatment

Medical management of shunt infections consists of systemic or intrathecal antimicrobial therapy. The success of antimicrobials as monotherapy is limited, as shown by James and colleagues.[116] In this study a combination of intravenous and intrathecal antibiotics showed a 30% efficacy with a 2- to 3-week course. The inability to remove bacteria from colonized hardware limits this approach to patients who are poor candidates for immediate surgical intervention; however, in all cases broad-spectrum antimicrobials are initiated until microbiological data are available. A standard regimen should include vancomycin, a broad-spectrum cephalosporin, and a third agent to cover anaerobic infections. Therapy is tailored as soon as antimicrobial identification and sensitivities are obtained.

Broad-spectrum antibiotics are often combined with temporary externalization of the distal catheter, particularly in ventriculoperitoneal shunts that present with infected pseudocysts or other intra-abdominal infections. Serial CSF sampling and serological markers can be used to determine resolution of the infection and timing for reinternalization.

The most efficacious intervention involves complete removal of the hardware with placement of a new temporary externalized ventriculostomy. Continuous microbiological and serological surveillance is maintained until the infection resolves, then a completely new shunt system is placed.[117] Recurrent infection following hardware removal and broad-spectrum antimicrobials ranges from 5 to 20%.[116,117]

Prophylactic Measures

Factors that have been associated with decreased rates of infection in single-institution series include reduction of the number of people in the operating room, performing shunt surgeries as the first cases of the day and with specially trained teams, decreasing the duration of surgery, avoiding contact between the shunt hardware and the skin, meticulous skin preparation, and use of prophylactic antibiotics.[118-120] The use of prophylactic antibiotics has been studied in detail with mixed results. A meta-analysis by Ratilal et al found significant benefit of prophylactic antibiotics in the first 24 hours after placement but did not find sufficient evidence of benefit after 24 hours.[121] Other factors previously considered include prevention of CSF leaks, postponing shunt placement in premature patients as long as possible, and use of double gloves.[93,94]

Antibiotic-Coated Catheters

Despite meticulous surgical technique, prophylactic pre- and postoperative antibiotics, and multiple targeted measures discussed above, complete eradication of colonizing organisms from the operative site and the shunt hardware with intravenous antibiotics alone is often inadequate and results in high rates of postoperative shunt infections.[83,94,122] To address this issue, controlled-release technology was used to develop antibiotic-impregnated shunt (AIS) systems capable of inhibiting biofilm formation on shunt hardware.[83,94,122-132] These systems are now readily available, and studies continue to validate their use in clinical practice.

Clinical Studies

Implementation of AIS systems has been shown to significantly decrease the incidence of early shunt infections (within 6 months of shunt implantation).[122,125,127,132] AIS systems decrease progression from catheter colonization to infection by enabling the sustained release of antibiotics into the catheter surface, which prevents staphylococcal colonization. The AIS system used at the authors' institution contains 0.054% rifampin (International Nonproprietary Name rifampicin) and 0.15% clindamycin,

which have been shown to be bactericidal against multiple species of staphylococci.[62,124,126,129] In 2003 Govender et al published the results of a prospective, randomized, controlled trial that evaluated the efficacy of an AIS system in preventing shunt infections when compared with an identical control shunt system.[125] One hundred ten patients were recruited; 60 patients were randomized to receive control shunt systems and 50 to receive AIS systems. Thirteen patients developed shunt infections, 10 in the control group and 3 in the AIS group. Staphylococcus species were identified in 83% of infected patients (whereas the 10 infected control shunts had positive cultures for staphylococci, none of the AIS shunts had any staphylococci). These results confirmed that AIS afforded antistaphylococcal protection, especially during the early postoperative period. In addition, in 2005 Sciubba et al conducted a retrospective study on 211 pediatric patients with hydrocephalus who underwent 353 shunt placement surgeries over a 3-year period.[122] The study compared patients before and after the introduction of AIS systems at their institution and included 6-month follow-ups for both groups. A multivariate regression analysis showed that AIS catheters were independently associated with a 2.4-fold decreased likelihood of shunt infection.

Despite the mounting evidence favoring AIS catheters, reluctance to use such systems in very young patients still exists due to concerns for antibiotic-related toxicity and for increased risk of colonization or infection in patients with an immature immune system by antibiotic-resistant organisms after prolonged exposure to the released antibiotics.

In an observational prospective study by the senior authors, 74 infants underwent 108 shunt surgeries with AIS catheters.[132] These patients were followed for over 9 months. Twenty-seven patients (36.5%) had received CSF diversion devices prior to the study. Five infections occurred in 5 patients (4.6% of procedures, 6.75% of patients), with 60% of these patients being > 32 weeks at birth. Thirty-three patients (44.6%) required shunt revision surgery, 5 (15%) for infection and 28 (85%) for malfunction. These results confirmed that AIS systems could be used safely in the treatment of patients younger than 1 year old and with a history of prematurity.

The results of that study propelled a follow-up study by the senior authors that compared the overall cost of regular shunts with the cost of AIS catheters.[130] The authors retrospectively reviewed data obtained in 211 pediatric patients who underwent 353 shunting procedures at their institution over a 3-year period and followed them for 12 months after surgery. The association between AIS catheter placement and subsequent shunt infection was assessed using a multivariate regression analysis, and potential factors contributing to the costs associated with treatment of postoperative shunt infections were analyzed. Two hundred eight shunts (59%) were placed with nonimpregnated catheters, and 145 shunts (41%) were placed with AIS catheters. Whereas 25 patients (12%) with non-AIS catheters developed a shunt infection, only 2 patients (1.4%) with AIS catheters became infected. Among infected patients, those with non-AIS catheters had longer hospital stays, more frequent complications related to the treatment regimen, and more frequent polymicrobial infections when compared with those implanted with AIS catheters. These results strongly suggested that despite the higher cost of individual AIS components, the rate of infection and the frequency and severity of related complications following postoperative infections are less when compared with patients implanted with non-AIS catheters.

Conclusion

Postoperative shunt infections constitute a major source of morbidity and cost and, despite considerable efforts, have not been eliminated. More studies are needed to further understand the risk factors and pathophysiology of this disease and to develop more effective treatment protocols and prevention strategies that could significantly reduce the frequency of these events. Newer techniques in microbiology and materials science may improve our understanding of the etiology of shunt infections and facilitate earlier diagnosis and more effective treatment. The development of antibiotic-impregnated catheters has had a significant impact in shunt infection rates and constitutes a safe and effective strategy to prevent these challenging complications.

♦ Lessons Learned

The use of fixed pressure-regulated valve systems for the treatment of hydrocephalus is in fact a success story over decades. Most of the clinical experience the community of pediatric neurosurgeons has is based on the use of this type of shunt valve. We also have the most experience with this type of valve when the issue is shunt-related complications, notably the excessive drainage of CSF and its consequences.

The thoughtful and pragmatic review by Sgouros reappraises fixed pressure valves and reminds us that little is proven in terms of improvement provided by other shunt valve designs such as flow-regulated valves, in particular, pressure-adjustable valve designs. It is clear that with the fixed pressure design we know best what to expect. Evidence is only slowly emerging about the real value of some improvements provided by adjustable valves, which we are only too eager to expect. The financial aspect is addressed in that the one determined thing about adjustable valves is that they are more expensive than "simple" valves. Clearly, this is important in both developed and developing countries.

The controversy is picked up elaborately by Benardete, who not only presents the available evidence about adjustable valve designs and their manufacturing varieties, but also shows the ability of adjustable models to change the opening pressure of a shunt valve without surgical revision. The concepts to treat large ventricles with a stepwise

decrease from an initially rather high valve setting and to treat slit ventricles with a stepwise increase from an initially low valve setting are intriguing and based on the objective to avoid sudden alterations to CSF dynamics. The evidence supports these concepts in that the number of shunt revisions appears to be significantly reduced by the use of adjustable valves. This constitutes a decrease in suffering, surgery, infection risk, length of hospital stay, and cost.

As practitioners, we must appreciate what we have and what we understand well, such as fixed pressure valves, and we must be critically open to new developments, such as adjustable valves, which may well be more widely used in the future once the evidence becomes firm and convinces many more in the pediatric neurosurgical community.

The Hopkins group discusses the benefits of antibiotic-impregnated catheters. They as well as several other centers have conducted retrospective studies that demonstrate the clinical efficacy in the reduction of shunt infections in children (particularly high-risk infants) since the introduction of these systems. These catheters prevent the colonization of gram-positive organisms and in turn decrease the risk for shunt infection. There have been no complications or resistant infections with these systems. Although many centers do not use these shunt systems, we will need prospective, randomized clinical studies to see the benefit of the shunt systems.

References

1. Nulsen FE, Spitz EB. Treatment of hydrocephalus by direct shunt from ventricle to jugular vein. Surg Forum 1952;2:399–403
2. Laurence KM, Coates S. The natural history of hydrocephalus: detailed analysis of 182 unoperated cases. Arch Dis Child 1962;37:345–362
3. Dennis M, Fitz CR, Netley CT, et al. The intelligence of hydrocephalic children. Arch Neurol 1981;38(10):607–615
4. Hirsch J-F. Consensus: long-term outcome in hydrocephalus. Childs Nerv Syst 1994;10(1):64–69

5. Keucher TR, Mealey J Jr. Long-term results after ventriculoatrial and ventriculoperitoneal shunting for infantile hydrocephalus. J Neurosurg 1979;50(2):179–186

6. Kokkonen J, Serlo W, Saukkonen A-L, Juolasmaa A. Long-term prognosis for children with shunted hydrocephalus. Childs Nerv Syst 1994;10(6):384–387

7. Riva D, Milani N, Giorgi C, Pantaleoni C, Zorzi C, Devoti M. Intelligence outcome in children with shunted hydrocephalus of different etiology. Childs Nerv Syst 1994;10(1):70–73

8. Sgouros S, Malluci CL, Walsh AR, Hockley AD. Long-term complications of hydrocephalus. Pediatr Neurosurg 1995;23(3):127–132

9. Drake JM, Sainte-Rose C. The Shunt Book. Cambridge, MA: Blackwell Science; 1995

10. Zemack G, Romner B. Do adjustable shunt valves pressure our budget? A retrospective analysis of 541 implanted Codman-Hakim programmable valves. Br J Neurosurg 2001;15(3):221–227

11. Warf BC. Comparison of 1-year outcomes for the Chhabra and Codman-Hakim Micro Precision shunt systems in Uganda: a prospective study in 195 children. J Neurosurg 2005;102(4, Suppl): 358–362

12. Aschoff A, Kremer P, Benesch C, Fruh K, Klank A, Kunze S. Overdrainage and shunt technology: a critical comparison of programmable, hydrostatic and variable-resistance valves and flow-reducing devices. Childs Nerv Syst 1995;11(4):193–202

13. Czosnyka Z, Czosnyka M, Richards HK, Pickard JD. Posture-related overdrainage: comparison of the performance of 10 hydrocephalus shunts in vitro. Neurosurgery 1998;42(2):327–333, discussion 333–334

14. Drake JM, da Silva MC, Rutka JT. Functional obstruction of an anti-siphon device by raised tissue capsule pressure. Neurosurgery 1993;32(1):137–139

15. Decq P, Barat J-L, Duplessis E, Leguerinel C, Gendrault P, Keravel Y. Shunt failure in adult hydrocephalus: flow-controlled shunt versus differential pressure shunts—a cooperative study in 289 patients. Surg Neurol 1995;43(4):333–339

16. Drake JM, Kestle JR, Milner R, et al. Randomized trial of cerebrospinal fluid shunt valve design in pediatric hydrocephalus. Neurosurgery 1998;43(2):294–303, discussion 303–305

17. Eymann R, Steudel W-I, Kiefer M. Pediatric gravitational shunts: initial results from a prospective study. J Neurosurg 2007;106(3, Suppl):179–184

18. Adeloye A. Management of infantile hydrocephalus in Central Africa. Trop Doct 2001;31(2):67–70

19. Blount JP, Campbell JA, Haines SJ. Complications in ventricular cerebrospinal fluid shunting. Neurosurg Clin N Am 1993;4(4): 633–656

20. Di Rocco C, Marchese E, Velardi F. A survey of the first complication of newly implanted CSF shunt devices for the treatment of nontumoral hydrocephalus: cooperative survey of the 1991–1992 Education Committee of the ISPN. Childs Nerv Syst 1994;10(5):321–327

21. Sainte-Rose C, Hoffman HJ, Hirsch JF. Shunt failure. Concepts Pediatr Neurosurg 1989;9:7–20

22. Sainte-Rose C, Piatt JH, Renier D, et al. Mechanical complications in shunts. Pediatr Neurosurg 1991–;17(1):2–9

23. Sainte-Rose C. Shunt obstruction: a preventable complication? Pediatr Neurosurg 1993;19(3):156–164

24. Kondageski C, Thompson D, Reynolds M, Hayward RD. Experience with the Strata valve in the management of shunt overdrainage. J Neurosurg 2007;106(2, Suppl):95–102

25. Pollack IF, Albright AL, Adelson PD; Hakim-Medos Investigator Group. A randomized, controlled study of a programmable shunt valve versus a conventional valve for patients with hydrocephalus. Neurosurgery 1999;45(6):1399–1408, discussion 1408–1411

26. Reinprecht A, Dietrich W, Bertalanffy A, Czech T. The Medos Hakim programmable valve in the treatment of pediatric hydrocephalus. Childs Nerv Syst 1997;13(11-12):588–593, discussion 593–594

27. Zemack G, Bellner J, Siesjö P, Strömblad LG, Romner B. Clinical experience with the use of a shunt with an adjustable valve in children with hydrocephalus. J Neurosurg 2003;98(3):471–476

28. Zemack G, Romner B. Seven years of clinical experience with the programmable Codman Hakim valve: a retrospective study of 583 patients. J Neurosurg 2000;92(6):941–948

29. Zemack G, Romner B. Adjustable valves in normal-pressure hydrocephalus: a retrospective study of 218 patients. Neurosurgery 2002;51(6):1392–1400, discussion 1400–1402

30. Hamid NA, Sgouros S. The use of an adjustable valve to treat overdrainage of a cyst-peritoneal shunt in a child with a large sylvian fissure arachnoid cyst. Childs Nerv Syst 2005;21(11):991–994

31. Aschoff A, Kremer P, Hashemi B, Kunze S. The scientific history of hydrocephalus and its treatment. Neurosurg Rev 1999;22(2-3): 67–93, discussion 94–95

32. Baru JS, Bloom DA, Muraszko K, Koop CE. John Holter's shunt. J Am Coll Surg 2001;192(1):79–85

33. Boockvar JA, Loudon W, Sutton LN. Development of the Spitz-Holter valve in Philadelphia. J Neurosurg 2001;95(1):145–147

34. Dandy WE, Blackfan KD. An experimental and clinical study of internal hydrocephalus. J Am Med Assoc 1913;61:2216–2217

35. Ransohoff J, Shulman K, Fishman RA. Hydrocephalus: a review of etiology and treatment. J Pediatr 1960;56:399–411

36. Egnor M, Zheng L, Rosiello A, Gutman F, Davis R. A model of pulsations in communicating hydrocephalus. Pediatr Neurosurg 2002; 36(6):281–303

37. Kestle J, Drake J, Milner R, et al. Long-term follow-up data from the Shunt Design Trial. Pediatr Neurosurg 2000;33(5):230–236

38. Rekate HL. The slit ventricle syndrome: advances based on technology and understanding. Pediatr Neurosurg 2004;40(6): 259–263

39. Kestle JR, Walker ML; Strata Investigators. A multicenter prospective cohort study of the Strata valve for the management of hydrocephalus in pediatric patients. J Neurosurg 2005;102(2, Suppl): 141–145

40. Arnell K, Eriksson E, Olsen L. The programmable adult Codman Hakim valve is useful even in very small children with hydrocephalus: a 7-year retrospective study with special focus on cost/benefit analysis. Eur J Pediatr Surg 2006;16(1):1–7

41. Reinprecht A, Czech T, Dietrich W. Clinical experience with a new pressure-adjustable shunt valve. Acta Neurochir (Wien) 1995; 134(3-4):119–124

42. Zemack G, Bellner J, Siesjö P, Strömblad LG, Romner B. Clinical experience with the use of a shunt with an adjustable valve in children with hydrocephalus. J Neurosurg 2003;98(3):471–476

43. Dietrich U, Lumenta C, Sprick C, Majewski B. Subdural hematoma in a case of hydrocephalus and macrocrania: experience with a pressure-adjustable valve. Childs Nerv Syst 1987;3(4):242–244

44. Lumenta CB, Roosen N, Dietrich U. Clinical experience with a pressure-adjustable valve SOPHY in the management of hydrocephalus. Childs Nerv Syst 1990;6(5):270–274

45. Chidiac A, Pelissou-Guyotat I, Sindou M. [Practical value of transcutaneous pressure adjustable valves (Sophy SU 8) in the treatment of hydrocephalus and arachnoid cysts in adults (75 cases)]. Neurochirurgie 1992;38(5):291–296

46. Kondageski C, Thompson D, Reynolds M, Hayward RD. Experience with the Strata valve in the management of shunt overdrainage. J Neurosurg 2007;106(2, Suppl):95–102

47. Rohde V, Weinzierl M, Mayfrank L, Gilsbach JM. Postshunt insertion CSF leaks in infants treated by an adjustable valve opening pressure reduction. Childs Nerv Syst 2002;18(12):702–704

48. Nomura S, Fujisawa H, Suzuki M. Effect of cell phone magnetic fields on adjustable cerebrospinal fluid shunt valves. Surg Neurol 2005;63(5):467–468

49. Miwa K, Kondo H, Sakai N. Pressure changes observed in Codman-Medos programmable valves following magnetic exposure and filliping. Childs Nerv Syst 2001;17(3):150–153

50. Fransen P, Dooms G, Thauvoy C. Safety of the adjustable pressure ventricular valve in magnetic resonance imaging: problems and solutions. Neuroradiology 1992;34(6):508–509

51. Schneider T, Knauff U, Nitsch J, Firsching R. Electromagnetic field hazards involving adjustable shunt valves in hydrocephalus. J Neurosurg 2002;96(2):331–334

52. Lüdemann W, Rosahl SK, Kaminsky J, Samii M. Reliability of a new adjustable shunt device without the need for readjustment following 3-Tesla MRI. Childs Nerv Syst 2005;21(3):227–229

53. McGirt MJ, Buck DW II, Sciubba D, et al. Adjustable vs set-pressure valves decrease the risk of proximal shunt obstruction in the treatment of pediatric hydrocephalus. Childs Nerv Syst 2007;23(3):289–295

54. Zemack G, Romner B. Do adjustable shunt valves pressure our budget? A retrospective analysis of 541 implanted Codman Hakim programmable valves. Br J Neurosurg 2001;15(3):221–227

55. Drake JM. The surgical management of pediatric hydrocephalus. Neurosurgery 2008;62(Suppl 2):633–640, discussion 640–642

56. Browd SR, Gottfried ON, Ragel BT, Kestle JR. Failure of cerebrospinal fluid shunts: 2. Overdrainage, loculation, and abdominal complications. Pediatr Neurol 2006;34(3):171–176

57. Browd SR, Ragel BT, Gottfried ON, Kestle JR. Failure of cerebrospinal fluid shunts: 1. Obstruction and mechanical failure. Pediatr Neurol 2006;34(2):83–92

58. Schreffler RT, Schreffler AJ, Wittler RR. Treatment of cerebrospinal fluid shunt infections: a decision analysis. Pediatr Infect Dis J 2002;21(7):632–636

59. Chien YW. Rate-control drug delivery systems: controlled release vs. sustained release. Med Prog Technol 1989;15(1-2):21–46

60. Jansen B, Kohnen W. Prevention of biofilm formation by polymer modification. J Ind Microbiol 1995;15(4):391–396

61. Kohnen W, Jansen B. Polymer materials for the prevention of catheter-related infections. Zentralbl Bakteriol 1995;283(2):175–186

62. Kohnen W, Schäper J, Klein O, Tieke B, Jansen B. A silicone ventricular catheter coated with a combination of rifampin and trimethoprim for the prevention of catheter-related infections. Zentralbl Bakteriol 1998;287(1-2):147–156

63. Garton HJ, Piatt JH Jr. Hydrocephalus. Pediatr Clin North Am 2004;51(2):305–325

64. Bajpai M. Congenital hydrocephalus occurs in approximately 1 case for every 2,000 live or stillborn births. Indian J Pediatr 1997;64(6, Suppl):1–3

65. Fernell E, Hagberg B, Hagberg G, von Wendt L. Epidemiology of infantile hydrocephalus in Sweden: 1. Birth prevalence and general data. Acta Paediatr Scand 1986;75(6):975–981

66. Persson EK, Hagberg G, Uvebrant P. Hydrocephalus prevalence and outcome in a population-based cohort of children born in 1989-1998. Acta Paediatr 2005;94(6):726–732

67. Van Landingham M, Nguyen TV, Roberts A, Parent AD, Zhang J. Risk factors of congenital hydrocephalus: a 10 year retrospective study. J Neurol Neurosurg Psychiatry 2009;80(2):213–217

68. Davidoff L. Treatment of hydrocephalus. Arch Surg 1929;18:1737–1762

69. Drake J, Sainte-Rose C. The Shunt Book. Cambridge, MA: Blackwell Science; 1995

70. Lifshutz JI, Johnson WD. History of hydrocephalus and its treatments. Neurosurg Focus 2001;11(2):E1

71. McCullough D. Hydrocephalus. Vol 3. Baltimore: Williams & Wilkiins; 1990

72. Milhorat T. Hydrocephalus: Historical Notes, Etiology, and Clinical Diagnosis. New York: Grune & Stratton; 1984

73. Matson DD. Current treatment of infantile hydrocephalus. N Engl J Med 1956;255(20):933–936

74. Pudenz RH. Experimental and clinical observations on the shunting of cerebrospinal fluid into the circulatory system. Clin Neurosurg 1957–1958;5:98–114, discussion 114–115

75. Pudenz RH. The surgical treatment of hydrocephalus—an historical review. Surg Neurol 1981;15(1):15–26

76. Pudenz RH, Russell FE, Hurd AH, Shelden CH. Ventriculo-auriculostomy: a technique for shunting cerebrospinal fluid into the right auricle—preliminary report. J Neurosurg 1957;14(2):171–179

77. Kennedy CR, Ayers S, Campbell MJ, Elbourne D, Hope P, Johnson A. Randomized, controlled trial of acetazolamide and furosemide in posthemorrhagic ventricular dilation in infancy: follow-up at 1 year. Pediatrics 2001;108(3):597–607

78. Whitelaw A. Repeated lumbar or ventricular punctures for preventing disability or shunt dependence in newborn infants with intraventricular hemorrhage. Cochrane Database Syst Rev 2000;2:CD000216

79. Whitelaw A. Repeated lumbar or ventricular punctures in newborns with intraventricular hemorrhage. Cochrane Database Syst Rev 2001;1:CD000216

80. Willis BK, Kumar CR, Wylen EL, Nanda A. Ventriculosubgaleal shunts for posthemorrhagic hydrocephalus in premature infants. Pediatr Neurosurg 2005;41(4):178–185

81. Karas CS, Baig MN, Elton SW. Ventriculosubgaleal shunts at Columbus Children's Hospital: neurosurgical implant placement in the neonatal intensive care unit. J Neurosurg 2007;107(3, Suppl):220–223

82. Rahman S, Teo C, Morris W, Lao D, Boop FA. Ventriculosubgaleal shunt: a treatment option for progressive posthemorrhagic hydrocephalus. Childs Nerv Syst 1995;11(11):650–654

83. Duhaime AC. Evaluation and management of shunt infections in children with hydrocephalus. Clin Pediatr (Phila) 2006;45(8):705–713

84. Chiou CC, Wong TT, Lin HH, et al. Fungal infection of ventriculoperitoneal shunts in children. Clin Infect Dis 1994;19(6):1049–1053

85. Filka J, Huttova M, Tuharsky J, Sagat T, Kralinsky K, Krcmery V Jr. Nosocomial meningitis in children after ventriculoperitoneal shunt insertion. Acta Paediatr 1999;88(5):576–578

86. Montero A, Romero J, Vargas JA, et al. *Candida* infection of cerebrospinal fluid shunt devices: report of two cases and review of the literature. Acta Neurochir (Wien) 2000;142(1):67–74

87. Kang JK, Lee IW. Long-term follow-up of shunting therapy. Childs Nerv Syst 1999;15(11-12):711–717

88. Dallacasa P, Dappozzo A, Galassi E, Sandri F, Cocchi G, Masi M. Cerebrospinal fluid shunt infections in infants. Childs Nerv Syst 1995;11(11):643–648, discussion 649

89. Etienne J, Charpin B, Grando J, Brun Y, Bes M, Fleurette J. Characterization of clinically significant isolates of *Staphylococcus epidermidis* from patients with cerebrospinal fluid shunt infections. Epidemiol Infect 1991;106(3):467–475

90. Rotim K, Miklic P, Paladino J, Melada A, Marcikic M, Scap M. Reducing the incidence of infection in pediatric cerebrospinal fluid shunt operations. Childs Nerv Syst 1997;13(11-12):584–587

91. Shapiro S, Boaz J, Kleiman M, Kalsbeck J, Mealey J. Origin of organisms infecting ventricular shunts. Neurosurgery 1988;22(5):868–872

92. Stamos JK, Kaufman BA, Yogev R. Ventriculoperitoneal shunt infections with gram-negative bacteria. Neurosurgery 1993;33(5):858–862

93. Duhaime AC, Bonner K, McGowan KL, Schut L, Sutton LN, Plotkin S. Distribution of bacteria in the operating room environment and its relation to ventricular shunt infections: a prospective study. Childs Nerv Syst 1991;7(4):211–214

94. Kulkarni AV, Drake JM, Lamberti-Pasculli M. Cerebrospinal fluid shunt infection: a prospective study of risk factors. J Neurosurg 2001;94(2):195–201

95. Mancao M, Miller C, Cochrane B, Hoff C, Sauter K, Weber E. Cerebrospinal fluid shunt infections in infants and children in Mobile, Alabama. Acta Paediatr 1998;87(6):667–670

96. Patriarca PA, Lauer BA. Ventriculoperitoneal shunt-associated infection due to *Haemophilus influenzae.* Pediatrics 1980;65(5):1007–1009

97. Baird C, O'Connor D, Pittman T. Late shunt infections. Pediatr Neurosurg 1999;31(5):269–273

98. Borges LF. Cerebrospinal fluid shunts interfere with host defenses. Neurosurgery 1982;10(1):55–60

99. Borgbjerg BM, Gjerris F, Albeck MJ, Børgesen SE. Risk of infection after cerebrospinal fluid shunt: an analysis of 884 first-time shunts. Acta Neurochir (Wien) 1995;136(1-2):1–7

100. Cochrane DD, Kestle J. Ventricular shunting for hydrocephalus in children: patients, procedures, surgeons and institutions in English Canada, 1989–2001. Eur J Pediatr Surg 2002;12(Suppl 1):S6–S11

101. Cochrane DD, Kestle JR. The influence of surgical operative experience on the duration of first ventriculoperitoneal shunt function and infection. Pediatr Neurosurg 2003;38(6):295–301

102. Pittman T, Williams D, Weber TR, Steinhardt G, Tracy T Jr. The risk of abdominal operations in children with ventriculoperitoneal shunts. J Pediatr Surg 1992;27(8):1051–1053

103. Miller PD, Pollack IF, Pang D, Albright AL. Comparison of simultaneous versus delayed ventriculoperitoneal shunt insertion in children undergoing myelomeningocele repair. J Child Neurol 1996;11(5):370–372

104. Tuli S, Drake J, Lamberti-Pasculli M. Long-term outcome of hydrocephalus management in myelomeningoceles. Childs Nerv Syst 2003;19(5-6):286–291

105. Lan CC, Wong TT, Chen SJ, Liang ML, Tang RB. Early diagnosis of ventriculoperitoneal shunt infections and malfunctions in children with hydrocephalus. J Microbiol Immunol Infect 2003; 36(1):47–50

106. Rekate HL, Yonas H, White RJ, Nulsen FE. The acute abdomen in patients with ventriculoperitoneal shunts. Surg Neurol 1979; 11(6):442–445

107. Gaskill SJ, Marlin AE. Pseudocysts of the abdomen associated with ventriculoperitoneal shunts: a report of twelve cases and a review of the literature. Pediatr Neurosci 1989;15(1):23–26, discussion 26–27

108. Roitberg BZ, Tomita T, McLone DG. Abdominal cerebrospinal fluid pseudocyst: a complication of ventriculoperitoneal shunt in children. Pediatr Neurosurg 1998;29(5):267–273

109. Bruinsma N, Stobberingh EE, Herpers MJ, Vles JS, Weber BJ, Gavilanes DA. Subcutaneous ventricular catheter reservoir and ventriculoperitoneal drain-related infections in preterm infants and young children. Clin Microbiol Infect 2000;6(4):202–206

110. Lo TY, Myles LM, Minns RA. Long-term risks and benefits of a separate CSF access device with ventriculoperitoneal shunting in childhood hydrocephalus. Dev Med Child Neurol 2003;45(1):28–33

111. Noetzel MJ, Baker RP. Shunt fluid examination: risks and benefits in the evaluation of shunt malfunction and infection. J Neurosurg 1984;61(2):328–332

112. Sood S, Canady AI, Ham SD. Evaluation of shunt malfunction using shunt site reservoir. Pediatr Neurosurg 2000;32(4):180–186

113. Tung H, Raffel C, McComb JG. Ventricular cerebrospinal fluid eosinophilia in children with ventriculoperitoneal shunts. J Neurosurg 1991;75(4):541–544

114. Kontny U, Höfling B, Gutjahr P, Voth D, Schwarz M, Schmitt HJ. CSF shunt infections in children. Infection 1993;21(2):89–92

115. Bayston R, Rodgers J. Role of serological tests in the diagnosis of immune complex disease in infection of ventriculoatrial shunts for hydrocephalus. Eur J Clin Microbiol Infect Dis 1994;13(5):417–420

116. James HE, Walsh JW, Wilson HD, Connor JD, Bean JR, Tibbs PA. Prospective randomized study of therapy in cerebrospinal fluid shunt infection. Neurosurgery 1980;7(5):459–463

117. Kulkarni AV, Rabin D, Lamberti-Pasculli M, Drake JM. Repeat cerebrospinal fluid shunt infection in children. Pediatr Neurosurg 2001;35(2):66–71

118. Choux M, Genitori L, Lang D, Lena G. Shunt implantation: reducing the incidence of shunt infection. J Neurosurg 1992;77(6):875–880

119. Faillace WJ. A no-touch technique protocol to diminish cerebrospinal fluid shunt infection. Surg Neurol 1995;43(4):344–350

120. Mottolese C, Grando J, Convert J, et al. Zero rate of shunt infection in the first postoperative year in children—dream or reality? Childs Nerv Syst 2000;16(4):210–212

121. Ratilal B, Costa J, Sampaio C. Antibiotic prophylaxis for surgical introduction of intracranial ventricular shunts. Cochrane Database Syst Rev 2006;3:CD005365

122. Sciubba DM, Stuart RM, McGirt MJ, et al. Effect of antibiotic-impregnated shunt catheters in decreasing the incidence of shunt infection in the treatment of hydrocephalus. J Neurosurg 2005;103(2, Suppl):131–136

123. Bayston R, Grove N, Siegel J, Lawellin D, Barsham S. Prevention of hydrocephalus shunt catheter colonisation in vitro by impregnation with antimicrobials. J Neurol Neurosurg Psychiatry 1989;52(5):605–609

124. Bayston R, Lambert E. Duration of protective activity of cerebrospinal fluid shunt catheters impregnated with antimicrobial agents to prevent bacterial catheter-related infection. J Neurosurg 1997;87(2):247–251

125. Govender ST, Nathoo N, van Dellen JR. Evaluation of an antibiotic-impregnated shunt system for the treatment of hydrocephalus. J Neurosurg 2003;99(5):831–839

126. Hampl J, Schierholz J, Jansen B, Aschoff A. In vitro and in vivo efficacy of a rifampin-loaded silicone catheter for the prevention of CSF shunt infections. Acta Neurochir (Wien) 1995;133(3-4):147–152

127. Hampl JA, Weitzel A, Bonk C, Kohnen W, Roesner D, Jansen B. Rifampin-impregnated silicone catheters: a potential tool for prevention and treatment of CSF shunt infections. Infection 2003; 31(2):109–111

128. Schierholz J, Jansen B, Jaenicke L, Pulverer G. In vitro efficacy of an antibiotic-releasing silicone ventricle catheter to prevent shunt infection. Biomaterials 1994;15(12):996–1000

129. Schierholz JM, Pulverer G. Development of a new CSF-shunt with sustained release of an antimicrobial broad-spectrum combination. Zentralbl Bakteriol 1997;286(1):107–123

130. Sciubba DM, Lin LM, Woodworth GF, McGirt MJ, Carson B, Jallo GI. Factors contributing to the medical costs of cerebrospinal fluid shunt infection treatment in pediatric patients with standard shunt components compared with those in patients with antibiotic impregnated components. Neurosurg Focus 2007;22(4):E9

131. Sciubba DM, McGirt MJ, Woodworth GF, Carson B, Jallo GI. Prolonged exposure to antibiotic-impregnated shunt catheters does not increase incidence of late shunt infections. Childs Nerv Syst 2007;23(8):867–871

132. Sciubba DM, Noggle JC, Carson BS, Jallo GI. Antibiotic-impregnated shunt catheters for the treatment of infantile hydrocephalus. Pediatr Neurosurg 2008;44(2):91–96

3 Noncommunicating Hydrocephalus

♦ Endoscopic Third Ventriculostomy

Shlomi Constantini and Jonathan Roth

Endoscopic third ventriculostomy (ETV) has become the treatment of choice for hydrocephalus originating from an intraventricular obstruction, usually at the level of the aqueduct. Despite widespread enthusiasm at being able to treat hydrocephalus without reliance on a foreign body and within the skull boundaries, inherent risks exist for this high-end procedure. The dilemma of how to treat a specific patient with hydrocephalus, whether with a shunt or with ETV, has to be resolved on an individual basis, taking into account factors such as age, etiology, anatomy, clinical behavior, the available technology, and the surgeon's experience. This chapter will discuss different patterns of hydrocephalus and the applicability of ETV.

Physiology and Advantages

In a third ventriculostomy, a hole is made using fiberoptic technology, under direct vision, on the floor of the third ventricle. The new opening allows cerebrospinal fluid (CSF) to exit downward to the interpeduncular cistern, continuing to the convexity of the brain, to be absorbed through "natural" pathways.

A patent third ventriculostomy converts an "obstructive" type of hydrocephalus into a communicating one. In contrast to the extracranial diversion produced by a ventriculoperitoneal shunt (VPS), ETV solves the problem of excess fluid within the brain boundaries through a more physiologic intracranial approach.[1,2] CSF drainage is therefore not significantly affected by position, gravity, or intra-abdominal pressure.

The lack of dependency on a foreign body is another advantage of ETV over shunting. The infections that frequently occur following VPS insertion usually mandate additional operative procedures for removing the hardware.[3] When infections do occur following ETV, they can be relatively easily resolved with antibiotic treatment only. In addition, shunts often malfunction due to tearing, blockage,

or misplacement. Shunt replacement, though dependent in part on original pathology and age, is required at an average rate of at least 10% per year.[4]

Early failure of ETV can occur either as a result of an insufficient opening on the floor of the third ventricle (due either to small diameter or lack of opening of the "second" membrane) or in situations where the final stage of CSF absorption, at the arachnoid granulations, is not functional.[5] Current methods attempting to test the absorption stage before an ETV are, unfortunately, not reliable.

Late failures of ETV do occur but are infrequent and rarely occur more than 6 months after surgery.[6] When compared with VPS, late failure rates following an initially successful ETV are probably rarer by more than an order of magnitude.[7] Late failures are usually attributed to scarring and closure of the stoma.[8,9] When a late failure does occur, a repeat ETV can be offered to patients who have no flow void on the floor of the third ventricle visible on magnetic resonance imaging (MRI).[8] Nevertheless, it is important to note that because late failures following ETV can and do occur, and may even cause "sudden death,"[10,11] patients should be warned that an ETV, even an initially successful one, does not cure hydrocephalus. Such patients should stay under supervision and follow-up and take symptoms associated with high intracranial pressure (ICP), if they do occur, very seriously.

Indications

The classic indication for ETV is primary or secondary aqueductal stenosis[1,2,12] (**Figs. 3.1** and **3.2**). When a tumor exists at the level of the pineal gland, or posterior third ventricle, ETV can be combined with an endoscopic biopsy. In hydrocephalus caused by tectal lesions, only an ETV is performed. In aqueductal stenosis, the MRI typically demonstrates a triventricular configuration, no flow at the level of the aqueduct, and displacement of the floor of the third ventricle downward.

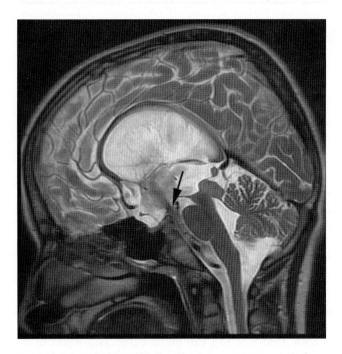

Fig. 3.1 Post-endoscopic third ventriculostomy (ETV) magnetic resonance imaging (MRI) reveals obstructive hydrocephalus caused by a tectal lesion compressing the aqueduct. A flow void is seen through the stoma in the floor of the third ventricle (*arrow*).

Age may be a factor in the success rates of ETV in aqueductal stenosis. Success rates in infants (measured as the resolution of symptoms with shunt freeness) were initially quoted as between 30 and 80%.[13] Recent publications have shown ~50% success rates.[14] Most, but not all, authors still believe that age (within the group of infants) is important for the prediction of success.[15,16] Because ETV in infants up to 2 years of age is so controversial, a randomized controlled study (under the auspices of the International Society for Pediatric Neurosurgery, International Study Group on Neuroendoscopy, and International Federation of Neuroendoscopy) is currently under way.[13] This international multicenter randomized clinical trial (the International Infant Hydrocephalus Study) focuses on neurobehavioral scoring as its primary outcome measure.

ETV has the potential to successfully treat situations where the fourth ventricle outlet is blocked (**Figs. 3.3** and **3.4**). Pathologies such as Chiari malformation and Dandy-Walker syndrome have been treated successfully with ETV in small series.[17] Further data are required for evidence-based decisions on ETV in these situations.

Similar decision patterns apply to chronically shunted patients who present with a shunt malfunction. This group seems to be ideal for ETV, as long as they show a primary or secondary blockage at the aqueduct when their shunt malfunctions.[18–20]

Initial enthusiasm for the role of ETV in children with a posterior fossa tumor has recently subsided.[21] ETV probably has a limited role to play as a temporary measure to control ICP until the tumor is removed.[22] After tumor removal, when the aqueduct is usually wide open, hydrocephalus, if present, is mostly absorptive.

Technique

ETV is done in patients under general anesthesia, usually through a right frontal, precoronal bur hole. The exact placement of the entry point is crucial, especially in complex cases such as combined ETV–biopsy procedures. Navigation may be helpful in choosing the placement of the bur hole, as well as for planning an optimal initial trajectory path to the ventricle and the foramen of Monro.[23,24] Once inside the ventricle, the procedure is determined by the individual anatomy, and navigation systems are less useful. Use of peel-away tubes has an advantage in establishing an open route that can be flushed as necessary and in preventing abrasions to the walls of the frontal lobe.

After a "tour" to identify the exact anatomy of the lateral ventricle, the neuroendoscope is advanced through the foramen of Monro to the third ventricle, taking care not to cause damage to the fornix and the choroid plexus. At this stage, the somewhat stereotypical anatomy of the third ventricle is revealed. The hole is aimed to be in front of the mammillary bodies, keeping to the midline, at the tuber cinereum and posterior to the median eminence and infundibulum. Special care is devoted to prevent perforations to the basilar artery bifurcation, situated on the other side of the membrane. The basilar pulsations may occasionally be seen through a thin membrane. Lasers are usually not used any more to create the hole. Most trained surgeons make the initial hole with a blunt monopolar electrode without current. Electricity is occasionally required when the membrane is tough. The hole is widened using a Fogarty catheter or the endoscopic forceps. The opening of the second membrane to fully visualize the content of the interpeduncular cistern and the subarachnoid space is very important (**Fig. 3.5**).

Complications

The most dreaded complication of ETV is basilar artery perforation.[25] Such an occurrence can be fatal. To prevent it, one should consider each patient's anatomy carefully, both on preoperative MRI and through the endoscope. The initial hole should be placed as anterior as possible, and only if a good view exists. Injury to the walls of the lateral ventricle occur mostly when the ventricles are not very big. Navigation systems can assist in choosing optimal trajectories and bur hole placement.[23,24] Small venous bleedings usually subside spontaneously with rinsing, using either Hartmann's solution or normal saline. Endocrinological complications have been described following ETV, but they are rare.[26] Chronic subdural hematomas have been reported

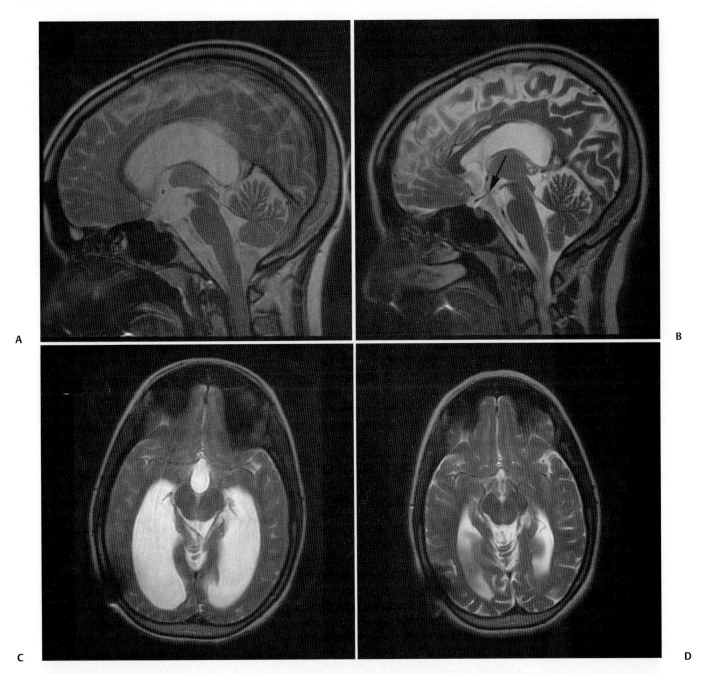

Fig. 3.2 (A,C) Obstructive hydrocephalus caused by aqueductal compression by a thalamic lesion. **(B,D)** After performing an ETV, the ventricles have decreased in size, and a flow void is apparent through the third ventricular floor (*arrow*).

and seem to occur more in those patients with very large fluid spaces to start with.[27] Infections may also occur and should be suspected when postoperative fever appears within 2 weeks of the procedure. Wound breakage may occur, especially in infants, and mandates special emphasis on closure techniques in this population.[5,28]

Ongoing hydrocephalus persists in some cases. Occasionally, the absorption systems of the brain require time to adapt. This temporary situation has led some to insert a continuous lumbar drain (CLD) or perform a lumbar tap following ETV procedures, thus allowing natural pathways to adapt and come into use gradually.[29] Others have advocated leaving Ommaya reservoirs to deal with early, as well as late, ETV failures.[30] In nonstraightforward cases, we also like to leave ICP monitoring for a few days. Pressure waves can be treated then with lumbar punctures or even CLDs.

Following an ETV, patients should spend the first postoperative night in an intensive care unit setting.

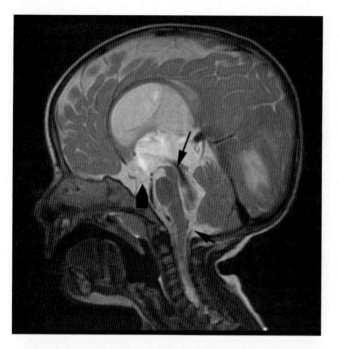

Fig. 3.3 Fourth ventricular outlet obstruction (FVOO), pre-ETV MRI. A flow void is seen through the aqueduct (*long arrow*) but not at the fourth ventricular outlet (*short arrow*). All the ventricles are enlarged, and the third ventricular floor bulges downward (*arrowhead*), suggesting a pressure gradient on it.

Technology

Most surgeons use rigid optical systems for ETV. Outer scope diameters range from 2.3 to 7.0 mm. Working channels > 2 mm allow the use of bipolar coagulation. Free hand scope manipulation is generally the rule for ETV. Arm holding and manipulation systems have been described and are available but have so far not gained widespread popularity.[24]

Results

ETV success rates have usually been measured in terms of "shunt freedom." Comparisons between centers and pathologic groups have been hampered by the lack of uniformity for both inclusion criteria and failure definitions. For noninfants, aqueductal stenosis (idiopathic or tumor-related) success rates of 50 to 90% are commonly described.[31-35]

Hydrocephalus Associated with Open Spina Bifida and Chiari Malformation

Open spina bifida and meningomyelocele are associated with a high incidence of hydrocephalus. Thirty-five to 90% of patients with meningomyelocele will have either clinical or radiologic evidence of hydrocephalus.[36] The etiology of hydrocephalus in these patients is multifactorial. However,

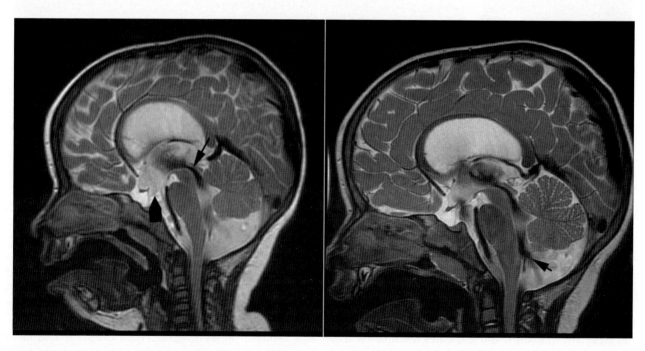

A

B

Fig. 3.4 (A) A suspected FVOO hydrocephalus. A flow void is present through the aqueduct (*arrow*), but the third ventricular floor is bulging downward (*arrowhead*), suggesting a pressure gradient. **(B)** After performing an ETV, a flow void is apparent through the stoma, and the third ventricular floor has less bulging. The flow void through the fourth ventricle outlet (*short arrow*) is much more obvious after the operation, suggesting that the diagnosis was not an FVOO. However, the patient improved after the ETV.

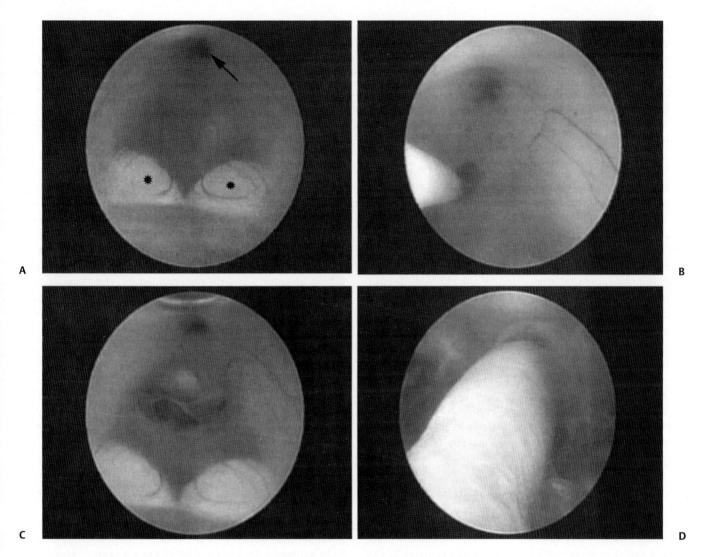

Fig. 3.5 (A) Intraoperative view of the tuber cinereum (mammillary bodies = asterisk, infundibular recess = *arrow*), **(B)** blunt poking of the floor, **(C)** the opening in the floor, and **(D)** a view of the basilar artery in the interpeduncular cistern.

most are secondary to a small posterior fossa with an associated Chiari (type II) malformation, causing an obstructive type of hydrocephalus. Other obstructing causes may be at the fourth ventricular outlet and aqueductal stenosis.[37–39] Low-grade ventriculitis and meningitis, as well as hypoplastic arachnoid villi, may also contribute with an absorptive component.[38] There is thus no single hydrocephalic-causing mechanism, and the communicating-obstructing nature depends on the predominating factors in an individual case.[12]

Some surgeons have excluded patients with meningomyelocele from ETV series based on the assumption that the hydrocephalus is not purely obstructive.[18,40] However, others have performed ETV in selected cases and achieved a reasonable success rate.[12,41]

In addition to the pathophysiologic basis of hydrocephalus in patients with meningomyelocele, these

patients have various cerebral anomalies and anatomical variations that may pose technical difficulties for performing the procedure, thus increasing the associated risk. These anomalies include an enlarged massa intermedia of the third ventricle, a distortion of the hypothalami, the absence of septum pellucidum, a small foramen of Monro, the presence of atypical veins on the third ventricular floor, arachnoidal adhesions and septations in the third ventricle, a narrow interpeduncular cistern, and the absence of the infundibulum.[37,40,42,43] Up to 70% of cases of myelomeningocele may have third ventricular floor anomalies.[43] In the largest series describing ETV in children with meningomyelocele, Teo and Jones described their experience with 78 patients.[12] These patients were carefully selected on the basis of imaging suggesting an obstructive hydrocephalus. The overall success rate was 72%. Three cases were aborted due to third ventricular anomalies precluding a safe procedure. The success rate for children younger than 2 years was 53%, and for elder children 80%. Further analysis showed that the low success rate was for ages less than 6 months (18%), whereas 6- to 26-month-old children had an 80% success rate. Warf described his results in 22 children with meningomyelocele younger than 1 year.[40] The success rate was 40%, and four cases were aborted due to distorted third ventricular anatomy. The 80% success rate in elder children, with no increased morbidity, places the outcome of ETV for patients with meningomyelocele at similar outcome rates as for aqueductal stenosis.[32,44] High rates (84%) were achieved for patients previously shunted who presented with shunt malfunction.[12] Shunted ventricles decrease the transmantle pressure, thus decompressing the subarachnoid space, while preserving CSF production by the choroid plexus of the fourth ventricle, thus enabling maturation of the arachnoid villi. Considering the ventricular distortion in patients with meningomyelocele, some surgeons prefer to first place a shunt, then offer an ETV at a shunt malfunction episode.[20]

Thus, MMC-related hydrocephalus is not an absolute contraindication for ETV. Selected patients with suitable anatomical configuration may undergo ETV with a high success rate. Meningomyelocele-related cerebral anomalies need to be addressed pre- and intraoperatively, to anticipate and prevent morbidity and mortality.

Fourth Ventricular Outlet Obstruction

Treatment of sole fourth ventricular outlet obstruction (FVOO) includes few options: supratentorial shunt placement, microsurgical opening of the fourth ventricular outlet, with or without stent placement, and ETV.[45–47]

Placement of a supratentorial shunt poses the basic risks of shunt systems. In addition, drainage of the supratentorial ventricles may cause secondary aqueductal stenosis and a trapped fourth ventricle, necessitating additional procedures.[48,49] Open fenestration of the fourth ventricle and stent placement when the aqueduct is stenotic are effective; however, stent failure may be fatal.[45]

FVOO is rarely a sole pathology. Most reported cases are related to myelomeningocele or Dandy-Walker syndrome.[37–39,50] Other associated malformations are Chiari I malformation and achondroplasia.[17,51,52] The etiology of acquired FVOO is multifactorial, either posthemorrhagic or postinfectious (including viral infections). The common resultant is adhesive arachnoiditis and occlusion of the ventricle outlet.

It is possible that some patients who are classified under the communicating hydrocephalus category have, in fact, an FVOO. The enlarged fourth ventricle does not help to differentiate the two situations. Some have claimed that in FVOO, the Luschka foramina should be enlarged.

ETV has seldom been reported as the treatment for FVOO.[46] Concerning the etiology related to adhesive arachnoiditis, the role of ETV is unclear. However, the few cases reported to date had good clinical outcome, with no failures. In addition, no patient developed a trapped fourth ventricle. This may be due to a more physiologic CSF drainage rate, obviating secondary aqueductal stenosis. Fenestration of the fourth ventricle outlet is a more physiologic treatment; however, the high success rate and more simple procedure make ETV the preferred treatment. Despite modern MRI techniques, this is the situation where contrast material ventriculography may have an added value in the selection process. We have successfully performed ETV for a few such patients with hydrocephalus, where, despite a clearly open aqueduct, the floor of the third ventricle has been downward displaced, a secondary sign of a pressure gradient between the third ventricle and the interpeduncular cistern.

Dandy-Walker Syndrome

Dandy-Walker syndrome is associated with a high rate of hydrocephalus. However, many patients do not have hydrocephalus at birth.[53] Hydrocephalus is caused by obstruction of the fourth ventricular outlet secondary to atresia of foramina of Luschka and Magendie.[50] The obstruction may be partial with a functional insufficiency, thus explaining the low rate of hydrocephalus at birth.[53] The sylvian aqueduct may be obstructed or open.[48,54] The treatment of Dandy-Walker syndrome has posed much debate. Microsurgical opening of the fourth ventricular outlet has been proposed for children older than 3 years.[55] However, success rates for the later procedure among younger children have been low (15%) and associated with high mortality (10%).[53] Thus, the main treatments consists of CSF diversion, from the supratentorial, infratentorial, or both compartments.[48,53,55,56] These treatments have several associated complications. Shunting the supratentorial ventricles may cause secondary aqueductal stenosis from pressure differentials between the supra- and infratentorium, causing an isolated fourth ventricle and necessitating additional shunt placements.[48] Thus, some surgeons suggest placing a fourth ventricular shunt primarily. Posterior fossa shunts have a high complication rate (42% morbidity directly associated with the proximal catheter).[57] Villavicencio et al have proposed an open fenestration for patients with symptomatic posterior fossa cysts after exhausting the shunt options.[58]

Thus, the deciding factor is aqueductal patency. A patent aqueduct enables placement of a supratentorial shunt (risking secondary aqueductal obstruction with a trapped fourth ventricle). An obstructed aqueduct necessitates drainage of both compartments.

Due to the obstructive nature of hydrocephalus, some surgeons have tried ETVs for patients with Dandy-Walker syndrome. These procedures have been performed alone, in addition to aqueductal stenting (between the third ventricle and the posterior fossa cyst), or in addition to fenestration of the posterior fossa cyst.[56,59–61] Mohanty et al published the largest series of ETV in patients with Dandy-Walker syndrome.[56] They used a rigid endoscope for the ETV and a flexible endoscope if needed for aqueductal procedures. After a standard ETV was performed, the aqueduct was inspected. If obstructed, the membrane was fenestrated, and a cystoventricular stent was placed, if needed. The overall ETV success rate in this study was 76%. No specific morbidity or mortality occurred in this group. Smaller series including patients with Dandy-Walker syndrome had success rates of 42 to 66%.[60,61]

Thus, despite the lack of large series, the current literature notes favorable results for ETV alone or in addition to an aqueductal procedure (membrane fenestration, with or without stent placement).

Postinfectious and Posthemorrhagic Hydrocephalus

Postinfectious and posthemorrhagic hydrocephalus is mostly thought to occur due to absorption insufficiency secondary to adhesions in the CSF pathways—basal cisterns, subarachnoid space, and intraventricular septations.[40,62] Thus, CSF flow is obstructed in the subarachnoid space and at the draining end point, the arachnoid villi. These mechanisms led to the concept that the preferred treatment is a shunt, and ETV was considered contraindicated in patients with a previous infection or hemorrhage.[41,63] Siomin et al performed a multicenter retrospective study analyzing the results in posthemorrhagic and/or postinfectious hydrocephalus patients undergoing an ETV.[64] Interestingly, the success rates in patients after either hemorrhage or infection who had a triventricular pattern were 60 to 64%; however, patients with previous central nervous system (CNS) infection and hemorrhage had only 23% success rates. The presence of an infection did not alter the high success rate for ETV in patients with aqueductal stenosis (90%). All premature infants with intraventricular hemorrhage who had their ETV as the first treatment failed. However, all patients who underwent the ETV at the time of a shunt failure were successful. This may be due to transformation of the hydrocephalus to an obstructive hydrocephalus by the shunt, while maintaining CSF production by the fourth ventricle that enables arachnoid granulation maturation. Warf presented his experience in ETV in Uganda.[40] In 300 cases of ETV, 60% had postinfectious hydrocephalus. Warf subdivided

the patients into four groups depending on age (younger than and older than 1 year) and whether the aqueduct was patent or obstructed. The success rate for postinfectious hydrocephalus according to the subgroups was 45% for children younger than 1 year and with a patent aqueduct; the remaining subgroups had success rates between 70 and 80%. The difference between children with a patent and obstructed aqueduct was not significant (50 vs 70%, respectively; $p = .064$), however, the difference between children younger and older than 1 year was significant (60 vs 80%, respectively; $p = .042$). Warf also mentions the technical difficulty in performing an ETV in patients with significant postinfectious changes, especially in the presence of scar tissue, hemosiderin, or inflammatory deposits. Warf's criteria for postinfectious hydrocephalus, however, are problematic. He defined as postinfectious hydrocephalus any case that fulfilled the following: (1) no hydrocephalus at birth and (2) either a history of a febrile disease and/or seizure preceding a clinically apparent hydrocephalus or radiologic and endoscopic evidence of prior ventriculitis. The endoscopic evidence of prior ventriculitis included intraventricular septations, scarring of the third ventricular floor, distortion of the third ventricle, studding of the ependyma with inflammatory exudates or hemosiderin, and obstruction of the foramen of Monro by inflammatory exudates or scar. As noted elsewhere, posthemorrhagic findings may overlap these endoscopic ones.[62] In addition, certain viral diseases may cause aqueductal stenosis, thus biasing the hydrocephalus etiology toward clear obstructive.[65–67] Warf did not mention the infectious cause of his cases but does note that cultures were negative at the time of endoscopy.

Neither Warf nor Siomin notified higher morbidity or mortality among the postinfectious or posthemorrhagic cases. The high success rate in these patients suggests that the subarachnoid space is not obliterated and the absorption capacity is not hampered as previously thought. Thus, the current literature supports ETV as the treatment of triventricular hydrocephalus in patients with a previous history of a CNS infection or hemorrhage, especially children older than 1 year.

Future Prospects

Neuroendoscopy faces challenges in expanding technology and conceptual boundaries, as well as in understanding better how to select the right patients and how to enhance procedure efficacy. This process has to be accomplished through collaborative work.

Acknowledgments We thank Sigal Freedman for her help with the figures.

◆ Ventriculoperitoneal Shunts

Gregory G. Heuer and Phillip B. Storm

Hydrocephalus is one of the most common conditions treated by pediatric neurosurgeons, with an incidence of 1 in 2000 births.[68] Hydrocephalus can result from several conditions, but in its most common form, it presents prenatally, at birth, or in the early neonatal period.

Although there have been several methods to describe and categorize hydrocephalus and the accumulation of CSF, one of the first classification schemes separated patients into those having communicating or absorptive hydrocephalus and those having noncommunicating or obstructive hydrocephalus. Patients with noncommunicating hydrocephalus are those that have enlargement of the ventricles because of an obstruction rather than the diffuse enlargement of all four ventricles seen in communicating hydrocephalus as a result of decreased absorption of CSF into the sagittal sinus. The causes of noncommunicating hydrocephalus include aqueductal stenosis, brainstem tumors, intraventricular tumors, intracranial cysts, postinfectious hydrocephalus, encephaloceles, and genetic/syndromic hydrocephalus.[69]

ETV was first described by William Mixter, a urologist.[70] In 1923 Mixter used a urethroscope to perform a third ventriculostomy in a patient with hydrocephalus. Walter Dandy, an early pioneer in many areas of neurosurgery, successfully used both primitive endoscopes and open techniques to perform third ventriculostomies.[71] However, these early approaches were associated with a high rate of complications and failure; therefore, this technique was not widely adopted. Although previous shunting devices had been attempted as early as 1905, in 1952 the modern shunt was developed by Nulsen, Spitz, and Holter at the Children's Hospital of Philadelphia.[72,73] With the development of these new shunts, the management of hydrocephalus dramatically changed, as a large number of patients could now be treated safely and effectively. Due to the development of more advanced surgical techniques in the early 1980s, a resurgence in the use of ETV occurred.

With two effective surgical procedures available to treat children who present with noncommunicating hydrocephalus, there now exists a controversy concerning the optimal treatment. There has not yet been a randomized trial comparing these two techniques. ETV can be a useful technique for the treatment of noncommunicating hydrocephalus in patients who have had multiple shunt revisions. VPS, however, is the most effective treatment and should be the first line of therapy. There are several factors for the surgeon to consider when deciding on the treatment of choice for each patient, including patient selection criteria, surgical technique, patient care, and complications.

Discussion

Patient Selection Criteria

VPS is safely preformed in patients of all ages and is indicated for all types and causes of hydrocephalus. Even in cases of slit ventricles, a ventricular catheter can be successfully placed, and only in rare instances are additional technologies, such as intraoperative ultrasound and stereotaxic image guidance, needed for this placement. In most instances, a single catheter is effective in treating patients with either communicating or noncommunicating hydrocephalus. However, in some cases of hydrocephalus associated with cysts or other obstructions, effective treatment may require the placement of multiple catheters or fenestration of the septations.

Whereas VPS is indicated for any patient with hydrocephalus, ETV is indicated only in a small percentage of patients with hydrocephalus. The most important factor in evaluating a patient for an ETV is anatomy. In a review by Jallo et al, a patient is considered a candidate for ETV if the patient has certain anatomical features, such as isolated enlargement of the lateral and third ventricles with a normal-sized or small fourth ventricle, an adequately sized third ventricle to allow safe movement of the endoscope, and the presence of adequate space between the basilar artery and the clivus to allow the ventriculostomy to be performed without damaging any vascular structures.[74] In patients who do not have this anatomy, ETV can be technically difficult, dangerous, or impossible.

Shunting, however, can be safely and effectively performed in patients of all ages, regardless of the etiology of the hydrocephalus. There is a higher rate of complications and failure in younger patients, particularly in patients younger than 6 months and in premature infants.[75–78] However, most studies on ETV have shown decreased effectiveness in children younger than 2 years, due to either reduced CSF absorption or the development of arachnoid membranes after the ETV.[79–81] There is currently disagreement as to the age limit for ETV, both as to what the age cutoff is and to whether this age limit exists,[82,83] but the vast majority of the literature on ETV demonstrates that ETV effectiveness is decreased in younger patients. Additionally, in infants and newborns, it can be difficult to determine if hydrocephalus is entirely noncommunicating.[69]

The studies on the relationship between age and both ETV and shunting indicate that both treatment modalities can be more difficult in younger patients. It is possible that the advent of new shunt technology may be able to overcome some problems that are intrinsic to the shunt mechanism itself,[84] but it is unclear if advances in ETV technology can overcome issues that are likely to be patient-related in the majority of cases.

The ability to properly select patients for ETV is thought to be essential to the success of the procedure. Overall, large studies indicate that only 16 to 20% of patients treated for hydrocephalus present with the type of diagnoses that even potentially could be treated with ETV,[76,78] and many of these patients will not be candidates for ETV due to age, anatomy, or some other factor. In those patients who are not candidates for ETV, shunting is the only option.

Surgical Technique and Patient Care

The surgical technique for placement of a standard VPS is well established and routinely performed at all neurosurgical centers. This technique can be used in a wide range of patients. Even in newborns, shunts can be safely placed normally in 20 minutes and almost always within 1 hour.

Other than the ventricular catheter and shunt device, no significant extra equipment is required for placement. During the operation, the surgeon knows that the CSF is flowing through the shunt prior to leaving the operating room.

Postoperatively, patients are observed for any signs or symptoms of immediate shunt malfunction. In the absence of these findings, patients are sent home on postoperative day 1.[68]

In contrast to shunt placement, third ventriculostomies are performed using specialized endoscopic equipment. This equipment may include an endoscope, control panel, irrigation pump, Bugbee wire, balloon catheter, laser, and endoscopic electrocautery device.[74] In centers that do not routinely perform endoscopic procedures, the expenditure for the purchase, upkeep, and upgrades that are unavoidable for this type of technology is significant. Even with the significant technical advances that have been made in this type of equipment, there still remains a significant learning curve for surgeons as they begin to use this technology. This learning curve is invariably higher than that for the more common shunt placement procedure. Furthermore, the number of patients who are appropriate candidates, even using liberal selection criteria, is still very small, making it even more difficult to become facile at ETV.

Even in the most experienced hands, serious periprocedural complications are more common in ETV than in shunting. The mortality rate in ETV is ~1%, resulting from serious complications such as vascular or hypothalamic injury, not to mention serious morbidity-related fornicial injury and oculomotor palsy.[85-90] The periprocedural mortality rate associated with shunting procedures is < 0.1%.[75,78]

Postoperative care in shunted patients routinely consists of observation alone. Because a correctly functioning shunt immediately reduces ICP, patients should have some immediate improvement in their signs and symptoms. In the rare incidence of suspected shunt failure in the immediate postoperative period, the shunt can be tested by tapping the shunt valve to assess the proximal and distal portions of the mechanism. In contrast, determining the success of ETV is problematic. Because the ventricular size may not change dramatically after surgery, in both ETV and shunting, it cannot be used as a reliable indicator of a successful procedure.[91]

Some authors propose the use of external ventricular drains to monitor ICP and confirm a pressure decrease, as a treatment for intraventricular hemorrhage that can occur during the procedure or in patients with prior shunts to "wean" them from CSF shunting.[74,92-95] This increases the overall complication rate of the ETV procedure, as the patient is now exposed to the complication of infection that is associated with external drains (a rate that is higher than that associated with internalized shunts). Other experts advocate placement of a subcutaneous reservoir after ETV so that CSF can be accessed for diagnostic or therapeutic purposes when patients acutely decompensate after ETV failure.[96] This technique adds time to an already longer procedure; additionally, it gives patients permanent hardware and exposes them to hardware infection. Patients are exposed not only to nearly the same risk of hardware infection as a shunt but also to the greater risk of the ETV itself.

Complications

The placement of a VPS is a very safe procedure. The periprocedural mortality rate associated with shunting procedures is < 0.1%.[75,78] However, a major frustration with shunting procedures involves the long-term complications related to these devices. These complications include suboptimal shunting (either over- or undershunting), mechanical failure, and infection. Overall, the failure rate of shunts is significant, with various studies showing a 1-year failure rate as high as 30 to 40%.[75,77,78] These numbers are misleading; however, because they are skewed by premature infants who have a myriad of medical problems, making VPS more difficult (in most of these patients, ETV is absolutely contraindicated). To be able to fully compare the two methods, patients who are not candidates for ETV would have to be removed from the analysis. This selected population consists of older patients with noncommunicating hydrocephalus. Although variable at different institutions, the infection and 1-year failure rates are much lower in this group.[76,77,97-99] Additionally, new designs may be able to overcome some of the mechanical failures and infections seen with shunts. The use of programmable shunts has been shown to decrease proximal obstructions, and the use of antibiotic-impregnated catheters has been shown to decrease the rate of infection significantly.[100-104]

The shunt mechanism does have several benefits in the management of many of the complications, particularly when compared with ETV. There are several readily available techniques to test the function of a shunt. First, the valve may be depressed and examined to determine if there is any refill of the valve and at what speed this occurs. Additionally, the valve may be tapped with a needle to determine if the shunt is functioning properly and in many instances to determine if the ICP is increased. In the event of a distal malfunction or an infection, the catheter may be externalized, effectively stabilizing the patient. Also, most malfunctions can be treated effectively with simple shunt revisions that normally take less time than the initial placement.

The long-term failure rate of ETV has been shown to be the same as the long-term failure rate of shunts.[105] The long-term failure rate of ETV is underreported because patients often have to go some distance for an ETV at a center with a significant volume and an experienced surgeon, then undergo shunting locally when the ETV fails. These patients are often reported as examples of long-term success despite failure. At our institution, we have treated several ETV failures with a redo ETV or placement of a shunt, just as some of our ETVs have undoubtedly been managed elsewhere and are not accurately reported as failures. As the ETV technology improves, making the procedure safer and more permanent, it is expected to make shunting obsolete in properly selected patients.

Conclusion

Shunting remains the treatment of choice for noncommunicating hydrocephalus. It is safer, faster, allows for easy evaluation of function, is not limited by age or anatomy of the prepontine cistern, does not have a steep learning curve, and fails at the same rate as the more dangerous ETV. ETV has a mortality rate that is an order of magnitude greater than a VPS, and the morbidity of an ETV is substantially higher at the time of the initial procedure. The high frequency of ETV failures both in the short and long term has caused many surgeons to leave a subcutaneous reservoir behind, thereby negating the benefit of decreased infection and lack of hardware. Externalized ventriculostomies after ETV also have a higher infection rate than placement/replacement of a shunt, and ventriculostomies are inserted in every ETV that has massive hemorrhaging as a complication. Externalized ventriculostomies are also placed when a shunt is removed and converted to a third ventriculostomy. This not only increases the infection rate but also extends the length of stay beyond a shunt revision and emphasizes the inability to evaluate the efficacy of the ETV immediately after the procedure. The only indication for an ETV is in the rare patient with noncommunicating hydrocephalus who presents later in life, has a favorable anatomy, and has had multiple shunt revisions.

◆ Lessons Learned

Hydrocephalus is the most common disease treated by pediatric neurosurgeons. Shunt systems and endoscopic procedures have existed since the infancy of neurosurgery. Unlike communicating hydrocephalus, this condition has two treatment modalities, each with proponents. Although ETV was performed as early as the 1920s, with the advent of shunt catheters and valves, this procedure fell out of favor. There was a revitalization in the endoscopic technique with the advances in optics and instrumentation. The placement of a shunt system is relatively straightforward, with minimal risks for the majority of children, whereas ETV is associated with an increased procedural risk, in particular injury

to a major arterial vessel. Aside from the surgical risks associated with the procedure, the success rate is slightly lower for ETV, as some children lack a resorptive ability for the CSF. This has been documented in the literature by age of the child, etiology of the noncommunicating hydrocephalus, and technique. Although the surgical techniques for shunt placement are well established and performed around the world, long-term complications, such as malfunction and infection, are significantly higher in this population. These children are dependent upon the shunt system for their CSF diversion, and it is well known that these systems do fail.

References

1. Jones RF, Kwok BC, Stening WA, Vonau M. Neuroendoscopic third ventriculostomy: a practical alternative to extracranial shunts in non-communicating hydrocephalus. Acta Neurochir Suppl (Wien) 1994;61:79–83
2. Pierre-Kahn A, Renier D, Bombois B, Askienay S, Moreau R, Hirsch JF. [Role of the ventriculocisternostomy in the treatment of non-communicating hydrocephalus.] Neurochirurgie 1975;21(7): 557–569
3. Kestle JR, Garton HJ, Whitehead WE, et al. Management of shunt infections: a multicenter pilot study. J Neurosurg 2006;105(3, Suppl): 177–181
4. Drake JM, Kestle JR, Milner R, et al. Randomized trial of cerebrospinal fluid shunt valve design in pediatric hydrocephalus. Neurosurgery 1998;43(2):294–303, discussion 303–305
5. Navarro R, Gil-Parra R, Reitman AJ, Olavarria G, Grant JA, Tomita T. Endoscopic third ventriculostomy in children: early and late

complications and their avoidance. Childs Nerv Syst 2006;22(5): 506–513

6. Drake J, Chumas P, Kestle J, et al. Late rapid deterioration after endoscopic third ventriculostomy: additional cases and review of the literature. J Neurosurg 2006;105(2, Suppl):118–126

7. Kramer U, Kanner AA, Siomin V, Harel S, Constantini S. No evidence of epilepsy following endoscopic third ventriculostomy: a short-term follow-up. Pediatr Neurosurg 2001;34(3):121–123

8. Siomin V, Weiner H, Wisoff J, et al. Repeat endoscopic third ventriculostomy: is it worth trying? Childs Nerv Syst 2001;17(9):551–555

9. Wagner W, Koch D. Mechanisms of failure after endoscopic third ventriculostomy in young infants. J Neurosurg 2005;103(1, Suppl): 43–49

10. Hader WJ, Drake J, Cochrane D, Sparrow O, Johnson ES, Kestle J. Death after late failure of third ventriculostomy in children: report of three cases. J Neurosurg 2002;97(1):211–215

11. Lipina R, Palecek T, Reguli S, Kovarova M. Death in consequence of late failure of endoscopic third ventriculostomy. Childs Nerv Syst 2007;23(7):815–819

12. Teo C, Jones R. Management of hydrocephalus by endoscopic third ventriculostomy in patients with myelomeningocele. Pediatr Neurosurg 1996;25(2):57–63, discussion 63

13. Sgouros S, Kulkharni AV, Constantini S. The International Infant Hydrocephalus Study: concept and rational. Childs Nerv Syst 2006;22(4):338–345

14. Baldauf J, Oertel J, Gaab MR, Schroeder HW. Endoscopic third ventriculostomy in children younger than 2 years of age. Childs Nerv Syst 2007;23(6):623–626

15. Cinalli G, Sainte-Rose C, Chumas P, et al. Failure of third ventriculostomy in the treatment of aqueductal stenosis in children. J Neurosurg 1999;90(3):448–454

16. Koch-Wiewrodt D, Wagner W. Success and failure of endoscopic third ventriculostomy in young infants: are there different age distributions? Childs Nerv Syst 2006;22(12):1537–1541

17. Decq P, Le Guérinel C, Sol JC, Brugières P, Djindjian M, Nguyen JP. Chiari I malformation: a rare cause of noncommunicating hydrocephalus treated by third ventriculostomy. J Neurosurg 2001;95(5):783–790

18. Cinalli G, Salazar C, Mallucci C, Yada JZ, Zerah M, Sainte-Rose C. The role of endoscopic third ventriculostomy in the management of shunt malfunction. Neurosurgery 1998;43(6):1323–1327, discussion 1327–1329

19. Nishiyama K, Mori H, Tanaka R. Changes in cerebrospinal fluid hydrodynamics following endoscopic third ventriculostomy for shunt-dependent noncommunicating hydrocephalus. J Neurosurg 2003;98(5):1027–1031

20. O'Brien DF, Javadpour M, Collins DR, Spennato P, Mallucci CL. Endoscopic third ventriculostomy: an outcome analysis of primary cases and procedures performed after ventriculoperitoneal shunt malfunction. J Neurosurg 2005;103(5, Suppl):393–400

21. Sainte-Rose C, Cinalli G, Roux FE, et al. Management of hydrocephalus in pediatric patients with posterior fossa tumors: the role of endoscopic third ventriculostomy. J Neurosurg 2001;95(5):791–797

22. Morelli D, Pirotte B, Lubansu A, et al. Persistent hydrocephalus after early surgical management of posterior fossa tumors in children: is routine preoperative endoscopic third ventriculostomy justified? J Neurosurg 2005;103(3, Suppl):247–252

23. Gil Z, Siomin V, Beni-Adani L, Sira B, Constantini S. Ventricular catheter placement in children with hydrocephalus and small ventricles: the use of a frameless neuronavigation system. Childs Nerv Syst 2002;18(1-2):26–29

24. Siomin V, Constantini S. Basic principles and equipment in neuroendoscopy. Neurosurg Clin N Am 2004;15(1):19–31

25. Abtin K, Thompson BG, Walker ML. Basilar artery perforation as a complication of endoscopic third ventriculostomy. Pediatr Neurosurg 1998;28(1):35–41

26. Schroeder HW, Niendorf WR, Gaab MR. Complications of endoscopic third ventriculostomy. J Neurosurg 2002;96(6):1032–1040

27. Beni-Adani L, Siomin V, Segev Y, Beni S, Constantini S. Increasing chronic subdural hematoma after endoscopic III ventriculostomy. Childs Nerv Syst 2000;16(7):402–405

28. Teo C, Rahman S, Boop FA, Cherny B. Complications of endoscopic neurosurgery. Childs Nerv Syst 1996;12(5):248–253, discussion 253

29. Cinalli G, Spennato P, Ruggiero C, et al. Intracranial pressure monitoring and lumbar puncture after endoscopic third ventriculostomy in children. Neurosurgery 2006;58(1):126–136, discussion 126–136

30. Mobbs RJ, Vonau M, Davies MA. Death after late failure of endoscopic third ventriculostomy: a potential solution. Neurosurgery 2003;53(2):384–385, discussion 385–386

31. Brockmeyer D, Abtin K, Carey L, Walker ML. Endoscopic third ventriculostomy: an outcome analysis. Pediatr Neurosurg 1998; 28(5):236–240

32. Hopf NJ, Grunert P, Fries G, Resch KD, Perneczky A. Endoscopic third ventriculostomy: outcome analysis of 100 consecutive procedures. Neurosurgery 1999;44(4):795–804, discussion 804–806

33. Li KW, Roonprapunt C, Lawson HC, et al. Endoscopic third ventriculostomy for hydrocephalus associated with tectal gliomas. Neurosurg Focus 2005;18(6A):E2

34. O'Brien DF, Hayhurst C, Pizer B, Mallucci CL. Outcomes in patients undergoing single-trajectory endoscopic third ventriculostomy and endoscopic biopsy for midline tumors presenting with obstructive hydrocephalus. J Neurosurg 2006;105(3, Suppl):219–226

35. Tisell M, Almström O, Stephensen H, Tullberg M, Wikkelsö C. How effective is endoscopic third ventriculostomy in treating adult hydrocephalus caused by primary aqueductal stenosis? Neurosurgery 2000;46(1):104–110, discussion 110–111

36. Wakhlu A, Ansari NA. The prediction of postoperative hydrocephalus in patients with spina bifida. Childs Nerv Syst 2004; 20(2):104–106

37. Rekate HL. Selecting patients for endoscopic third ventriculostomy. Neurosurg Clin N Am 2004;15(1):39–49

38. Yamada H, Nakamura S, Tanaka Y, Tajima M, Kageyama N. Ventriculography and cisternography with water-soluble contrast media in infants with myelomeningocele. Radiology 1982;143(1): 75–83

39. Gilbert JN, Jones KL, Rorke LB, Chernoff GF, James HE. Central nervous system anomalies associated with meningomyelocele, hydrocephalus, and the Arnold-Chiari malformation: reappraisal of theories regarding the pathogenesis of posterior neural tube closure defects. Neurosurgery 1986;18(5):559–564

40. Warf BC. Hydrocephalus in Uganda: the predominance of infectious origin and primary management with endoscopic third ventriculostomy. J Neurosurg 2005;102(1, Suppl):1–15

41. Fukuhara T, Vorster SJ, Luciano MG. Risk factors for failure of endoscopic third ventriculostomy for obstructive hydrocephalus. Neurosurgery 2000;46(5):1100–1109, discussion 1109–1111

42. Kawamura T, Morioka T, Nishio S, Mihara F, Fukui M. Cerebral abnormalities in lumbosacral neural tube closure defect: MR imaging evaluation. Childs Nerv Syst 2001;17(7):405–410

43. Pavez A, Salazar C, Rivera R, et al. Description of endoscopic ventricular anatomy in myelomeningocele. Minim Invasive Neurosurg 2006;49(3):161–167

44. Gangemi M, Donati P, Maiuri F, Longatti P, Godano U, Mascari C. Endoscopic third ventriculostomy for hydrocephalus. Minim Invasive Neurosurg 1999;42(3):128–132

45. Chai WX. Long-term results of fourth ventriculo-cisternostomy in complex versus simplex atresias of the fourth ventricle outlets. Acta Neurochir (Wien) 1995;134(1–2):27–34

46. Mohanty A, Anandh B, Kolluri VR, Praharaj SS. Neuroendoscopic third ventriculostomy in the management of fourth ventricular outlet obstruction. Minim Invasive Neurosurg 1999;42(1):18–21

47. Rifkinson-Mann S, Sachdev VP, Huang YP. Congenital fourth ventricular midline outlet obstruction: report of two cases. J Neurosurg 1987;67(4):595–599

48. Asai A, Hoffman HJ, Hendrick EB, Humphreys RP. Dandy-Walker syndrome: experience at the Hospital for Sick Children, Toronto. Pediatr Neurosci 1989;15(2):66–73

49. Hawkins JC III, Hoffman HJ, Humphreys RP. Isolated fourth ventricle as a complication of ventricular shunting: report of three cases. J Neurosurg 1978;49(6):910–913

50. Glasauer FE. Isotope cisternography and ventriculography in congenital anomalies of the central nervous system. J Neurosurg 1975;43(1):18–26

51. Milhorat TH, Chou MW, Trinidad EM, et al. Chiari I malformation redefined: clinical and radiographic findings for 364 symptomatic patients. Neurosurgery 1999;44(5):1005–1017

52. Ryken TC, Menezes AH. Cervicomedullary compression in achondroplasia. J Neurosurg 1994;81(1):43–48

53. Hirsch JF, Pierre-Kahn A, Renier D, Sainte-Rose C, Hoppe-Hirsch E. The Dandy-Walker malformation: a review of 40 cases. J Neurosurg 1984;61(3):515–522

54. Carmel PW, Antunes JL, Hilal SK, Gold AP. Dandy-Walker syndrome: clinico-pathological features and re-evaluation of modes of treatment. Surg Neurol 1977;8(2):132–138

55. Kumar R, Jain MK, Chhabra DK. Dandy-Walker syndrome: different modalities of treatment and outcome in 42 cases. Childs Nerv Syst 2001;17(6):348–352

56. Mohanty A, Biswas A, Satish S, Praharaj SS, Sastry KV. Treatment options for Dandy-Walker malformation. J Neurosurg 2006;105(5, Suppl):348–356

57. Lee M, Leahu D, Weiner HL, Abbott R, Wisoff JH, Epstein FJ. Complications of fourth-ventricular shunts. Pediatr Neurosurg 1995;22(6):309–313, discussion 314

58. Villavicencio AT, Wellons JC III, George TM. Avoiding complicated shunt systems by open fenestration of symptomatic fourth ventricular cysts associated with hydrocephalus. Pediatr Neurosurg 1998;29(6):314–319

59. Mohanty A. Endoscopic third ventriculostomy with cystoventricular stent placement in the management of Dandy-Walker malformation: technical case report of three patients. Neurosurgery 2003;53(5):1223–1228, discussion 1228–1229

60. Buxton N, MacArthur D, Mallucci C, Punt J, Vloeberghs M. Neuroendoscopic third ventriculostomy in patients less than 1 year old. Pediatr Neurosurg 1998;29(2):73–76

61. O'Brien DF, Seghedoni A, Collins DR, Hayhurst C, Mallucci CL. Is there an indication for ETV in young infants in aetiologies other than isolated aqueduct stenosis? Childs Nerv Syst 2006;22(12):1565–1572

62. Handler LC, Wright MG. Postmeningitic hydrocephalus in infancy: ventriculography with special reference to ventricular septa. Neuroradiology 1978;16:31–35

63. Cinalli G. Alternatives to shunting. Childs Nerv Syst 1999; 15(11–12):718–731

64. Siomin V, Cinalli G, Grotenhuis A, et al. Endoscopic third ventriculostomy in patients with cerebrospinal fluid infection and/or hemorrhage. J Neurosurg 2002;97(3):519–524

65. Cinalli G, Spennato P, Ruggiero C, Aliberti F, Maggi G. Aqueductal stenosis 9 years after mumps meningoencephalitis: treatment by endoscopic third ventriculostomy. Childs Nerv Syst 2004; 20(1):61–64

66. Viola L, Chiaretti A, Castorina M, et al. Acute hydrocephalus as a consequence of mumps meningoencephalitis. Pediatr Emerg Care 1998;14(3):212–214

67. Rotilio A, Salar G, Dollo C, Ori C, Carteri A. Aqueductal stenosis following mumps virus infection: case report. Ital J Neurol Sci 1985;6(2):237–239

68. Wiswell TE, Tuttle DJ, Northam RS, Simonds GR. Major congenital neurologic malformations: a 17-year survey. Am J Dis Child 1990; 144(1):61–67

69. Beni-Adani L, Biani N, Ben-Sirah L, Constantini S. The occurrence of obstructive vs absorptive hydrocephalus in newborns and infants: relevance to treatment choices. Childs Nerv Syst 2006;22(12): 1543–1563

70. Mixter TH. Ventriculoscopy and puncture of the third ventricle. Boston Med Surg J 1923;188:277–278

71. Rachel RA. Surgical treatment of hydrocephalus: a historical perspective. Pediatr Neurosurg 1999;30(6):296–304

72. Boockvar JA, Loudon W, Sutton LN. Development of the Spitz-Holter valve in Philadelphia. J Neurosurg 2001;95(1):145–147

73. Nulsen FE, Spitz EB. Treatment of hydrocephalus by direct shunt from ventricle to jugular vain. Surg Forum 1951;(2):399–403

74. Jallo GI, Kothbauer KF, Abbott IR. Endoscopic third ventriculostomy. Neurosurg Focus 2005;19(6):E11

75. Di Rocco C, Marchese E, Velardi F. A survey of the first complication of newly implanted CSF shunt devices for the treatment of nontumoral hydrocephalus. Cooperative survey of the 1991–1992 Education Committee of the ISPN. Childs Nerv Syst 1994; 10(5): 321–327

76. McGirt MJ, Leveque JC, Wellons JC III, et al. Cerebrospinal fluid shunt survival and etiology of failures: a seven-year institutional experience. Pediatr Neurosurg 2002;36(5):248–255

77. Piatt JH Jr, Carlson CV. A search for determinants of cerebrospinal fluid shunt survival: retrospective analysis of a 14-year institutional experience. Pediatr Neurosurg 1993;19(5):233–241, discussion 242

78. Drake JM, Kestle JR, Milner R, et al. Randomized trial of cerebrospinal fluid shunt valve design in pediatric hydrocephalus. Neurosurgery 1998;43(2):294–303, discussion 303–305

79. Etus V, Ceylan S. Success of endoscopic third ventriculostomy in children less than 2 years of age. Neurosurg Rev 2005; 28(4): 284–288

80. Gorayeb RP, Cavalheiro S, Zymberg ST. Endoscopic third ventriculostomy in children younger than 1 year of age. J Neurosurg 2004; 100(5, Suppl Pediatrics):427–429

81. Wagner W, Koch D. Mechanisms of failure after endoscopic third ventriculostomy in young infants. J Neurosurg 2005;103(1, Suppl): 43–49

82. Yadav YR, Jaiswal S, Adam N, Basoor A, Jain G. Endoscopic third ventriculostomy in infants. Neurol India 2006;54(2):161–163

83. Fritsch MJ, Kienke S, Ankermann T, Padoin M, Mehdorn HM. Endoscopic third ventriculostomy in infants. J Neurosurg 2005; 103(1, Suppl):50–53

84. Drake JM, Kestle JR, Tuli S. CSF shunts 50 years on—past, present and future. Childs Nerv Syst 2000;16(10-11):800–804

85. Abtin K, Thompson BG, Walker ML. Basilar artery perforation as a complication of endoscopic third ventriculostomy. Pediatr Neurosurg 1998;28(1):35–41

86. Schroeder HWS, Niendorf W-R, Gaab MR. Complications of endoscopic third ventriculostomy. J Neurosurg 2002;96(6):1032–1040

87. Di Rocco C, Massimi L, Tamburrini G. Shunts vs endoscopic third ventriculostomy in infants: are there different types and/or rates of complications? A review. Childs Nerv Syst 2006;22(12):1573–1589

88. Cinalli G, Salazar C, Mallucci C, Yada JZ, Zerah M, Sainte-Rose C. The role of endoscopic third ventriculostomy in the management of shunt malfunction. [Review]. Neurosurgery 1998;43(6):1323–1327, discussion 1327–1329

89. Vandertop PW. Traumatic basilar aneurysm after endoscopic third ventriculostomy: case report. Neurosurgery 1998;43(3):647–648

90. McLaughlin MR, Wahlig JB, Kaufmann AM, Albright AL. Traumatic basilar aneurysm after endoscopic third ventriculostomy: case report. Neurosurgery 1997;41(6):1400–1403, discussion 1403–1404

91. Schwartz TH, Yoon SS, Cutruzzola FW, Goodman RR. Third ventriculostomy: post-operative ventricular size and outcome. Minim Invasive Neurosurg 1996;39(4):122–129

92. Bellotti A, Rapanà A, Iaccarino C, Schonauer M. Intracranial pressure monitoring after endoscopic third ventriculostomy: an effective method to manage the "adaptation period." Clin Neurol Neurosurg 2001;103(4):223–227

93. Hopf NJ, Grunert P, Fries G, Resch KD, Perneczky A. Endoscopic third ventriculostomy: outcome analysis of 100 consecutive procedures. Neurosurgery 1999;44(4):795–804, discussion 804–806

94. Frim DM, Goumnerova LC. Telemetric intraventricular pressure measurements after third ventriculocisternostomy in a patient with noncommunicating hydrocephalus. Neurosurgery 1997; 41(6):1425–1428, discussion 1428–1430

95. Rapanà A, Bellotti A, Iaccarino C, Pascale M, Schönauer M. Intracranial pressure patterns after endoscopic third ventriculostomy. Preliminary experience. Acta Neurochir (Wien) 2004;146(12):1309–1315, discussion 1315

96. Mobbs RJ, Vonau M, Davies MA. Death after late failure of endoscopic third ventriculostomy: a potential solution. Neurosurgery 2003;53(2):384–385, discussion 385–386

97. Ammirati M, Raimondi AJ. Cerebrospinal fluid shunt infections in children: a study on the relationship between the etiology of hydrocephalus, age at the time of shunt placement, and infection rate. Childs Nerv Syst 1987;3(2):106–109

98. Tuli S, Drake J, Lawless J, Wigg M, Lamberti-Pasculli M. Risk factors for repeated cerebrospinal shunt failures in pediatric patients with hydrocephalus. J Neurosurg 2000;92(1):31–38

99. Enger PO, Svendsen F, Wester K. CSF shunt infections in children: experiences from a population-based study. Acta Neurochir (Wien) 2003;145(4):243–248, discussion 248

100. McGirt MJ, Buck DW II, Sciubba DM, et al. Adjustable vs set-pressure valves decrease the risk of proximal shunt obstruction in the treatment of pediatric hydrocephalus. Childs Nerv Syst 2007; 23(3):289–295

101. Sciubba DM, Stuart RM, McGirt MJ, et al. Effect of antibiotic-impregnated shunt catheters in decreasing the incidence of shunt infection in the treatment of hydrocephalus. J Neurosurg 2005;103(2, Suppl):131–136

102. Sciubba DM, Lin LM, Woodworth GF, McGirt MJ, Carson B, Jallo GI. Factors contributing to the medical costs of cerebrospinal fluid shunt infection treatment in pediatric patients with standard shunt components compared with those in patients with antibiotic impregnated components. Neurosurg Focus 2007;22(4):E9

103. Pattavilakom A, Xenos C, Bradfield O, Danks RA. Reduction in shunt infection using antibiotic impregnated CSF shunt catheters: an Australian prospective study. J Clin Neurosci 2007;14(6): 526–531

104. Aryan HE, Meltzer HS, Park MS, Bennett RL, Jandial R, Levy ML. Initial experience with antibiotic-impregnated silicone catheters for shunting of cerebrospinal fluid in children. Childs Nerv Syst 2005;21(1):56–61

105. Tuli S, Alshail E, Drake J. Third ventriculostomy versus cerebrospinal fluid shunt as a first procedure in pediatric hydrocephalus. Pediatr Neurosurg 1999;30(1):11–15

4 Compartmentalized Hydrocephalus

♦ Endoscopic Fenestration

Rick Abbott

Compartmentalized hydrocephalus, also referred to as multiloculated or multicystic hydrocephalus, is a known and dreaded complication of an inflammatory process within the cerebrospinal fluid (CSF) compartments of the brain. Although rare, when present it significantly increases the complexity in treating the associated hydrocephalus. Until the reintroduction of the endoscope to neurosurgeons in the mid-1980s, the two treatments available were multiple shunt catheters and craniotomy. As neurosurgeons have become more facile with endoscopy, the management of this condition has increasingly been dependent on fenestration of these spaces endoscopically. What follows is a discussion of this entity, its management with the endoscope, the complications seen, and the outcome.

Pathophysiology

Fluid spaces can become trapped or isolated in response to an inflammatory process within the CSF compartments of the brain. The most common sources for this process, or ventriculitis, are infection and hemorrhage.[1-3] Small passageways between the ventricles, such as the foramina of Monro, Magendie, and Luschka, and the sylvian aqueduct can scar over, entrapping the upstream ventricular space(s). Additionally, hemorrhage within the germinal matrix of a premature infant or a severe infectious ventriculitis, such as is seen with gram-negative or fungal organisms, can cause the subependymal layers to dissociate from adjacent parenchyma, thus giving rise to one or more sequestered spaces that grow into the adjacent ventricle. Further complicating this process is that over time this dissociative process can evolve, leading to new cysts forming months after the offending force has been dealt with.[4] Finally, an infection that is extremely pyogenic will create a turbid CSF that will result in an extremely inflamed ependyma, which will scar when in contact with adjacent ependymal surfaces, leading to entrapped CSF spaces.

The end result of the processes described above is one or more CSF spaces that are no longer in communication with the normal CSF circulatory pathways or that are no longer in communication with a shunted CSF space. These trapped spaces can accumulate fluid over time either from choroid plexus residing within the trapped space or from transudate from the walls of the space. As the fluid accumulates, the size of the space increases, and it becomes a mass that causes the intracranial pressure to rise. It is at that point that the patient begins to deteriorate clinically.

Treatment

Fenestration of multiple intraventricular cysts has come to be favored over the use of catheters. Managing a ventricular drainage system that incorporates multiple proximal catheters can be complicated, and when such a system is used to drain multiple subependymal cysts, there is a tendency for the cysts to collapse down around the catheters and occlude them. Before endoscopy became widely available, managing such a patient usually ended in craniotomy to fenestrate the cysts into one large fluid space after multiple trips to the operating room for addition and revision of proximal catheters.[5] Consequently, neurosurgeons welcomed the addition of the endoscope to their armamentarium. Their excitement, however, was soon blunted when they realized that these cysts typically lacked landmarks. Only with the addition of image guidance systems did the endoscope become a truly effective tool for managing multiloculated ventricles.

Over the past several decades, there has been a tremendous advance in the use of neuroendoscopy for managing various intraventricular pathologies, including multiloculated ventricles. This is due to improvements in the optics of the endoscope, improved imaging technology, and the marriage of image-guided surgery with neuroendoscopy.[6] Also important has been the development of instruments such as microforceps, lasers, saline torches, and microballoons.[7–11] With these advancements have come increasing reports of their use for fenestration of septations within hydrocephalic ventricles or the septum pellucidum in isolated ventricles, fenestration of arachnoid cysts and tumor cysts such as seen with craniopharyngioma, and placement of catheters in ventricles or intratumor cystic cavities. Of these it could be argued that the management of multiloculated ventricles has experienced the greatest change due to the introduction of the endoscope.

In approaching multiloculated ventricles with the endoscope, the surgeon should first consider the type of scope to use. Available are fiberoptic scopes with deflectable tips, semirigid or rigid fiberoptic scopes, and rigid glass rod or lens scopes. The advantage of a rigid lens scope is the superior visualization of structures that it provides. The image that this system projects to the camera is a perfect reflection of the surgical field, and it can be magnified to infinity with crystal clarity. The disadvantage of this type of scope is that, because it is a rod, its tip cannot be deflected to inspect a wider field of view. The view can be widened only by changing the scope to another with a different angulation in its tip's lens (e.g., exchanging a 0-degree scope for a 30-degree scope to see the margins of the field better).

Flexible fiberoptic scopes with deflectable tips will allow for greater fields of view, but the conduction of the image from the tip to the camera degrades the image quality, resulting in a poorer image as compared with a lens scope (so-called pixilation). Semirigid or rigid fiberoptic scopes' main advantage is their size; they suffer the same disadvantage as flexible fiberoptic endoscopes. One option for the surgeon is to use both a rigid lens scope and a flexible fiberoptic scope to manage multiloculated ventricles, as advocated by Oi.[12] The superior image of the rod scope can be used to familiarize the surgeon with the anatomy present, and the flexible scope can be used to better navigate the environment to accomplish the surgical goals.

There is a growing list of instruments available to the endoscopist to manage multiloculated ventricles. For fenestration, there are monopolar and bipolar cautery units, as well as lasers. Fogarty catheters or specially developed microballoons can be used for enlargement of small fenestrations. Tissue can be cut with specialty knives or scissors that fit the endoscope's working channels, and tissue can be removed with various types of forceps that work with the endoscope. Increasingly sophisticated holding devices for endoscopes have been developed; some even include micromanipulators that allow for precise, small movements of the scope once on site in the surgical field.[6] The use of these devices is somewhat controversial in that they limit large movements of the scope, tending to confine the surgeon's field of interest. An important aspect of multiloculated ventricles is that normal anatomical landmarks are frequently masked or absent. Consequently, targeting a fenestration can be difficult. The introduction of intraoperative ultrasound and image-guided surgery has been an effective answer to this problem. A second bur hole will allow for the use of ultrasonography during an endoscopic procedure. The ultrasound can be used to visualize the turbulence of irrigation as it leaves the tip of the endoscope, allowing the endoscopist to understand just where in the fluid space the scope's tip is.[13] The difficulty with this technique, however, is that the image is two dimensional, and the ultrasonic head must be rotated to see the scope's tip in a different plane. If the jet of fluid emerging from the tip is not parallel to the image's plane, it will not be seen. Image guidance is a better answer for the orientation problem. For rigid scopes, tracking devices can be affixed to the scope, allowing tracking of the tip during the surgery (**Fig. 4.1**). When projected onto preoperative imagery, targeting of the fenestrations becomes very straightforward. If flexible scopes are to be used, a tracking device can be attached to the channel through which the scope will be delivered to the target. Tracking probes can be used as obturators for the scope's channel to orient the placement of the channel at the intended fenestration site.

Potentially, all the instruments mentioned above may be needed during the procedure, so steps should be taken to ensure they are compatible with the scopes planned for use. Assisting personnel should be familiar with the instrumentation to be used and how to troubleshoot any problems. They should also be aware of the flow of the case and anticipate the surgeon's needs during the operation. This is critical in endoscopy, as the surgeon is commonly working in tight spaces near critical structures. Time on site should be kept to a minimum to avoid surgeon fatigue that will occur as a result of controlling the scope in such an environment. It is not a bad idea to rehearse the surgery mentally or at least to go through the steps of the procedure in advance with the assisting personnel. The surgeon should be familiar with his or her instrumentation, their capabilities, and their appropriateness for the demands that will be present during the procedure. He or she should also be aware of what backup equipment is available, how to use it, and where it is located.

It is useful to spend some time studying the patient's radiographs. First, goals for the surgery are set. When multiple cysts are present, it may be impossible to fenestrate them all through a single bur hole. As the cysts are fenestrated and the CSF drained, there will be an expected shift in the anatomy, making the preoperative films irrelevant. Thought should be given to the anatomy underlying the walls of a fluid space that is being fenestrated, particularly if that space is narrow. The planned

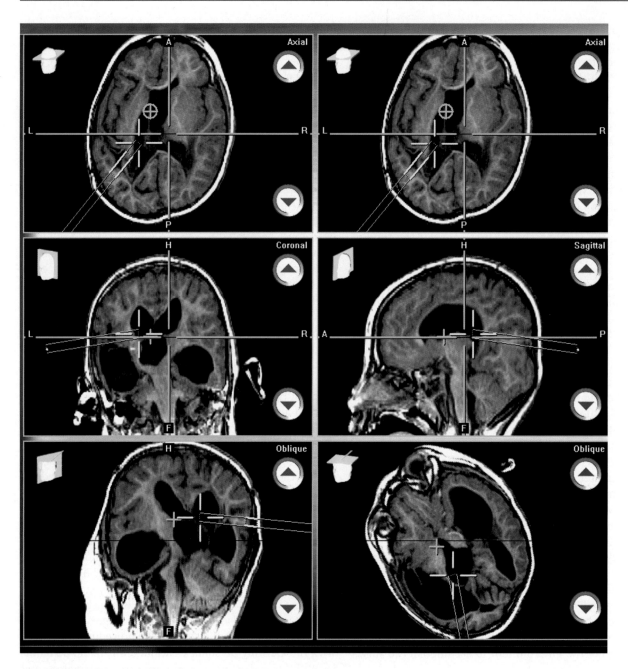

Fig. 4.1 Endoscope's guide sleeve being tracked as it moves to the target.

surgery should occur along a straight line, as it is much simpler to stay oriented in this situation than it is when multiple turns must be taken. Computer-assisted navigational equipment can be useful for this by establishing a line of targeted cysts and points for their fenestration, then drawing the line out to the skull's edge to locate the bur hole. Also, by studying the anatomy as seen on the image set, the surgeon can anticipate where visible landmarks might be that will help with orientation during the procedure. Finally, it is important during planning to acknowledge that in many cases all the cysts cannot be fenestrated in a single setting. There is nothing wrong with sharing this with the patient's family and telling them that instead of one large craniotomy, several relatively minor surgeries may be needed. Postoperative imagery can be used to determine what has been accomplished and what is left to fenestrate. A postoperative computed tomography (CT) scan with contrast injected into the ventricles to determine what has been communicated can be very helpful in this regard (**Fig. 4.2**).

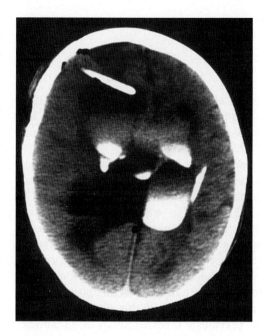

Fig. 4.2 Contrast injection via a shunt into the ventricles showing which have been successfully communicated.

Once a surgical plan has been made, the patient is brought to the operating room. Ideally, the patient should be positioned in such a manner that the planned bur hole will be at the apex of the surgical field. This will minimize loss of CSF during the procedure. Sometimes this can be difficult, though, as another requirement of patient positioning is the need to reference to the guidance system. With careful planning and forethought, these two goals can be accomplished. After drilling the bur hole, the guidance system is used to place the endoscope's working sleeve at the first fenestration target. The system can be used for placement at other fenestration targets, but it must be remembered that the accuracy of the guidance system degrades with fenestration of cysts that are under pressure and the loss of CSF. With each fenestration the surgeon should become increasingly conservative and more reliant on landmarks in the operative field. If there are no landmarks, and the surgeon is concerned about shifting anatomy, then the procedure should be stopped and postoperative imagery obtained to assess what remains to be done.

There are several ways to perform fenestrations. Monopolar cautery can be used to make a series of punctate holes that are then connected using scissors, or it can be scrolled to outline the intended fenestration, with forceps used to remove any tissue fragments. Lasers can also be used to cut a fenestration. When using an instrument that cuts using energy, the surgeon must be thoughtful of what lies hidden on the other side of the wall being fenestrated. Ideally, the energy source should confine the delivered energy to the wall itself, and the instrument should not deflect the wall into underlying structures. Once the fenestration is made, the scope is advanced through it to confirm that the fenestration is complete. By doing this, not only is the completeness of the fenestration checked, but the fenestration is also enlarged as the scope is moved to inspect the cyst it has just entered.

After such a surgery, there is usually a major decompression, with a resulting drop in intracranial pressure. Not uncommonly the brain becomes mobile in such a setting, with the patient experiencing nausea and dysequilibrium, particularly with movement. Families should be warned of this, and intravenous fluids should be provided until things stabilize for the patient.

Outcome and Complications

There are relatively few articles that report on outcome after managing multiloculated ventricles endoscopically. Spennato et al report on 23 of their patients, 12 of whom had multiloculated ventricles.[14] Six required only a single endoscopic procedure, four required two procedures, one four procedures, and one seven. One avoided shunting altogether, and eight required one shunt, with one of these patients' systems having two proximal catheters. The remaining three required two or more shunts. The authors also reported that most required one or no revisions during the follow-up period (3–51 months). There were four cases of infection in these 23 patients, one postoperative thalamic hematoma and one case of CSF leakage. Lewis et al reported on 34 cases of loculated ventricles managed endoscopically.[13] Thirteen of these patients had multiloculated ventricles, and six required more than one endoscopic procedure. Three of these patients had one or more shunt malfunctions following the endoscopic procedure, but this represented an improvement over the 52 revisions this group required prior to the procedure. Lewis et al reported one CSF leak and one ventriculitis in their 23 patients. The results of these two reports compare favorably to the study by Nida and Haines of six patients whose multiloculated ventricles were managed with an open craniotomy for cyst fenestration.[5] Five of these patients required a total of 86 shunt revisions prior to the endoscopic procedure (median of 8) and only 8 following the procedure (median of 1) (average follow-up of 44.5 months before the procedure and 27 months after).

Conclusion

Neuroendoscopy has become an effective tool in the management of compartmentalized hydrocephalus, and the treatment of the condition has been simplified. The time in hospital for such patients should be lessened because of fewer shunt malfunctions; consequently, the quality of life for them and their families has improved.

♦ Open Craniotomy or Shunting

David I. Sandberg, J. Gordon McComb, and Mark D. Krieger

Compartmentalized hydrocephalus, also called multilocu-lated hydrocephalus, is a condition in which patients have multiple CSF compartments in the brain that are divided by septations and do not communicate with one another. Treatment is required when signs and symptoms of elevat-ed intracranial pressure are associated with progressive enlargement of one or more compartments. Neurosurgical management of these patients is often extremely challenging, and outcomes are often poor despite multiple operations. Following, we briefly review the etiologies of compartmen-talized hydrocephalus, then focus on treatment options. We present the rationale for open craniotomy and microsurgi-cal fenestration as an effective means of creating communi-cation between various CSF compartments and enabling CSF diversion to be achieved without multiple shunt catheters.

Compartmentalized Hydrocephalus: Etiologies

Compartmentalized hydrocephalus is most commonly asso-ciated with a prior history of central nervous system (CNS) infection and/or intraventricular hemorrhage.[15–21] These and other insults to the brain most frequently occur during the neonatal period, particularly in premature infants.[18,20,22,23] In an early report describing this phenomenon, Schultz and Leeds proposed that the formation of intraventricular septations is likely due to the organization of exudate and debris that accompany ventriculitis.[21] Pathologically, the septations separating abnormal ventricular compartments are composed of fibroglial elements, small areas of denuded ependyma, subependymal gliosis, and associated inflam-matory cells.[21] Septations can create artificial divisions within a single ventricular compartment and/or occlude the foramen of Monro, the cerebral aqueduct, and the outlets of the fourth ventricle.[19] Production of CSF within cystic compartments that do not communicate with other CSF spaces can cause progressive enlargement of one or more compartments.

Infection causing compartmentalized hydrocephalus may be attributed to neonatal meningitis in children with no prior history of hydrocephalus.[20,23] Additionally, compart-mentalized hydrocephalus may occur following CNS infec-tions in shunted children whose ventricular compartments were enlarged but not loculated prior to the infection.[19] When CNS infection is implicated as a cause, gram-negative organisms are particularly prominent. In a review of patients with postinfectious compartmentalized hydrocephalus, 9 of 13 patients were noted to have gram-negative infections.[20]

In a separate review of 12 patients with compartmentalized hydrocephalus attributed to CNS shunt infections, 8 had documented gram-negative infections, 2 had gram-positive infections, and 2 had fungal infections.[19]

Intraventricular hemorrhage, particularly in premature infants, is also frequently associated with compartmental-ized hydrocephalus. Loculated, noncommunicating CSF compartments can be noted in patients with intraventricu-lar hemorrhage in the absence of associated CNS infection.[17] However, because so many patients with loculated hydro-cephalus have a history of both CNS infection and intraven-tricular hemorrhage associated with prematurity, it is often difficult to determine which of these factors played a dom-inant role in the pathogenesis of this phenomenon. For example, in our previously reported series of 33 patients who underwent craniotomy for compartmentalized hydro-cephalus, the majority had a history of both CNS infection (*n* = 23; 70%) and prematurity with intraventricular hemorrhage (*n* = 20; 61%).[15]

Although nearly all patients with compartmentalized hydrocephalus had documented CNS infections, premature germinal matrix hemorrhage, or both of these entities, rare cases are associated with neither of these conditions. For example, compartmentalized hydrocephalus has been reported in association with birth trauma and brain tumors in a very small number of patients.[18]

Management Options

Shunting

The vast majority of patients with compartmentalized hydrocephalus, regardless of fenestration procedures, will require CSF diverting shunts. Prior to fenestration proce-dures, many patients have undergone multiple revisions of ventriculoperitoneal shunts. Despite a functioning shunt, additional intervention is warranted when progressive enlargement of one or more compartments that are not adequately drained by the shunt is associated with signs or symptoms of elevated intracranial pressure. At this point, one option is to place additional ventricular catheters con-nected to the previous shunt system or to place additional separate shunt systems.

Multiple ventricular catheters can be used to treat com-partmentalized hydrocephalus and alleviate symptoms,[24] but most neurosurgeons currently try to avoid placing addi-tional intracranial catheters for several reasons. First, because multiple CSF compartments are often present, two or more proximal catheters may not adequately decompress all of the enlarging CSF compartments. Moreover, additional operations with added shunt hardware will increase the risk of subsequent shunt malfunctions and infections. Finally, the management of shunt malfunction or infection in patients with multiple shunt catheters or systems can be quite complicated.

Rather than placing multiple shunt systems when treating compartmentalized hydrocephalus, a fenestration procedure is recommended, via either endoscopic techniques or open craniotomy. Regardless of which means is chosen, the vast majority of patients will still require a shunt to adequately treat hydrocephalus. The goal of fenestration is to reduce the number of shunt systems to one. In the most recent published reports describing fenestration for compartmentalized hydrocephalus via endoscopy or craniotomy, only a small minority of patients in each series were shunt-free after fenestration.[15,25]

Neuroendoscopic Management

Neuroendoscopic techniques are increasingly being used for a variety of neurosurgical conditions, including compartmentalized hydrocephalus. Several authors have reported endoscopic procedures to create communication between isolated CSF compartments.[25–32] These reports describe successful communications created between previously isolated CSF compartments with a subsequent decrease in shunt revisions and avoidance of multiple shunt catheters in the majority of patients. The rationale for endoscopic management of compartmentalized hydrocephalus is presented separately by Dr. Abbott in the preceding section of this chapter.

Neuroendoscopy is routinely used by all three authors. We have found that endoscopic fenestration is very effective when only a single loculation or very few loculations are present, and endoscopic management in this circumstance should be considered the procedure of choice. However, in complex cases with multiple loculations, we have achieved greater success via open minicraniotomy than endoscopy. Below we present our rationale for this approach.

Craniotomy for Fenestration

In complex cases of compartmentalized hydrocephalus, we believe there are multiple advantages of craniotomy over endoscopy. First, the operating microscope provides better visualization of the various loculated compartments and membranes than the endoscope. Second, because of the limited instrumentation currently available with endoscopy compared with microsurgical techniques, fenestrations tend to be smaller and would logically be more likely to close over time. The operating microscope provides higher magnification as well as a wider and deeper field of view than the endoscope, which facilitates the creation of a wide opening of septations. We believe that

multiple large communications created between the various CSF compartments offers the greatest possibility of avoiding the need for repeated fenestrations or additional intracranial catheters over time.

We have also found that it is easier to "get lost" regarding anatomical landmarks with endoscopy in these complex cases than with the operating microscope. Frameless stereotaxy, in our opinion, provides little help in this regard because of the profound shift that occurs during surgery as multiple cysts are fenestrated and subsequently deflate. Finally, bleeding is much easier to control with standard techniques under the operating microscope than with endoscopy, during which even a small amount of bleeding can significantly hamper visualization. The only disadvantages of minicraniotomy compared with endoscopy are a larger incision and the need for elevation of a small bone flap, usually 3 to 4 cm in diameter. The craniotomy is often performed simultaneously with a shunt revision, and only a small extension of the existing shunt incision is typically required to create a small bone flap. The amount of time required for these steps is probably equivalent to the time spent for an endoscopic procedure.

Typically, a minicraniotomy for fenestration of compartmentalized hydrocephalus is performed via a posterior parietal approach. The patient is positioned in the supine or lateral decubitus position with the body well taped to the operating room table to facilitate rotation of the table in various directions to obtain different views. Surgery is often performed on the side with the thinnest cortical mantle if no shunt is present. If a shunt is present, the previous shunt incision is opened and extended several centimeters to allow enough bone exposure for a small craniotomy (typically 3–4 cm in diameter). A small cortical incision enables entry into the most superficial CSF compartment. Standard microsurgical techniques enable wide fenestration between as many CSF compartments as possible. Via a supratentorial approach, communication can be achieved not only among loculated collections on both sides supratentorially but also with posterior fossa loculated cysts, which often protrude through the tentorial notch. Septations are typically divided with a combination of bipolar cautery, suction, microscissors, and various dissectors. Most frequently, after completion of the fenestration, a new proximal catheter is placed under direct vision into the compartment most likely to remain patent and keep open communication with other compartments. This catheter is then connected to existing shunt systems. The dura is closed in a watertight fashion around the catheter, and the intradural space is filled with irrigation prior to closure to prevent subsequent brain collapse. **Figures 4.3, 4.4,** and **4.5** demonstrate pre- and postoperative imaging studies and intraoperative findings in a typical patient.

Only two studies describing craniotomy for compartmentalized hydrocephalus have been published. Nida and Haines

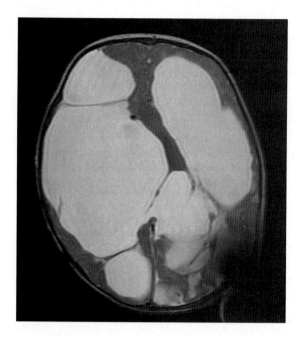

Fig. 4.3 Preoperative axial T2-weighted magnetic resonance imaging scan in a 6-month-old patient with a history of prematurity, grade IV intraventricular hemorrhage, and ventriculitis. Multiple ventricular compartments separated by septations are noted.

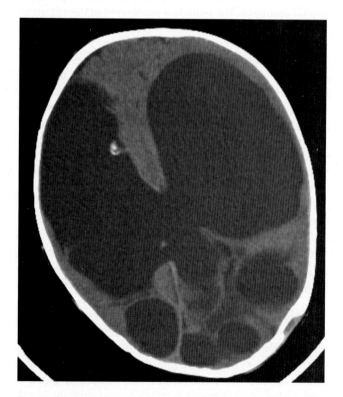

Fig. 4.5 Postoperative computed tomography scan in the same patient demonstrating communication between several previously loculated cerebrospinal fluid–filled compartments. (From Sandberg DI, McComb JG, Krieger MD. Craniotomy for fenestration of multiloculated hydrocephalus in pediatric patients. Neurosurgery 2005 Jul;57(1 Suppl):100–6, discussion 100–6. Reprinted by permission.)

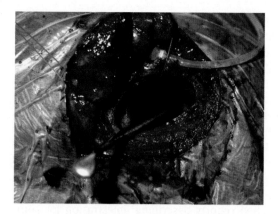

Fig. 4.4 Intraoperative photograph taken during a craniotomy for fenestration of compartmentalized hydrocephalus in this patient. The shunt valve is visualized beneath the skin flap, and clear Silastic tubing is attached to the proximal end of the valve to prevent entry of blood or debris. A Penfield no. 1 dissector is visualized that has been placed from the posterior parietal incision and now rests on the frontal bone after communication of previously loculated compartments.

reported a series of 10 patients, 4 of whom were treated by shunting alone, and 6 of whom underwent craniotomy for fenestration followed by shunt placement.[22] In this series, a craniotomy was performed to allow fenestration via a transcallosal approach. The authors describe a decrease in the number of shunt revisions required in patients who underwent craniotomy compared with preoperatively, and fewer shunt revisions were subsequently required in these patients than in those who were shunted without fenestration.

In 2005 we reported on our series of 33 patients who underwent craniotomies for compartmentalized hydrocephalus.[15] Thirty-one of these procedures were performed via a posterior parietal approach, and two were performed via a posterior fossa craniotomy and upper cervical laminectomies. There were no new neurologic deficits noted in any patients, and no patient required a blood transfusion intraoperatively. As expected, neurologic status was extremely poor in the vast majority of patients both pre- and postoperatively. Over a median follow-up of 3.7 years, the majority of patients ($n = 25$) maintained shunt systems with only one catheter, and one patient did not require a shunt. Six patients required two shunt catheters, and one required three shunt catheters. During this period, many patients (19 of 33) required additional fenestration procedures (ranging from one to six procedures), a finding that has also been noted in reports on endoscopic fenestration procedures in this challenging patient population.[25]

Conclusion

Compartmentalized hydrocephalus is an extremely challenging condition to manage. The vast majority of patients will require a shunt. The goal of fenestration is to reduce the number of shunting systems required to treat the hydrocephalus, ideally to only one. Fenestrations may be performed endoscopically or via craniotomy. In the authors' experience, craniotomy and microsurgical techniques most effectively create wide communications between loculated compartments in complex cases. Fenestration procedures may reduce the number of shunt revisions required, but the rate of shunt revision and/or repeat fenestration, either endoscopic or open, is high in this patient population. Unfortunately, despite aggressive interventions to treat compartmentalized hydrocephalus, neurologic outcomes tend to be very poor in this population, as most patients have severely damaged brains due to prior intraventricular hemorrhage and/or CNS infection.

♦ Lessons Learned

Compartmentalized or multiloculated hydrocephalus is one of the more difficult conditions treated by pediatric neurosurgeons, as it requires multiple procedures and the need for multiple shunt systems. As the authors report, the difficulties arise from the anatomy and the effect of the multiple loculated fluid collections or ventricles. The diagnostic modalities include magnetic resonance imaging and CT scans with dye to help elucidate the lack of communication between the fluid collections and the ventricular system. The treatment for this condition can be microsurgical or endoscopic. The chapter illustrates the advantages of each approach. The endoscopic route is minimally invasive but more difficult as the anatomy is distorted and visualization blurred from previous hemorrhage or infectious process. The microsurgical approach provides better visualization and control of the potential bleeding sources, but it is more invasive and requires a potentially longer hospital stay.

References

1. Albanese V, Tomasello F, Sampaolo S. Multiloculated hydrocephalus in infants. Neurosurgery 1981;8(6):641–646
2. Miner ME. Posthemorrhagic hemispheric cysts in neonates: treatment by cystoventriculostomy. Neurosurgery 1987;21(1):105–107
3. Schultz P, Leeds NE. Intraventricular septations complicating neonatal meningitis. J Neurosurg 1973;38(5):620–626
4. Brown LW, Zimmerman RA, Bilaniuk LT. Polycystic brain disease complicating neonatal meningitis: documentation of evolution by computed tomography. J Pediatr 1979;94(5):757–759
5. Nida TY, Haines SJ. Multiloculated hydrocephalus: craniotomy and fenestration of intraventricular septations. J Neurosurg 1993;78(1):70–76
6. Siomin V, Constantini S. Basic principles and equipment in neuroendoscopy. In: Abbott R, ed. Clinical Neuroendoscopy. Vol 15. Philadelphia: WB Saunders; 2004:19–32
7. Bucholz RD, Pittman T. Endoscopic coagulation of the choroid plexus using the Nd:YAG laser: initial experience and proposal for management. Neurosurgery 1991;28(3):421–426, discussion 426–427
8. Cohen AR. Endoscopic ventricular surgery. Pediatr Neurosurg 1993;19(3):127–134
9. Heilman CB, Cohen AR. Endoscopic ventricular fenestration using a "saline torch." J Neurosurg 1991;74(2):224–229
10. Levy ML, Lavine SD, Mendel E, McComb JG. The endoscopic stylet: technical notes. Neurosurgery 1994;35(2):335–336, discussion 335–336
11. Vries JK. An endoscopic technique for third ventriculostomy. Surg Neurol 1978;9(3):165–168
12. Oi S, Abbott R. Loculated ventricles and iosolated compartments in hydrocephalus: their pathophysiology and the efficacy of neuroendoscopic surgery. In: Abbott R, ed. Clinical Neuroendoscopy. Vol 15. Philadelphia: WB Saunders; 2004:77–87
13. Lewis AI, Keiper GL Jr, Crone KR. Endoscopic treatment of loculated hydrocephalus. J Neurosurg 1995;82(5):780–785
14. Spennato P, Cinalli G, Ruggiero C, et al. Neuroendoscopic treatment of multiloculated hydrocephalus in children. J Neurosurg 2007;106(1, Suppl):29–35
15. Sandberg DI, McComb JG, Krieger MD. Craniotomy for fenestration of multiloculated hydrocephalus in pediatric patients. Neurosurgery 2005;57(1, Suppl):100–106, discussion 100–106
16. Brown LW, Zimmerman RA, Bilaniuk LT. Polycystic brain disease complicating neonatal meningitis: documentation of evolution by computed tomography. J Pediatr 1979;94(5):757–759
17. Eller TW, Pasternak JF. Isolated ventricles following intraventricular hemorrhage. J Neurosurg 1985;62(3):357–362
18. Handler LC, Wright MG. Postmeningitic hydrocephalus in infancy: ventriculography with special reference to ventricular septa. Neuroradiology 1978;16:31–35
19. Jamjoom AB, Mohammed AA, al-Boukai A, Jamjoom ZA, Rahman N, Jamjoom HT. Multiloculated hydrocephalus related to cerebrospinal fluid shunt infection. Acta Neurochir (Wien) 1996;138(6):714–719
20. Kalsbeck JE, DeSousa AL, Kleiman MB, Goodman JM, Franken EA. Compartmentalization of the cerebral ventricles as a sequela of neonatal meningitis. J Neurosurg 1980;52(4):547–552
21. Schultz P, Leeds NE. Intraventricular septations complicating neonatal meningitis. J Neurosurg 1973;38(5):620–626
22. Nida TY, Haines SJ. Multiloculated hydrocephalus: craniotomy and fenestration of intraventricular septations. J Neurosurg 1993;78(1):70–76

23. Albanese V, Tomasello F, Sampaolo S. Multiloculated hydrocephalus in infants. Neurosurgery 1981;8(6):641–646

24. Kaiser G. The value of multiple shunt systems in the treatment of nontumoral infantile hydrocephalus. Childs Nerv Syst 1986;2(4):200–205

25. Spennato P, Cinalli G, Ruggiero C, et al. Neuroendoscopic treatment of multiloculated hydrocephalus in children. J Neurosurg 2007;106(1, Suppl):29–35

26. Kleinhaus S, Germann R, Sheran M, Shapiro K, Boley SJ. A role for endoscopy in the placement of ventriculoperitoneal shunts. Surg Neurol 1982;18(3):179–180

27. Lewis AI, Keiper GL Jr, Crone KR. Endoscopic treatment of loculated hydrocephalus. J Neurosurg 1995;82(5):780–785

28. Heilman CB, Cohen AR. Endoscopic ventricular fenestration using a "saline torch." J Neurosurg 1991;74(2):224–229

29. Fritsch MJ, Mehdorn M. Endoscopic intraventricular surgery for treatment of hydrocephalus and loculated CSF space in children less than one year of age. Pediatr Neurosurg 2002;36(4):183–188

30. Nowosławska E, Polis L, Kaniewska D, et al. Effectiveness of neuroendoscopic procedures in the treatment of complex compartmentalized hydrocephalus in children. Childs Nerv Syst 2003;19(9):659–665

31. Oi S, Hidaka M, Honda Y, et al. Neuroendoscopic surgery for specific forms of hydrocephalus. Childs Nerv Syst 1999;15(1):56–68

32. Powers SK. Fenestration of intraventricular cysts using a flexible, steerable endoscope. Acta Neurochir Suppl (Wien) 1992;54:42–46

5   Slit Ventricle Syndrome

♦ Surgical Management

Jonathan P. Miller and Alan R. Cohen

The development of the ventriculoperitoneal (VP) shunt has dramatically improved the prognosis for patients with hydrocephalus, but it has produced problems of its own. Slit ventricle syndrome (SVS) represents one of the more difficult shunt-related diseases to treat largely because there is no consensus and little evidence as to what exactly it is, why it occurs, and how best to treat it. Even the nomenclature is confusing: the syndrome has been variously named normal volume hydrocephalus,[1,2] noncompliant ventricle syndrome,[3,4] shunt-related pseudotumor cerebri,[5] and small ventricle–induced cerebrospinal fluid (CSF) shunt dysfunction.[6] Some have questioned whether the syndrome even exists at all.[7]

Although small "slitlike" ventricles are a frequent occurrence in long-standing shunted hydrocephalus, it does appear that there is a subset of shunted patients who have symptoms of shunt dysfunction with elevated intracranial pressure (ICP) and no evidence of ventricular dilation. The formal definition of SVS involves the clinical triad of intermittent transient symptoms of shunt dysfunction (defined as headaches lasting 10–90 minutes), small ventricles on computed tomography (CT), and slow shunt valve refill.[8] This condition has been estimated to affect between 6 and 22% of all patients who have radiologic slit ventricles and headaches.[4,9] In one series of 370 shunted patients, 11.5% developed SVS, and 6.5% required surgical intervention, despite the finding of radiographic slit ventricles in > 60%.[10] SVS does not present during infancy[11] or when hydrocephalus occurs in adults.[2] Most commonly, it presents between 5 and 10 years of age in patients who had been shunted during infancy (**Fig. 5.1**).[11,12]

Because headache is common in shunt patients, SVS must be differentiated from other conditions that can cause headaches in patients with radiologic slit ventricles, such as CSF overdrainage, intermittent proximal shunt dysfunction, and migraine.[4,13] One study used invasive ICP monitoring to differentiate five subtypes of "slit ventricle syndromes":

low-pressure headaches due to overdrainage, intermittent proximal shunt obstruction, true shunt failure without ventriculomegaly, intracranial hypertension with a working shunt, and headaches unrelated to shunt function.[2]

Etiology

In SVS, the ventricles do not enlarge in response to elevated ICP produced by shunt malfunction. Intermittent symptoms are presumed to be caused by catheter obstruction produced by small ventricles that leads to increased pressure, marginal

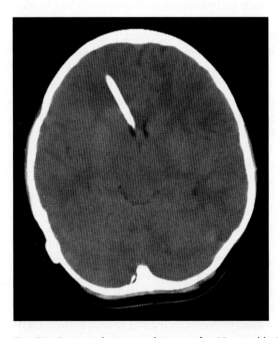

Fig. 5.1 Computed tomography scan of a 10-year-old girl who had been shunted during infancy. Despite small ventricles, lumbar puncture demonstrated high opening pressure, and a proximal shunt malfunction was found during surgical exploration.

dilation, and restoration of catheter function.[2,4,9] Patients with SVS have noncompliant ventricles that remain very small even in the face of markedly elevated ICP. Three theories have been advanced as to why this is the case, and it is possible that more than one or even all three are correct.

The first theory to explain noncompliant ventricles is that there is increased ventricular wall stiffness in SVS that prevents expansion in response to pressure changes. This is thought to be due to chronic changes in the ventricular wall, such as subependymal gliosis in patients with long-term ventricular drainage. Direct measurement of ventricular compliance demonstrated increased ventricular elastance in four SVS patients.[1] A canine model of long-standing shunted hydrocephalus with overdrainage has shown histologic evidence of subependymal and periventricular gliosis that presumably led to increased elastance,[14] although these findings were not confirmed in autopsy examination of one patient with small ventricles and a long-standing ventricular shunt.[15]

A second proposed mechanism for noncompliant ventricles in SVS argues that overshunting of infantile hydrocephalus leads to craniocerebral disproportion with microcephaly and synostosis that produces very small ventricles that are unable to expand. Dampening of cerebral pressure waves might cause understimulation of growth of the calvaria and premature ossification of sutures.[16,17] It has long been known that chronic shunting produces dramatic changes in the skull, especially thickness,[18] and one study of 400 patients shunted in infancy found overdrainage associated with microcephaly and synostosis in > 8%.[19] Microcephaly does occur in SVS,[12] histologic evidence of craniosynostosis has been observed,[16] and subtemporal decompression and other cranial expansion techniques have been used with some therapeutic success.[9,17]

A third theory about etiology of SVS postulates that the problem is with venous hypertension leading to poor absorption of CSF at the level of the arachnoid granulations. It is known that CSF is not absorbed until ICP is 3 to 6 mm Hg higher than pressure in the venous sinuses, particularly the superior sagittal sinus.[20] High venous pressure can lead to hydrocephalus in achondroplasia.[21,22] Venous bypass has been used successfully to treat selected cases of hydrocephalus,[23] and other intracranial hypertension syndromes (particularly pseudotumor cerebri) are believed to occur because of elevated venous pressure.[20] Chronic shunting of hydrocephalus in patients with distensible heads could lead to uncoupling of ventricular and venous pressure due to dampening of the normal intraventricular pulse pressure. High venous pressure in SVS patients could then prevent appropriate absorption of CSF, leading to distention of cortical subarachnoid spaces as well as increased cerebral elastance due to venous congestion.[9,20] SVS patients may therefore have an acquired form of shunt-related pseudotumor cerebri.[5]

Treatment Options

Conservative Treatment

A significant number of SVS patients will improve without surgical intervention.[24] Conservative treatment options include observation, hydration, diuresis, and corticosteroid treatment. Antimigraine therapy has been successfully used to treat SVS patients, possibly by reducing venous congestion or improving coupling of CSF absorption to ICP.[25,26] It is unclear whether patients who improve without surgical intervention truly have SVS or simply small ventricles with shunt-associated headaches that are not related to ICP.[5]

Shunt Revision/Removal

In the setting of slit ventricles and low-pressure headaches, it is possible that the problem involves simple CSF overdrainage. In this case, increasing the valve pressure or adding an antisiphon device can be very effective.[8] Clinical improvement is not always accompanied by reexpansion of the ventricles.[8] Some patients with overdrainage syndromes in fact will not require a shunt at all. One trial of externalization with ICP monitoring in 22 patients with SVS demonstrated that 5 did not require shunting and underwent removal of the shunt without further treatment.[27]

Cranial Expansion Procedures

Increasing intracranial volume could be an effective treatment for SVS by reducing the effects of decreased compliance, especially if synostosis and microcephaly are present. Subtemporal decompression was first performed by Cushing for raised ICP and later by Dandy to treat pseudotumor cerebri and was popularized as a treatment for intermittent shunt obstruction due to small ventricles by Epstein et al.[28] The procedure involves removal of part of the temporal bone to create an artificial fontanelle. This allows release of pressure and can vent pressure waves that presumably occur as a result of abnormal buffering capacity.[3] One study of 22 SVS patients treated with ipsilateral subtemporal decompression with the dura left open found that shunt-related admissions were decreased by 75% and shunt revisions by nearly 80%.[29] Subtemporal decompression by itself can dramatically reduce ICP[6,30] and seems to work even if the ventricle does not enlarge postoperatively.[31] In a study of 32 SVS patients, subtemporal decompression was associated with an early increase in the number of shunt revisions in the early postoperative period, but the number of admissions for raised ICP was reduced.[3]

Other more extensive calvarial expansion techniques have also been used to treat SVS based on the observation that widespread pathologic suture fusion occurs in this condition. In one report, 14 patients with intracranial hypertension in spite of a functioning shunt were treated with craniotomy and morcellation of bone from the coronal suture to the transverse sinus and to the squamosal sutures on either side, and symptoms were improved in all patients.[9] Another study involved three patients treated with a biparietal craniotomy with reorientation of the bone flap to provide more intracranial volume. In this study, ICP was monitored invasively before and after the operation and was observed to be dramatically improved in each patient.[17] In a study of five SVS patients treated with cranial expansion and removal of sclerotic sutures, all were asymptomatic at 24 months postoperatively.[16]

Lumboperitoneal Shunt

Lumboperitoneal (LP) shunting is postulated to be an effective treatment for SVS because it allows for drainage of the cortical subarachnoid space as well as the ventricles.[5,32,33] LP shunts are often avoided in the pediatric population due to fear of scoliosis, pain, neurologic changes, and hindbrain herniation.[34] However, if valves are used, and LP shunts are placed only in older children, these complications are rare.[5] Reestablishment of a pressure gradient from the ventricles to the subarachnoid space allows normalization of ventricular size, and subarachnoid drainage prevents distention of cortical subarachnoid spaces. In one early report, a patient with SVS and progressive shunt dysfunction was confirmed to have communicating hydrocephalus by cisternogram, then underwent placement of an LP shunt that alleviated his symptoms.[35] A more recent series of LP shunt insertion showed clinical improvement in seven SVS patients.[32] Each patient had symptoms of intermittent shunt malfunction and a functioning shunt demonstrated by shunt tap or surgical exploration, and the VP shunts were not removed. In three of these patients who now had VP and LP shunts, subsequent VP shunt dysfunction actually led to ventriculomegaly,[36] supporting the hypothesis that LP shunting allows a pressure gradient from the ventricles to the subarachnoid space.

If communication of CSF can be demonstrated using radiographic techniques, LP shunting can be used by itself with permanent removal of the VP shunt.[33] In a series of 27 patients with severe SVS, incapacitating headaches, and recurrent proximal shunt malfunction, CT scan after intraventricular injection of iohexol verified communicating hydrocephalus in 24 patients. These patients underwent VP shunt removal and placement of an LP shunt with resolution of symptoms and normalization of ventricular size. There were no cases of hindbrain herniation or other complications.[33] Another series of 33 patients with SVS possibly due to an isolated ventricle underwent replacement of the VP shunt with an LP shunt. Postoperatively, all patients had resolution of symptoms, there were fewer subsequent shunt revisions and infections, and no patient experienced hindbrain herniation.[7] For patients with lumbar anatomy that

precludes LP shunt placement, cisterna magna-ventricle-peritoneum shunts have been used with good results.[37]

Endoscopic Third Ventriculostomy

Endoscopic third ventriculostomy (ETV) is an appealing treatment for hydrocephalus because patients can become shunt-free even after prolonged shunt reliance (**Fig. 5.2**).[38] ETV for SVS seems counterintuitive, as ventricular enlargement is one of the principal requirements for safe ventriculoscopy. As a result, early attempts were mainly performed as a last resort in patients for whom other treatments had failed. In one study, five patients with aqueductal stenosis underwent ETV after failure of valve upgrade and subtemporal decompression, and all five had encouraging results.[39] In another series including seven SVS patients undergoing ETV, two were rendered shunt-free, and the other five had improvement of symptoms.[10]

More recently, several techniques have been used to produce ventricular enlargement in preparation for ETV, such as externalization of the shunt with[40] or without[27] controlled intracranial hypertension, or placement of a programmable valve[41,42] or high-pressure antisiphon device.[43] In one study of 22 patients with SVS, patients underwent shunt externalization and invasive ICP monitoring, and all 16 patients who demonstrated a need for continued shunting underwent ETV regardless of the putative cause of hydrocephalus.[27] Ten of these patients became shunt-free. Of the six failures, four were apparent prior to discharge from the hospital, and the other two had scarring over the ventriculostomy defect. In a series of four patients with SVS and small ventricles, VP shunts were externalized, and the external ventricular drainage bag was gradually elevated to an average of 18.8 cm above head level over an average of 5.8 days to render the ventricles navigable. Three of the four patients were successfully rendered shunt-free.[40] In another study, 15 patients with SVS underwent ventricular cannulation using a very small flexible endoscope to measure compliance.[42] In 4 patients, compliance was low, and ETV was performed using a larger endoscope; in the other 11 patients, a shunt with a programmable valve was inserted and the pressure slowly increased over an average of 16.3 months, after which ETV was performed. All 15 patients in this study became shunt-free with no symptoms.

ETV for SVS is not without risks, as these patients frequently have adhesions that make ventricular cannulation and navigation difficult and potentially hazardous. Additionally, two studies have identified transient short-term memory loss as a risk of ETV in SVS patients.[27,39]

Management Plan

Any attempt to formulate a treatment plan for patients with SVS should include a careful assessment of symptoms and

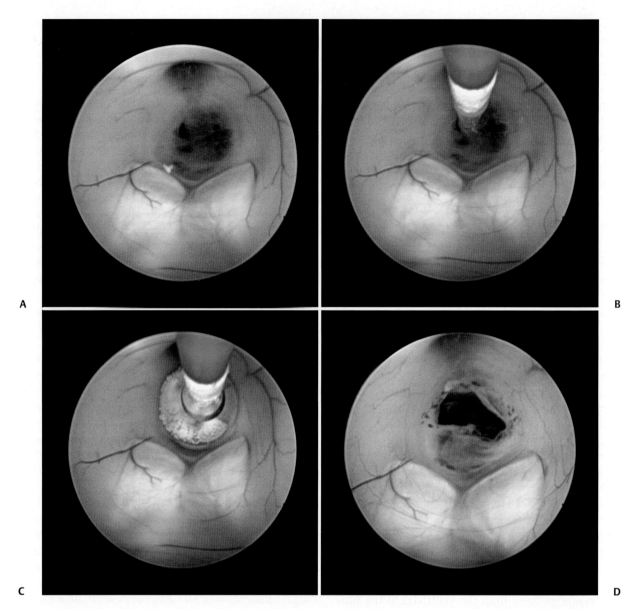

Fig. 5.2 Intraoperative photographs showing the steps of endoscopic third ventriculostomy in a patient with ventriculomegaly. **(A)** The thinned floor of the third ventricle is visible between the infundibular recess and the mammillary bodies. **(B)** A no. 4 French Fogarty balloon catheter is used to perforate the floor of the third ventricle, **(C)** then inflated to produce **(D)** an opening. This operation may be difficult to perform if the ventricles are small and do not enlarge with controlled shunt occlusion.

measurement of ICP by means of intraparenchymal fiberoptic monitor placement or lumbar puncture. Conservative treatment is a good first step for any patient who does not have disabling symptoms. If a patient presents with symptoms of low-pressure headaches and low pressure on monitoring, valve upgrade can often be helpful. Evidence of intermittent shunt malfunction can usually be effectively treated by replacing the shunt in a different location, using stereotactic guidance if necessary. Subtemporal decompression is reserved for patients who have not responded to other treatments. Cranial expansion surgery may be effective in cases

of synostosis. ETV is difficult in patients with SVS, and our general technique is to externalize the shunt and occlude it transiently with ICP monitoring in an attempt to enlarge the ventricles. Frameless stereotactic image guidance is useful in cannulating small ventricles with the endoscope. We perform LP shunting infrequently in the pediatric population.

Conclusion

SVS is a difficult entity to treat because of uncertainty regarding both the etiology and the most effective treatment for this condition. The principal theories as to the etiology of SVS involve decreased brain compliance, cephalocranial disproportion, and venous hypertension. Several treatments have been used successfully, including ventricular shunt revision, cranial expansion techniques, LP shunting, and ETV. With patience and careful application of these approaches, most SVS patients can be managed successfully with a satisfactory long-term outcome.

◆ Lumboperitoneal Shunting

Harold L. Rekate

The term slit ventricle syndrome is a catch-all term that refers to a severe headache disorder in patients with ventricular shunts and chronic headaches. Our original definition of the term defined the condition as a triad of small ventricles on imaging studies, severe headaches lasting 10 to 90 minutes, and slow or no refill of a shunt-flushing device.[44] Many reports of the syndrome followed, but there was no consensus about its definition or evidence about the cause of the headaches. It was assumed that SVS was related to chronic overdrainage of CSF by the shunt system and that the resulting long-term changes in the brain or skull led to the headaches.[45-47]

Based on a retrospective review of patients with chronic headaches and shunts, we defined five distinct pathophysiologies that had been incorporated into the concept of SVS,[48] including intermittent proximal obstruction; severely low ICP analogous to spinal headaches; cephalocranial disproportion, which occurs only in the context of genetic craniofacial syndromes (i.e., the patient has increased ICP despite a working shunt); and intracranial hypertension associated with nonresponsive ventricles and shunt failure. The latter has been called normal volume hydrocephalus (NVH) by Engel and colleagues, who originally described it.[49] The fifth pathophysiology is shunt-related migraine, which is a diagnosis of exclusion. It requires definitive evidence of normal ICP dynamics. These patients usually have a family history positive for migraine headaches.

Patients with low-pressure headaches and intermittent proximal obstruction are best managed by upgrading the valve and ascertaining that the valve mechanism includes a device that minimizes the gravitational effects caused by the height differential between the ventricular catheter in the lateral ventricles and the peritoneal catheter terminis. Patients with Crouzon or Pfeiffer syndrome and hydrocephalus have a complex problem that includes hindbrain herniation and obstruction of venous outflow.[50,51] In such cases, the only functional strategy is a surgical approach that involves enlarging the intracranial compartment.[52-54]

NVH and shunt-related migraine are the most persistent and troubling conditions to manage. Without ICP monitoring, possibly on multiple occasions, it is often impossible to differentiate the two conditions. These patients are frequent visitors to emergency rooms and are often admitted to the neurosurgical service. On each occasion, they undergo imaging studies. The cost of missing a shunt failure could mean new neurologic deficits or even the patient's death. Considerable energy and money can be consumed, and these patients likely undergo several unnecessary surgical interventions. We have found it valuable to assess whether such patients can function without their shunt and thereby avoid these constant interventions. As we gained experience using ETV to manage shunt failure, we decided to attempt shunt removal in patients with frequent shunt failure or intractable headaches in an effort to improve their quality of life.[55]

Shunt Removal Protocol

Patients with chronic severe headaches and demonstrably working shunts have their shunt system removed and replaced with an external ventricular drain (EVD). The patient is taken to the intensive care unit, where the EVD is closed to ICP monitoring. A new imaging study is obtained 12 to 24 hours later. If the patient's ICP is > 30 mm Hg, the EVD is opened at 30 cm above the level of the head to ensure the patient's safety.

This protocol (**Fig. 5.3**)[55] is associated with three possible outcomes. In ~25% of the cases, ventricular size increases minimally to moderately without symptoms or an increase in ICP. The EVD is removed from these patients who have shunt-independent arrest of their hydrocephalus. Typically, these patients developed hydrocephalus from neonatal intraventricular hemorrhage or were shunted when diagnosed with a brain tumor that was later treated. The results were expected in about half of the patients: ICP increased, the patients were symptomatic, and their ventricles expanded. Except patients with hydrocephalus associated with spina bifida, 80% of patients with ventricles that expand will respond to ETV and can become shunt-independent. We presume that the outcome is not as predictable in patients with spina bifida because their Chiari II malformation is associated with multiple sites of obstruction to CSF flow not found in other forms of SVS.[56,57]

In the remaining 25%, ICP increases considerably, but ventricular size increases little if at all. These patients have NVH.

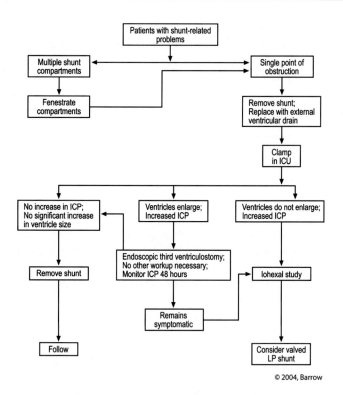

Fig. 5.3 Algorithm of treatment of patients with severe headache disorders and a shunt (slit ventricle syndrome). ICP, intracranial pressure; ICU, intensive care unit; LP, lumboperitoneal. (From Barrow Neurological Institute. Reprinted by permission.)

All of our patients in this group were shunted during infancy, regardless of the age at which they became symptomatic. Typically, they had developed triventricular hydrocephalus associated with asymptomatic but excessive growth in head circumference and normal developmental milestones. The 25% incidence in our patients is consistent with the findings of McComb's retrospective analysis of shunted infants (McComb JG, personal communication, 2000).

We injected iohexol 180 in these patients. In our initial report of this experience, the ventricular system communicated with the spinal subarachnoid space in 24 of 27 patients. The remaining three patients had a history of severe ventriculitis that led to a secondary obstruction of their CSF pathways. Overall, the patients in this series were neurologically normal and bright. In this group of patients, LP shunts have successfully managed their condition.[58–60]

Normal Volume Hydrocephalus, Slit Ventricle Syndrome, and Pseudotumor Cerebri

The patients described above had a presumptive diagnosis of hydrocephalus secondary to aqueductal stenosis. What has happened? NVH is the most troubling and confusing of the subsets of SVS. If these patients had no history of overt hydrocephalus during infancy, they would be diagnosed with pseudotumor cerebri, which is also called idiopathic intracranial hypertension. The pathophysiology underlying these two conditions is the same, and their management is similar.

Our work on a mathematical model of CSF dynamics in hydrocephalus led us to study patients with pseudotumor cerebri using retrograde venographic measurement of ICP. Based on these measurements, we postulated that all cases of pseudotumor cerebri are caused by increased intracranial venous sinus pressure.[61,62] We have performed this study in more than 150 patients with various forms of pseudotumor cerebri, including 15 patients with NVH. All of the latter have showed increased pressure in the superior sagittal sinus. NVH is pseudotumor cerebri that begins before the fontanelle and sutures close.[63]

Explaining the relationship of pseudotumor cerebri to aqueductal stenosis requires a few steps. Except in the context of the sex-linked form of the condition that is inherited only in male offspring, aqueductal stenosis is an effect of hydrocephalus and not a general cause. Care should be taken when equating triventricular hydrocephalus with aqueductal stenosis. In naturally occurring animal models of congenital hydrocephalus, the hydrocephalus develops before the secondary closure of the aqueduct. Based on the injection of iodinated dyes in humans, shunting opens the aqueduct mechanically.[64] Recently, we have shown that adult patients with triventricular hydrocephalus and chronic compensated hydrocephalus or long-standing overt ventriculomegaly of the adult (LOVA) have secondary opening of the aqueduct after ETV.[65] In such cases, the initial step is ventriculomegaly, which increases the size of the temporal horns of the lateral ventricles. This increase exerts pressure inward on the midbrain. Functionally, the aqueduct is closed but reopens with adequate treatment of the hydrocephalus.

Even in babies with isolated triventricular hydrocephalus, ventricular size is unlikely to stabilize after ETV.[66] Several reasons may account for this finding. A brain with an open fontanelle is in communication with atmospheric pressure. Pressure high enough to lead to the absorption of spinal fluid may not be possible. This discussion could lead to the conclusion that aqueductal stenosis is related to a terminal CSF absorption defect that leads to ventriculomegaly and would not be expected to respond to ETV.

We recently reported a case of a young woman who was shunted as an adult for LOVA and who suffered from multiple shunt complications. Eventually, she underwent ETV, which failed to relieve her symptoms and did not decrease the size of her ventricles. ICP monitoring led to the realization that her ICP remained elevated to 35 mm Hg despite the free flow of CSF through the stoma of the ETV and through a subsequently opened aqueduct. Retrograde venography showed that both transverse sinuses were stenotic. After venous stenting, ICP and CSF flow normalized.[65]

NVH therefore is a form of pseudotumor cerebri that begins in infancy. The hydrocephalus results from the distensibility of the infant's skull. Effective treatments for the management of pseudotumor cerebri usually require surgical strategies that access the CSF in both the cortical subarachnoid space and cerebral ventricles. In most instances, this strategy is best served by placing an LP shunt. After shunting, the ventricles become smaller than normal (slitlike). In patients with an intact septum pellucidum, the shunted lateral ventricle ends up smaller than the unshunted ventricle.[67–69] Work in our laboratory has shown that this ventricular asymmetry is caused by the septum pellucidum lying against the head of the caudate nucleus. A pressure differential can be recorded between the two lateral ventricles. The lateral ventricle with the shunt is isolated. CSF from the contralateral ventricle and the cortical subarachnoid space cannot flow into the shunted ventricle,[69] leading to reversible obstruction of the ventricular catheter.

Lumboperitoneal Shunts in the Treatment of Slit Ventricle Syndrome

At the annual meeting of the Joint Section on Pediatric Neurological Surgery of the American Association of Neurological Surgeons and the Congress of Neurological Surgeons in New York in December 2001, two presentations were given on the use and utility of LP shunts in the management of SVS.[59,60] However, the approaches of the two presenting groups differed significantly. The work of the Chicago group treated symptomatic patients with severe difficulties with symptomatic slit ventricles by adding an LP shunt to an existing shunt system. In contrast, our use of LP shunts resulted from our shunt-removal protocol. LP shunts were placed in patients who had previously had their shunts removed and not replaced. Patients of the Chicago group had two separate shunts, whereas our patients were treated only with the LP shunts.

Later the Chicago group reported on a group of patients with symptomatic ventricular enlargement after placement of an LP shunt. Based on these observations, these authors suggested that LP shunts preferentially drained the subarachnoid space rather than the ventricle.[70] My own discussion of the pathophysiology of the SVS that followed that report postulated a lack of communication between the ventricle and cortical subarachnoid space. When the LP shunts were placed, ICP decreased below the opening pressure of the ventricular valve. Because no CSF could drain through the valve in the ventricle, ventriulomegaly developed. The patient had intraventricular obstructive hydrocephalus.[71] If the subarachnoid space is to be drained by a second shunt system, the ventricle and the subarachnoid space must be in communication.

Operative Procedure

Preoperatively, an imaging study using CT or magnetic resonance imaging is obtained for the purpose of applying frameless stereotactic techniques for placement of an intraventricular reservoir. Determining whether LP shunts are functional is difficult, especially in this group of patients, because shunt failure cannot be diagnosed on the basis of imaging studies. Even the routine use of reservoirs incorporated into the LP shunt does not make the assessment of these shunts simple. Therefore, we routinely implant a ventricular reservoir when an LP shunt is placed. The patient is placed in a lateral decubitus position with the side of the previous peritoneal shunt up. The head is placed in a head holder, and the frameless stereotactic system is registered. The head and the LP shunt site are prepared separately and draped appropriately. We use a 9.5 mm Rickham Reservoir (Codman Corp., Raynham, Massachusetts) because it is easy to access later.

A 2 cm vertical incision is made at the L3–L4 interspace. The spinal subarachnoid space is accessed with a 14-gauge Tuohy needle (Codman) and a lumbar catheter inserted at least 10 cm into the subarachnoid space. The needle is withdrawn, and free flow of CSF is determined. A transverse incision, usually the preexisting VP shunt incision, is reopened and carried down to the peritoneum with a muscle-splitting technique.

We prefer a variant of a Codman Hakim programmable valve with SiphonGuard (Codman). A magnetic instrument can be used to change the opening pressure of this valve between 30 and 200 mm H_2O. The SiphonGuard prevents overdrainage using a flow-restriction mechanism. It has little to do with siphoning. Rather, it prevents sudden rushes of CSF when patients assume the erect position or at the time of sudden Valsalva maneuvers. Valves employing diaphragm mechanisms are inappropriate for LP shunts. However, other flow-restricting valves and gravity-compensating mechanisms can be used for this purpose.

The ability to program the valve requires that the valve not rotate. A modified form of the valve therefore incorporates a flat-bottom stage to prevent rotation (**Fig. 5.4**). For the valve to be reprogrammed, it must be placed superficially in an accessible area and not deep in the soft tissues. Typically, we set all valves at 100 mm H_2O. If the operative report is not immediately available, and the valve has not been changed, the pressure setting is known.

At the time of the initial implantation of an LP shunt and reservoir, we typically monitor ICP for 48 hours. Recumbent ICP should be between 5 and 15 mm Hg, and upright ICP should be between −5 and +5 mm Hg. In our experience with this valve, these readings have been obtained in all patients who have undergone the procedure. In this group of patients, all CSF compartments communicate with all others (**Fig. 5.5**). From the perspective of CSF dynamics,

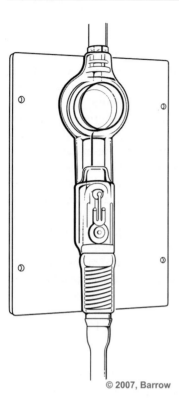

© 2007, Barrow

Fig. 5.4 Illustration of the modified programmable valve in a lumboperitoneal shunt with a flat stage that prevents rotation in the subcutaneous tissue. (From Barrow Neurological Institute. Reprinted by permission.)

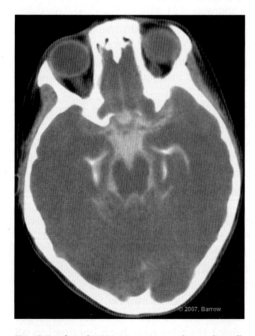

© 2007, Barrow

Fig. 5.5 Iohexol 180 cisternogram shows that all cerebrospinal fluid compartments communicate with each other. (From Barrow Neurological Institute. Reprinted by permission.)

these pressure profiles are normal. ICP can be monitored using an intraparenchymal transducer or by affixing a 23-gauge butterfly needle transcutaneously into the reservoir.

Postoperative Management

Patients with this severe subset of SVS have had severe headache disorders for a long time and may have received narcotic medications for their chronic daily headaches. Their headache disorder may not resolve completely despite normal ICP, normal CSF dynamics, and drainage of all CSF compartments through a common pathway. Four percent of the world's population has a headache at least 15 days per month, which is the definition of chronic daily headaches.[72–74] Just under half of the adult patients shunted during infancy report severe or disabling headaches. Therefore, successful treatment must be defined with an objective end point; it cannot depend completely on the severity of the headache.

Before initiating the treatment protocol, my discussion with these patients includes a commitment to ensure that their ICP and ICP dynamics are normal but not freedom from headache. Patients are informed that ~80% of those undergoing placement of an LP shunt for SVS have complete or near complete resolution of their severe headache disorder. For the remainder, it will likely be necessary to measure ICP through the implanted reservoir to convince yourself, the patient, and the other physicians managing the patient's pain that the problem is unrelated to the shunt.

A full description of the management of chronic daily headaches is beyond the scope of this discussion. In general, however, patients often treated with pain medication must be withdrawn from these medicines carefully. The use of medication for chronic headaches leads to a condition known as medication overuse headaches, which requires management by an established pain management team.

Concerns about the Use of Lumboperitoneal Shunts

For several reasons, neurosurgeons, particularly pediatric neurosurgeons, are reluctant to use LP shunts to manage either hydrocephalus or pseudotumor cerebri. In the first place, the one-piece LP shunts in common usage rely on the small diameter of the tubing and distal slit valves to prevent overdrainage. These shunts effectively lower ICP. However, the hydrostatic forces created when a fully grown individual stands up tend to overwhelm the valvular mechanism. Consequently, severe postural headaches are common in such patients. A valve mechanism must be added to these shunts to prevent this problem. The valve system described above can be manipulated to prevent this complication.

The second problem relates to the potential for the development of secondary hindbrain herniation (i.e., an acquired Chiari I malformation). This condition, which can be lethal, is reportedly common in patients undergoing LP shunting.[75,76] Patients reported to have this severe complication were infants with growing brains when their LP shunt was placed via laminectomy with no add-on valves. However, there have been no cases of acquired Chiari I malformations among children who received LP shunts in which valves were used rather than straight tubes with distal slits.[59] The careful use of valves with LP shunts will at least minimize this complication.

There is a strong sense that LP shunts are unreliable. The proximal catheter is thin and fragile, and the likelihood of breakage at the connector is greater than with ventricular shunts with no connector at or below the nuchal line. In general, however, the reputation of LP shunts as fragile and likely to suffer mechanical failure primarily relates to the disease processes commonly treated with lumbar shunts. The management of pseudotumor cerebri with LP shunts often means that treated patients are morbidly obese. Therefore, they have high intraperitoneal pressure, which makes the placement of peritoneal catheters difficult.

It is also difficult to determine whether the shunt is working at all, much less whether it is functioning correctly. In this condition, shunt failure cannot be diagnosed on the basis of imaging studies. Therefore, a physical measurement of ICP is needed. Typically, patients with LP shunts would have to undergo a lumbar puncture to determine ICP. Especially in obese patients or anxious children, pressure measured by lumbar puncture may be unreliable. Furthermore, negative ICP cannot be measured via lumbar pressure. These problems can be overcome by implanting ventricular tapping reservoirs. Pressure can then be measured accurately with minimal discomfort in relaxed patients whenever a complaint suggests shunt failure. Negative ICP can be measured by a fluid-coupled transducer without surgical intervention.

Management of Slit Ventricle Syndrome in Patients Who Are Not Candidates for Lumboperitoneal Shunts

LP shunts cannot be placed in all patients with SVS. There are relative and absolute contraindications to their placement. Spina bifida (i.e., a Chiari II malformation) and achondroplasia are absolute contraindications to the use of LP shunts. LP shunting is contraindicated in patients with spina bifida for three reasons. The most obvious is the problem of the attachment of the neural placode to the scar at the level of the initial repair and tethering of the spinal cord to the placode. This situation makes implantation of the lumbar catheter problematic and probably dangerous. The generalized arachnoiditis associated with this condition tends to interfere with CSF flow from the intracranial compartment to the spinal subarachnoid space. Finally, the Chiari II malformation tends to prevent CSF flow through the region of the foramen magnum and upper cervical spine.

Patients with achondroplasia are most likely to suffer from the severe form of SVS. In these patients, hydrocephalus relates to obstruction of venous outflow at the stenotic jugular foramina.[77–79] These cases are complicated by a very small foramen magnum, which is likely to prevent the flow of CSF from the cortical to the spinal subarachnoid space. These patients also have severe generalized spinal stenosis often with little or no CSF flow to the lumbar theca. The severe stenosis also makes placement of the lumbar catheter problematic.

Two categories of patients with SVS represent relative contraindications to the use of LP shunts. Patients with coexistent SVS and a Chiari I malformation may undergo successful LP shunting if two conditions are met: prior decompression of the hindbrain hernia and demonstrably adequate unimpeded CSF flow across the foramen magnum. LP shunts will lead to ventricular dilatation in patients with an intraventricular obstruction to the flow of CSF and NVH.[70] This problem is actually quite rare. It primarily occurs in patients who develop hydrocephalus during infancy due to venous hypertension but whose course was severely complicated by an intercurrent severe shunt infection; the resulting ventriculitis leads to secondary obstruction of CSF flow within the ventricles.[80] In such cases, all of these compartments must communicate with each other proximal to the valve so that there is no differential change in the solid geometry of the system. The cortical subarachnoid space must be included in any strategy used to treat the severe form of SVS.

Johnston and Sheridan managed pseudotumor cerebri by using shunts from the cisterna magna to the peritoneum.[81] My own experiences in this situation have not been encouraging. Catheters placed in the cisterna magna and then connected to a valve to the peritoneal catheter have connectors at or below the level of the nuchal line. They are difficult to assess, and they tend to break relatively quickly. In these cases, the cisterna magna is still a fixed reservoir of CSF that accesses the cortical subarachnoid space.

The fragility of the system is improved greatly by splicing a catheter in the cisterna magna to an existing shunt system, thereby creating a cisterna magna–ventricle–peritoneum shunt (**Fig. 5.6**).[82,83] Because LP shunt tubing is

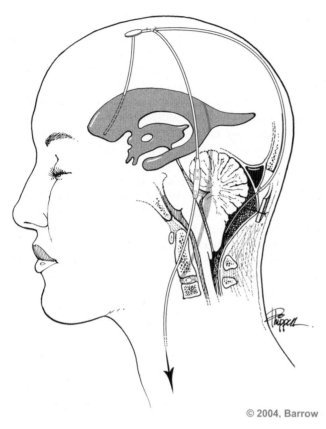

© 2004, Barrow

Fig. 5.6 Illustration of a cisterna magna–ventricle–peritoneum shunt. (From Barrow Neurological Institute. Reprinted by permission.)

soft, we use it in the cisterna magna. If a standard ventricular catheter is used, it will eventually rest on the upper cervical or cranial nerves or within the brainstem and cause lower cranial nerve dysfunction or severe pain. Once this catheter is located extracranially, a step-down connector is used to connect it to a standard bore peritoneal catheter. It is then drawn up to the reservoir of an existing VP shunt and thence to a valve. This configuration allows extracranial mixing of the various CSF compartments, and a programmable valve allows ICP and CSF dynamics to be fine-tuned.

Conclusion

The goal of treatment of patients with shunt-related headaches should be to normalize ICP and CSF dynamics. That is, all CSF compartments should communicate freely with each other. After this goal is accomplished, it is possible and necessary to ensure that ICP dynamics are normal. That is, recumbent ICP should be 5 to 15 mm Hg, and erect ICP should be between −5 and +5 mm Hg. Strategies to accomplish these goals may require that the shunt system access both the ventricular and subarachnoid space CSF. In most patients, such access can be provided by placing a valve-regulated LP shunt. Management of this condition is facilitated by the concurrent use of a ventricular reservoir.

◆ Lessons Learned

Slit ventricle syndrome is the bane of all pediatric neurosurgeons. As Drs. Miller and Cohen state in their introduction, the development of the ventriculoperitoneal shunt has resulted in prolonged survival of infants. There is no consensus and little evidence, however, as how to best prevent and treat this condition. The authors outline the etiology

and treatment options for SVS. Dr. Rekate's contribution clearly outlines the management of this condition with lumboperitoneal shunts. There is a protocol illustration that guides neurosurgeons on how to manage this rare but potentially devastating condition.

References

1. Engel M, Carmel PW, Chutorian AM. Increased intraventricular pressure without ventriculomegaly in children with shunts: "normal volume" hydrocephalus. Neurosurgery 1979;5(5):549–552
2. Rekate HL. Classification of slit-ventricle syndromes using intracranial pressure monitoring. Pediatr Neurosurg 1993;19(1):15–20
3. Buxton N, Punt J. Subtemporal decompression: the treatment of noncompliant ventricle syndrome. Neurosurgery 1999;44(3):513–518, discussion 518–519
4. Olson S. The problematic slit ventricle syndrome: a review of the literature and proposed algorithm for treatment. Pediatr Neurosurg 2004;40(6):264–269
5. Rekate HL. The slit ventricle syndrome: advances based on technology and understanding. Pediatr Neurosurg 2004;40(6):259–263
6. Walsh JW, James HE. Subtemporal craniectomy and elevation of shunt valve opening pressure in the management of small ventricle-induced cerebrospinal fluid shunt dysfunction. Neurosurgery 1982;10(6 Pt 1):698–703
7. Sood S, Barrett RJ, Powell T, Ham SD. The role of lumbar shunts in the management of slit ventricles: does the slit-ventricle syndrome exist? J Neurosurg 2005;103(2, Suppl):119–123
8. Hyde-Rowan MD, Rekate HL, Nulsen FE. Reexpansion of previously collapsed ventricles: the slit ventricle syndrome. J Neurosurg 1982;56(4):536–539

9. Epstein F, Lapras C, Wisoff JH. "Slit-ventricle syndrome": etiology and treatment. Pediatr Neurosci 1988;14(1):5–10

10. Walker ML, Fried A, Petronio J. Diagnosis and treatment of the slit ventricle syndrome. Neurosurg Clin N Am 1993;4(4):707–714

11. Cardoso ER, Del Bigio MR, Schroeder G. Age-dependent changes of cerebral ventricular size: 1. Review of intracranial fluid collections. Acta Neurochir (Wien) 1989;97(1-2):40–46

12. Oi S, Matsumoto S. Infantile hydrocephalus and the slit ventricle syndrome in early infancy. Childs Nerv Syst 1987;3(3):145–150

13. Foltz EL, Blanks JP. Symptomatic low intracranial pressure in shunted hydrocephalus. J Neurosurg 1988;68(3):401–408

14. Oi S, Matsumoto S. Morphological findings of postshunt slit-ventricle in experimental canine hydrocephalus: aspects of causative factors of isolated ventricles and slit-ventricle syndrome. Childs Nerv Syst 1986;2(4):179–184

15. Del Bigio MR. Neuropathological findings in a child with slit ventricle syndrome. Pediatr Neurosurg 2002;37(3):148–151

16. Albright AL, Tyler-Kabara E. Slit-ventricle syndrome secondary to shunt-induced suture ossification. Neurosurgery 2001;48(4):764–769, discussion 769–770

17. Eide PK, Helseth E, Due-Tonnessen B, Lundar T. Changes in intracranial pressure after calvarial expansion surgery in children with slit ventricle syndrome. Pediatr Neurosurg 2001;35(4): 195–204

18. Kaufman B, Weiss MH, Young HF, Nulsen FE. Effects of prolonged cerebrospinal fluid shunting on the skull and brain. J Neurosurg 1973;38(3):288–297

19. Faulhauer K, Schmitz P. Overdrainage phenomena in shunt treated hydrocephalus. Acta Neurochir (Wien) 1978;45(1-2):89–101

20. Karahalios DG, Rekate HL, Khayata MH, Apostolides PJ. Elevated intracranial venous pressure as a universal mechanism in pseudotumor cerebri of varying etiologies. Neurology 1996;46(1):198–202

21. Pierre-Kahn A, Hirsch JF, Renier D, Metzger J, Maroteaux P. Hydrocephalus and achondroplasia: a study of 25 observations. Childs Brain 1980;7(4):205–219

22. Steinbok P, Hall J, Flodmark O. Hydrocephalus in achondroplasia: the possible role of intracranial venous hypertension. J Neurosurg 1989;71(1):42–48

23. Sainte-Rose C, LaCombe J, Pierre-Kahn A, Renier D, Hirsch JF. Intracranial venous sinus hypertension: cause or consequence of hydrocephalus in infants? J Neurosurg 1984;60(4):727–736

24. Benzel EC, Reeves JD, Kesterson L, Hadden TA. Slit ventricle syndrome in children: clinical presentation and treatment. Acta Neurochir (Wien) 1992;117(1-2):7–14

25. Obana WG, Raskin NH, Cogen PH, Szymanski JA, Edwards MS. Antimigraine treatment for slit ventricle syndrome. Neurosurgery 1990;27(5):760–763, discussion 763

26. Nowak TP, James HE. Migraine headaches in hydrocephalic children: a diagnostic dilemma. Childs Nerv Syst 1989;5(5):310–314

27. Baskin JJ, Manwaring KH, Rekate HL. Ventricular shunt removal: the ultimate treatment of the slit ventricle syndrome. J Neurosurg 1998;88(3):478–484

28. Epstein FJ, Fleischer AS, Hochwald GM, Ransohoff J. Subtemporal craniectomy for recurrent shunt obstruction secondary to small ventricles. J Neurosurg 1974;41(1):29–31

29. Holness RO, Hoffman HJ, Hendrick EB. Subtemporal decompression for the slit-ventricle syndrome after shunting in hydrocephalic children. Childs Brain 1979;5(2):137–144

30. Allan R, Chaseling R. Subtemporal decompression for slit-ventricle syndrome: successful outcome after dramatic change in intracranial

31. Linder M, Diehl J, Sklar FH. Subtemporal decompressions for shunt-dependent ventricles: mechanism of action. Surg Neurol 1983; 19(6):520–523

32. Le H, Yamini B, Frim DM. Lumboperitoneal shunting as a treatment for slit ventricle syndrome. Pediatr Neurosurg 2002;36(4): 178–182

33. Rekate HL, Wallace D. Lumboperitoneal shunts in children. Pediatr Neurosurg 2003;38(1):41–46

34. Chumas PD, Armstrong DC, Drake JM, et al. Tonsillar herniation: the rule rather than the exception after lumboperitoneal shunting in the pediatric population. J Neurosurg 1993;78(4):568–573

35. Ide T, Aoki N, Miki Y. Slit ventricle syndrome successfully treated by a lumboperitoneal shunt. Neurol Res 1995;17(6):440–442

36. Khorasani L, Sikorski CW, Frim DM. Lumbar CSF shunting preferentially drains the cerebral subarachnoid over the ventricular spaces: implications for the treatment of slit ventricle syndrome. Pediatr Neurosurg 2004;40(6):270–276

37. Rekate HL, Nadkarni T, Wallace D. Severe intracranial hypertension in slit ventricle syndrome managed using a cisterna magna-ventricle-peritoneum shunt. J Neurosurg 2006;104(4, Suppl):240–244

38. Boschert J, Hellwig D, Krauss JK. Endoscopic third ventriculostomy for shunt dysfunction in occlusive hydrocephalus: long-term follow up and review. J Neurosurg 2003;98(5):1032–1039

39. Reddy K, Fewer HD, West M, Hill NC. Slit ventricle syndrome with aqueduct stenosis: third ventriculostomy as definitive treatment. Neurosurgery 1988;23(6):756–759

40. Butler WE, Khan SA. The application of controlled intracranial hypertension in slit ventricle syndrome patients with obstructive hydrocephalus and shunt malfunction. Pediatr Neurosurg 2001;35(6):305–310

41. Kamikawa S, Kuwamura K, Fujita A, Ohta K, Eguchi T, Tamaki N. [The management of slit-like ventricle with the Medos programmable Hakim valve and the ventriculofiberscope.] No Shinkei Geka 1998;26(4):349–356

42. Chernov MF, Kamikawa S, Yamane F, Ishihara S, Hori T. Neurofiberscope-guided management of slit-ventricle syndrome due to shunt placement. J Neurosurg 2005;102(3, Suppl): 260–267

43. Boschert JM, Krauss JK. Endoscopic third ventriculostomy in the treatment of shunt-related over-drainage: preliminary experience with a new approach how to render ventricles navigable. Clin Neurol Neurosurg 2006;108(2):143–149

44. Hyde-Rowan MD, Rekate HL, Nulsen FE. Reexpansion of previously collapsed ventricles: the slit ventricle syndrome. J Neurosurg 1982;56(4):536–539

45. Di Rocco C. Is the slit ventricle syndrome always a slit ventricle syndrome? Childs Nerv Syst 1994;10(1):49–58

46. Bruce DA, Weprin B. The slit ventricle syndrome. Neurosurg Clin N Am 2001;12(4):709–717

47. Kan P, Walker ML, Drake JM, Kestle JR. Predicting slitlike ventricles in children on the basis of baseline characteristics at the time of shunt insertion. J Neurosurg 2007;106(5, Suppl):347–349

48. Rekate HL. Classification of slit-ventricle syndromes using intracranial pressure monitoring. Pediatr Neurosurg 1993;19(1):15–20

49. Engel M, Carmel PW, Chutorian AM. Increased intraventricular pressure without ventriculomegaly in children with shunts: "normal volume" hydrocephalus. Neurosurgery 1979;5(5):549–552

pressure wave morphology. Report of two cases. J Neurosurg 2004; 101(2, Suppl):214–217

50. Bristol RE, Lekovic GP, Rekate HL. The effects of craniosynostosis on the brain with respect to intracranial pressure. Semin Pediatr Neurol 2004;11(4):262–267

51. Francis PM, Beals S, Rekate HL, Pittman HW, Manwaring K, Reiff J. Chronic tonsillar herniation and Crouzon's syndrome. Pediatr Neurosurg 1992;18(4):202–206

52. Albright AL, Tyler-Kabara E. Slit-ventricle syndrome secondary to shunt-induced suture ossification. Neurosurgery 2001;48(4):764–769, discussion 769–770

53. Cohen SR, Dauser RC, Newman MH, Muraszko K. Surgical techniques of cranial vault expansion for increases in intracranial pressure in older children. J Craniofac Surg 1993;4(3):167–176, discussion 174–176

54. Martínez-Lage JF, Ruiz-Espejo Vilar A, Pérez-Espejo MA, Almagro MJ, Ros de San Pedro J, Felipe Murcia M. Shunt-related craniocerebral disproportion: treatment with cranial vault expanding procedures. Neurosurg Rev 2006;29(3):229–235

55. Baskin JJ, Manwaring KH, Rekate HL. Ventricular shunt removal: the ultimate treatment of the slit ventricle syndrome. J Neurosurg 1998;88(3):478–484

56. Rekate H. Neurosurgical management of the child with spina bifida. In: Rekate H, ed. Comprehensive Management of Spina Bifida. Boca Raton, FL: CRC Press; 1991:93–112

57. Rekate H. Neurosurgical management of adults with spina bifida. In: Wyszynski D, ed. Neural Tube Defects: From Origin to Treatment. New York: Oxford University Press; 2006:241–249

58. Ide T, Aoki N, Miki Y. Slit ventricle syndrome successfully treated by a lumboperitoneal shunt. Neurol Res 1995;17(6):440–442

59. Le H, Yamini B, Frim DM. Lumboperitoneal shunting as a treatment for slit ventricle syndrome. Pediatr Neurosurg 2002;36(4):178–182

60. Rekate HL, Wallace D. Lumboperitoneal shunts in children. Pediatr Neurosurg 2003;38(1):41–46

61. Karahalios DG, Rekate HL, Khayata MH, Apostolides PJ. Elevated intracranial venous pressure as a universal mechanism in pseudotumor cerebri of varying etiologies. Neurology 1996;46(1):198–202

62. Rekate HL, Brodkey JA, Chizeck HJ, el Sakka W, Ko WH. Ventricular volume regulation: a mathematical model and computer simulation. Pediatr Neurosci 1988;14(2):77–84

63. Rekate HL, Nadkarni TD, Wallace D. The importance of the cortical subarachnoid space in understanding hydrocephalus. J Neurosurg Pediatr 2008;2(1):1–11

64. Nugent GR, Al-Mefty O, Chou S. Communicating hydrocephalus as a cause of aqueductal stenosis. J Neurosurg 1979;51(6):812–818

65. Rekate HL. Long-standing overt ventriculomegaly in adults: pitfalls in treatment with endoscopic third ventriculostomy. Neurosurg Focus 2007;22(4):E6

66. Buxton N, Macarthur D, Mallucci C, Punt J, Vloeberghs M. Neuroendoscopic third ventriculostomy in patients less than 1 year old. Pediatr Neurosurg 1998;29(2):73–76

67. Kaufman B, Weiss MH, Young HF, Nulsen FE. Effects of prolonged cerebrospinal fluid shunting on the skull and brain. J Neurosurg 1973;38(3):288–297

68. Linder M, Diehl JT, Sklar FH. Significance of postshunt ventricular asymmetries. J Neurosurg 1981;55(2):183–186

69. Rekate HL, Williams FC Jr, Brodkey JA, McCormick JM, Chizeck HJ, Ko W. Resistance of the foramen of Monro. Pediatr Neurosci 1988;14(2):85–89

70. Khorasani L, Sikorski CW, Frim DM. Lumbar CSF shunting preferentially drains the cerebral subarachnoid over the ventricular spaces: implications for the treatment of slit ventricle syndrome. Pediatr Neurosurg 2004;40(6):270–276

71. Rekate HL. The slit ventricle syndrome: advances based on technology and understanding. Pediatr Neurosurg 2004;40(6):259–263

72. Colás R, Muñoz P, Temprano R, Gómez C, Pascual J. Chronic daily headache with analgesic overuse: epidemiology and impact on quality of life. Neurology 2004;62(8):1338–1342

73. Cupini LM, Calabresi P. Medication-overuse headache: pathophysiological insights. J Headache Pain 2005;6(4):199–202

74. Dowson AJ, Dodick DW, Limmroth V. Medication overuse headache in patients with primary headache disorders: epidemiology, management and pathogenesis. CNS Drugs 2005;19(6):483–497

75. Chumas PD, Armstrong DC, Drake JM, et al. Tonsillar herniation: the rule rather than the exception after lumboperitoneal shunting in the pediatric population. J Neurosurg 1993;78(4):568–573

76. Chumas PD, Kulkarni AV, Drake JM, Hoffman HJ, Humphreys RP, Rutka JT. Lumboperitoneal shunting: a retrospective study in the pediatric population. Neurosurgery 1993;32(3):376–383, discussion 383

77. Pierre-Kahn A, Hirsch JF, Renier D, Metzger J, Maroteaux P. Hydrocephalus and achondroplasia: a study of 25 observations. Childs Brain 1980;7(4):205–219

78. Sainte-Rose C, LaCombe J, Pierre-Kahn A, Renier D, Hirsch JF. Intracranial venous sinus hypertension: cause or consequence of hydrocephalus in infants? J Neurosurg 1984;60(4):727–736

79. Steinbok P, Hall J, Flodmark O. Hydrocephalus in achondroplasia: the possible role of intracranial venous hypertension. J Neurosurg 1989;71(1):42–48

80. Siomin V, Cinalli G, Grotenhuis A, et al. Endoscopic third ventriculostomy in patients with cerebrospinal fluid infection and/or hemorrhage. J Neurosurg 2002;97(3):519–524

81. Johnston IH, Sheridan MM. CSF shunting from the cisterna magna: a report of 16 cases. Br J Neurosurg 1993;7(1):39–43

82. Nadkarni TD, Rekate HL. Treatment of refractory intracranial hypertension in a spina bifida patient by a concurrent ventricular and cisterna magna-to-peritoneal shunt. Childs Nerv Syst 2005;21(7):579–582

83. Rekate HL, Nadkarni T, Wallace D. Severe intracranial hypertension in slit ventricle syndrome managed using a cisterna magna-ventricle-peritoneum shunt. J Neurosurg 2006;104(4, Suppl):240–244

6 Craniopharyngioma

♦ Radical Resection

Jeffrey H. Wisoff and Robert E. Elliott

Craniopharyngiomas comprise roughly 3% of all intracranial neoplasms[1,2] and are the most common nonglial brain tumor of childhood, constituting 6 to 8% of all pediatric brain tumors.[3–5] On a population scale, however, they are relatively rare lesions, with an incidence of only 0.13 per 100,000 person years.[6] Fewer than 350 combined adult and pediatric craniopharyngiomas are diagnosed each year in the United States, and less than half of these occur in children.[6,7] Thought to arise from embryological remnants of the craniopharyngeal duct, these benign epithelial neoplasms with solid, cystic, and calcified components can arise anywhere along an axis from the third ventricle to the pituitary gland.[8–12]

The benign histology of craniopharyngiomas, however, belies their rather malignant clinical course in children. Described by Harvey Cushing as "one of the most baffling problems to the neurosurgeon,"[13] their close proximity to the visual apparatus, circle of Willis, pituitary stalk, and hypothalamus predisposes these patients to severe adverse sequelae both at presentation and following treatment. Common findings include headache, vision loss, diabetes insipidus, panhypopituitarism, short stature, hypothalamic dysfunction with behavioral and memory disturbances, hyperphagia, and obesity.

Treatment Philosophy

Debate persists regarding the optimal management of craniopharyngiomas. Regardless of selected management strategy, however, definitive tumor control or cure should be the goal of any treatment for pediatric craniopharyngiomas. Two critical factors for potential cure are extent of surgical excision and cranial irradiation. Some centers advocate radical resection for surgical cure, whereas others favor limited resection followed by radiation therapy to limit injury to the hypothalamus. Both major paradigms provide similar rates of disease control and overall survival.[14–30] Although radical resection may have a higher potential for immediate perioperative morbidity,[14,20,31–36] limited resection and radiation therapy cause more delayed morbidity, including panhypopituitarism, visual deterioration, cognitive and attentional dysfunction, secondary central nervous system neoplasms, and cerebrovasculopathy, namely moyamoya disease.[22,37–45] Palliative procedures, such as stereotactic cyst aspiration and Ommaya reservoir drainage, may provide relief from compression of neural and visual structures, but these effects are invariably transient. Progressive solid and cystic tumor recurrence and growth are inevitable. We believe such therapies should not be considered definitive or adequate treatment early in the course of disease.

The relative scarcity of craniopharyngiomas, the persistent lack of consensus regarding optimal treatment, and the potential morbidity of all forms of treatment combine to make evaluations of the optimal management strategy difficult, if not impossible. Given similar rates of disease control and survival with the two main treatment strategies, the focus of outcome assessment has shifted to quality of life metrics.[22,34,46–50] However, detailed quality of life outcomes from large series of uniformly treated patients are scarce. Here, we describe our preferred treatment paradigm for craniopharyngiomas in children—radical resection with the aim of surgical cure.

Preoperative Evaluation

Depending on the clinical status and age of the patient prior to surgery, we prefer a complete evaluation by various specialists that includes opthalmologic, endocrinologic, and neuropsychological testing. Parents and families are counseled as to the expected short- and long-term postoperative course.

Our preoperative imaging protocol consists of magnetic resonance imaging (MRI) with frameless stereotactic image acquisition and computed tomography (CT). CT provides detailed information about the extent and location of tumoral calcification. Careful evaluation of multiplanar MRI is essential to understand the often complex relationship that craniopharyngiomas have to the visual apparatus, hypothalamus, and surrounding vasculature and will lead to improved outcomes.

First, the location of the tumor in relation to the optic apparatus must be determined. Tumors can be entirely subchiasmatic primarily within the sella, prechiasmatic with or without subfrontal extension, retrochiasmatic involving the floor of the third ventricle and hypothalamus, or have a complex relationship to the chiasm with both pre- and retrochiasmatic components. Second, attention must be paid to the relationship of the dorsal aspect of the tumor and the hypothalamus. Increased involvement and deformation of the hypothalamus have been shown to predict the level of preoperative hypothalamic dysfunction, as well as the operative morbidity of resection. Third, as craniopharyngiomas enlarge, they can form multilobulated cysts that extend along the pathways of least resistance and invade nearby anatomical spaces in the anterior, middle, and posterior fossae. These extensions must be recognized to optimize the surgical approach and minimize retraction injury to normal brain parenchyma.

Surgical Approaches

Given the variability of the precise location and size of craniopharyngiomas, a variety of approaches have been described by different surgeons. These include the subfrontal,[3,5,51–54] pterional,[14,17,36,55,56] combined,[15,28,30,32,34] bifrontal interhemispheric,[57,58] transcallosal,[59] subtemporal,[60] transpetrosal,[61] and transsphenoidal approaches.[62–65]

We prefer a modified pterional exposure that includes removal of the supraorbital rim, anterior orbital roof, and zygomatic process of the frontal bone. This approach provides the shortest, most direct route to the suprasellar region. It minimizes frontal and temporal lobe retraction with wide splitting of the sylvian fissure, allows early release of cerebrospinal fluid (CSF) from the sylvian and carotid cisterns to aid in brain relaxation, and provides early visualization of the carotid arteries and optic apparatus. Tumors extending from the pontomedullary junction to above the foramen of Monro can be successfully and safely removed using this approach without the need for corticectomy, sacrifice of the olfactory nerve, or potential cognitive dysfunction from retraction of both frontal lobes.

Surgical adjuncts include the Cavitron Ultrasonic Surgical Aspirator (CUSA; Tyco Healthcare, Mansfield, Massachusetts), frameless stereotaxy, and rigid and flexible endoscopes and should be used when appropriate. Recently, we have found that endoscopic visualization during dissection of tumor from the ventral surface of the chiasm and floor of the third ventricle greatly enhances the safety of

tumor removal in this critical region and allows complete removal of small fragments of tumor and/or calcium deposits that may or may not contain viable tumor cells. The endoscope is also useful for intraventricular visualization and potential resection of tumor that lies within the third or lateral ventricles not accessible via the transsylvian approach. We reserve the transsphenoidal approach for tumors that are primarily or completely within the sella turcica.

Operative Technique

Following induction and intubation, patient positioning, and stereotaxy registration, dexamethasone (0.1 mg/kg), phenytoin (15 mg/kg), and cephalexin (25 mg/kg) are administered. Mannitol (0.25 g/kg) is than given at the time of skin incision to aid in brain relaxation. The diuretic effect is maximal within 1 hour of infusion and will ideally have its maximal effect at the time of brain and tumor manipulation. Hyperventilation and progressive drainage of CSF from the sylvian and basal cisterns will usually provide excellent brain relaxation, even in the presence of hydrocephalus. Ventricular drainage is reserved for cases refractory to these maneuvers or in cases of severe, increased intracranial pressure unresponsive to medical management. However, if severe hydrocephalus is present or if there is a significant solid tumor component superiorly within the third ventricle, a 4 mm endoscope is placed into the lateral ventricle and held in place with a rigid retractor. This maneuver allows for alternation of visualization and dissection of tumor from the endoscopic, intraventricular, or microscopic transsylvian routes.

A Z-plasty skin incision posterior to the hairline is performed from the tragus to just beyond the midline. The temporalis fascia and muscle are sharply incised with a no. 15 blade and bluntly dissected off the underlying calvarium with a periosteal elevator to allow for excellent reapproximation at the end of the case and minimize temporalis muscle atrophy. A one-piece, modified pterional craniotomy with removal of the anterior orbital roof, supraorbital rim, and zygomatic process of the frontal bone is then performed with the craniotome and chisel and mallet. A brain retractor is used to prevent injury to the orbital contents or lacerate the periorbita during the orbital and supraorbital osteotomies. The dura is dissected from the sphenoid bone, which is removed with rongeurs down to the supraorbital fissure.

The dura is then elevated with a dural hook and incised in a C-shaped fashion. Especially for large tumors that distort the anatomy of or extend beyond the suprasellar cisterns, identification of the vascular anatomy provides critical internal landmarks for safe navigation. Laterally, the sylvian fissure is widely split, and the branches of the middle cerebral artery are identified. The arachnoidal dissection of

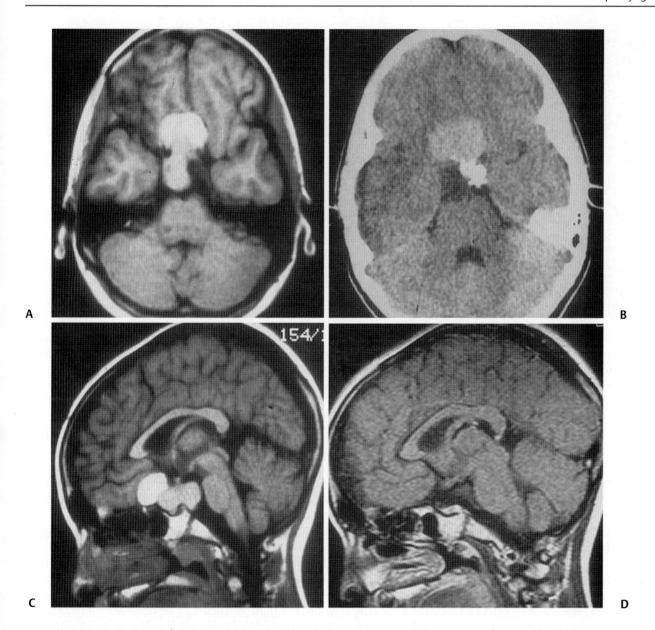

Fig. 6.1 This 9-year-old girl presented with severe, progressive headache. On examination, the child was found to have a partial left cranial nerve III palsy and 20/40 visual acuity on the left. **(A,C)** Following administration of gadolinium, magnetic resonance imaging (MRI) revealed a 4 cm, mixed cystic and solid tumor with a postfixed chiasm. **(B)** Solid calcification in the left suprasellar region was demonstrated on computed tomography (CT). **(D)** Via right pterional craniotomy, she underwent gross total resection (GTR) of the adamantinomatous craniopharyngioma with transient worsening but eventual improvement in her CN III palsy. Her visual acuity improved to 20/25 following surgery. Despite stalk preservation, she developed diabetes insipidus (DI) and requires DDAVP. She is now 18 years following GTR, has been without disease recurrence and completed graduate school after college.

the fissure proceeds medially to bifurcation of the internal cerebral artery. Once the carotid artery comes into view, careful inspection of the anterior cerebral artery, optic nerve, chiasm, and/or tracts is performed to understand the relationship of these structures to the tumor (**Figs. 6.1** and **6.2**).

We caution against early decompression of the cystic portion of the tumor, as this can result in redundancy of the tumor capsule and the overlying attenuated arachnoid. This loss of turgor can obscure the planes of dissection. The overarching strategy for craniopharyngioma resection is to develop an arachnoid plane circumferentially around the tumor within the suprasellar cisterns followed by stalk inspection and possible sectioning. The last and most critical step is manipulation and excision of the dorsal portion of the tumor involving the hypothalamus.

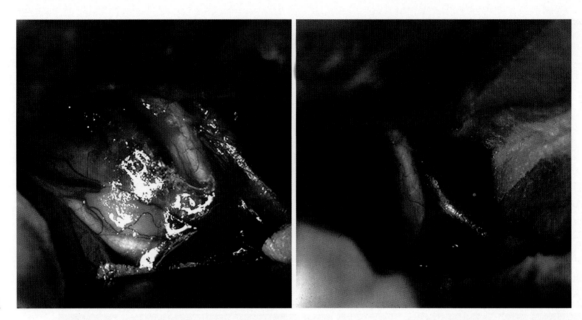

A

B

Fig. 6.2 (**A**) Intraoperative photograph following splitting of the right sylvian fissure confirming the prechiasmatic nature of the craniopharyngioma seen in **Fig. 6.1A.** The left optic nerve is elevated by tumor, rotated into view, and exhibits pallor. (**B**) Following GTR of the tumor, the optic nerves are decompressed, and vasospasm is evident in the right internal carotid artery and the A1 segment of the anterior cerebral artery.

Working in the opticocarotid, prechiasmatic, and carotidotentorial triangles, an arachnoidal plane is developed between the tumor capsule and the arteries of the circle of Willis. Careful attention must be paid to ensure the preservation of the basal perforators. This plane is developed in a posterior direction until the basilar artery is identified through the usually intact membrane of Lilliquist. This extracapsular dissection is usually facilitated by well-demarcated and preserved arachnoidal planes. In the case of recurrent tumors, these planes can be heavily scarred and may require increased use of sharp microdissection.

Following separation of the cerebral vasculature from the tumor capsule, the cyst can now be aspirated and solid components debulked. All attempts should be made to preserve the capsule of the tumor to allow gentle traction for eventual dissection of the tumor from its remaining attachments, especially the floor of the hypothalamus. Continuing to respect arachnoidal planes, the tumor is then dissected free of the optic chiasm, the contralateral carotid arteries, and its branches. Although an attempt is always made to identify and preserve the pituitary stalk, we have found this successful in only 30% of patients. We recommend sectioning the stalk as distal as possible without compromising negative margins to limit the severity of diabetes insipidus. Following separation of tumor from the entire circle of Willis, pituitary stalk, and optic apparatus, the capsule is grasped, and using a combination of gentle traction and blunt dissection, a gliotic plane is developed between the dorsal aspect of the tumor and the floor of the third ventricle and hypothalamus in the region of the tuber cinereum. Following tumor removal, the entire tumor bed must be inspected for residual disease with either a micromirror or an angled endoscope. Papaverine-soaked Gelfoam pledgets are then placed around the arteries of the circle of Willis to help ameliorate vasospasm (**Fig. 6.2**) and are removed prior to dural closure.

If the tumor has a significant retrochiasmatic or intraventricular component, the lamina terminalis must be fenestrated (**Fig. 6.3**). The lamina terminalis is distinguished from the chiasm by its pale, avascular appearance and is often distended and attenuated by the underlying tumor. Tumor within the third ventricle can be delivered simultaneously through the lamina terminalis, as well as from below the chiasm. We find the use of a 4 mm endoscope inserted into the third or lateral ventricle to be extremely helpful to assist in the delivery of the intraventricular component of the tumor, obviating the need for a transcallosal approach to achieve complete resection. For tumors with significant extension into the sella turcica, removal of the tuberculum sellae and posterior planum sphenoidale may be necessary to gain adequate exposure of the intrasellar space. Following tumor removal, all bony defects into the sinuses must be repaired to prevent postoperative CSF fistulas.

Postoperative Care

Following surgery and neurologic examination, all children are transferred immediately to the pediatric intensive care unit. A multidisciplinary team of pediatric endocrinologists,

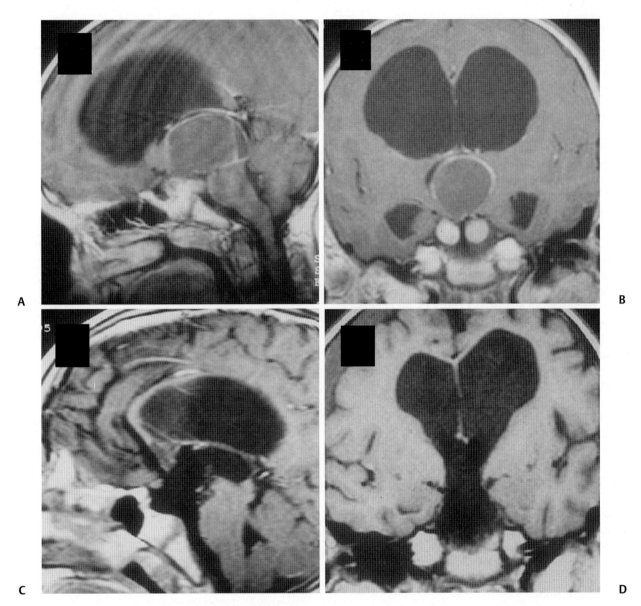

Fig. 6.3 (A,B) This 7-year-old boy presented with headache and behavioral outbursts. MRI revealed a 5 cm retrochiasmatic tumor with significant extension into the third ventricle, causing obstructive hydrocephalus. **(C,D)** Following GTR of his adamantinomatous craniopharyngioma via a right pterional approach and fenestration of the lamina terminalis, he remained neurologically, visually, and hormonally intact, and his hydrocephalus resolved following tumor removal. He did, however, experience slight worsening of his short-term memory but was able to do well in school and currently attends college. He remains disease-free 14 years following resection.

neuro-oncologists, and intensivists collaborate in the postoperative care. Frequent urine and electrolyte analyses are performed to monitor for and aggressively treat electrolyte disturbances, namely diabetes insipidus. Dexamethasone is tapered over the course of 1 week, and Dilantin is continued for 3 weeks following surgery. Dilantin is continued for extended periods only if seizures occur that are not attributable to electrolyte disturbances.

Postoperative MRI and CT are performed within 48 hours following surgery to ensure complete resection. Surveillance MRI and clinical follow-up occur every 3 months during the first year, every 4 months during the second year, every 6 months for the next 3 years, and every year for the next 5 years. Frequent imaging allows for early detection of recurrence while tumors are small and preferably asymptomatic. However, long-term imaging and follow-up are important, as late recurrences have been reported. Regular evaluations by dedicated pediatric endocrinologists, ophthalmologists, and neuro-oncologists are essential in managing these children long term.

Outcomes and Complications

In the MRI era, radiographically confirmed complete resection is possible in 80 to 100% of patients. Perioperative mortality following aggressive surgery has also declined substantially over the past 2 decades secondary to advances in neuroimaging and microsurgical techniques from over 10% down to 0 to 4% in most current series.[3,14–17,20,21,23,30,31,34,36,53,55,56,66–72] Multiple authors have reported surgeon experience with craniopharyngiomas has a significant impact on the likelihood of achieving complete resection and good functional outcomes.[26,34] Surgeons performing more than two operations per year for radical resection had good outcomes in 87% of children compared with only 52% in those performing fewer.[26]

Numerous centers have reported excellent rates of disease control and functional outcomes with the strategy of radical resection. In a large series by Zucarro,[30] complete resection was achieved in 69% of 153 children. All children who underwent complete resection were in school and no more than 1 year behind in grade level, in contrast to only 62% of children who had limited resection and radiation. Di Rocco et al[16] reported complete resection in 78% of 54 children treated with curative surgical intent. Overall improvement in intelligence quotient (IQ) occurred following resection in their series with a mean postoperative IQ of 112 (range 95–130). All but 2 of 50 surviving patients enjoy normal social interactions. In a series by Hoffman et al,[53] 26 of 27 children who underwent aggressive resection had IQ scores at or above average levels. Although 16 children had memory deficits, 14 of them attended regular schools. The authors contended that "memory impairment did not interfere with school progress if intelligence was adequate." Yasargil et al[36] reported good outcomes in 72.5% of children after initial surgery, and Fahlbusch et al[55] reported functional independence in 78% of adult and pediatric patients following radical resection.

In our series of 86 children who underwent radical resection of craniopharyngiomas, gross total resection (GTR) was accomplished in all 57 (100%) of primary tumors and in 18 of 29 (62%) of recurrent tumors with acceptably low morbidity (**Table 6.1**). In contrast to the findings of other centers of increased morbidity, mortality, and worse functional outcomes at reoperation,[14,20,21,23,30,55,73–77] we found no such differences in our series. Good and excellent functional outcomes were achieved in 80% of children, and over 60% of college-aged patients either attended or graduated from college—a clear indication of the high functionality of the majority of these children. New hypothalamic morbidity occurred in 25% of children and was mild or moderate in all but one case. Fewer than 20% of our patients developed obesity, and only two patients developed severe or morbid obesity. These results contrast greatly with those from a German multicenter study that reported severe obesity in

Table 6.1 Morbidity and Mortality in 86 Children after Radical Resection of Craniopharyngioma

	No. of Patients (%)	
	Primary	Recurrent
Perioperative mortality	2 (3.5%)	1 (3.4%)
Neurologic morbidity		
Stroke	2 (4.0%)	2 (9.0%)
Mild hemiparesis	1 (2.0%)	0 (0%)
Transient CN palsy	8 (16.0%)	1 (4.0%)
Permanent CN palsy	1 (2.0%)	1 (4.0%)
Lethargy/abulia	2 (4.0%)	1 (4.0%)
Visual acuity		
Preoperative deficit	14 (27.0%)	15 (60.0%)
Improved	10 (19.0%)	3 (12.0%)
Stable	35 (67.0%)	17 (68.0%)
Worse	7 (13.0%)	5 (20.0%)
Visual fields		
Preoperative deficit	23 (43.0%)	22 (85.0%)
Improved	13 (25.5%)	7 (27.0%)
Stable	25 (49.0%)	12 (46.0%)
Worse	13 (25.5%)	7 (27.0%)
Diabetes insipidus		
Preoperative	6 (12.0%)	19 (73.0%)
Postoperative, new	33 (73.0%)	6 (67.0%)
Postoperative, total	39 (78.0%)	25 (89.0%)
Anterior pituitary dysfunction		
Mean number hormones required ± SD	2.5 ± 1.1	2.1 ± 0.9

Note: There were no significant differences in operative mortality, neurologic, visual, or endocrinologic morbidity rates between patients with primary and recurrent tumors ($p > .05$).

CN, central nerve; SD, standard deviation.

44% of 185 children treated for craniopharyngiomas using various treatment modalities.[48] Although some centers contend that increasing tumor size limits the extent of resection and local disease control,[29,31,55,78–84] we agree with other authors[30,51,56,85] that size has no impact on the ability to achieve GTR—at least for virgin tumors. Nevertheless, given the large size and multicompartmental nature of giant craniopharyngiomas, a flexible and at times staged approach may be required for successful and safe extirpation of these tumors (**Fig. 6.4**).

Although our data did corroborate prior studies reporting worse overall survival rates for children with recurrent tumors,[25,29,36,55,73,86] subgroup analysis revealed excellent survival rates for children with nonirradiated recurrent tumors and those of smaller size at reoperation. Thus, prior

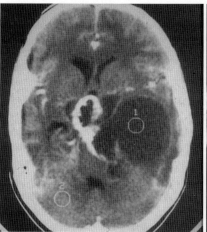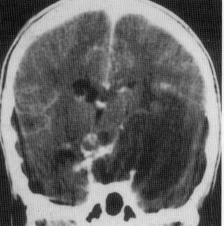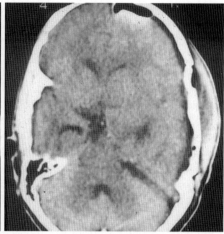

C

Fig. 6.4 (A,B) This 12-year-old boy who presented with headache was found on CT to have a giant, mixed cystic and solid tumor with extensive calcification in the suprasellar region and cystic extension into the left middle fossa. **(C)** Following GTR of this adamantinomatous craniopharyngioma, he experienced a stroke that left him with a mild right hemiparesis that improved over time. He did not suffer diabetes insipidus but was left with a new right superior quadrantanopia, likely from retraction of the left side of the optic chiasm during tumor removal. He experienced a 2 cm recurrence that was also treated with GTR 5 months following initial surgery. He received passing grades at appropriate level in school, required no adjuvant therapy, and has been disease-free for 23 months following his last surgery.

failed radiation therapy and large size at recurrence significantly limited our ability to achieve complete resection—the only remaining option for potential cure for these patients—and resulted in worse overall survival rates. In contrast, prior radical resection, per se, did not diminish the chance of achieving complete resection at reoperation, leading to improved disease control and survival rates. Fourteen children experienced a total of 15 recurrences following GTR at our hospital. All underwent reoperation at the time of recurrence except one child, who had radiosurgery, given the presence of fusiform dilatation of the internal carotid artery. GTR was achieved in 79% with no surgical morbidity or mortality. One patient had slight deterioration in vision, but no child experienced hypothalamic or memory dysfunction. Overall survival for this cohort was 92% at mean follow-up of 8 years, markedly higher than the rate of survival of recurrent tumors reported in the literature.

Recurrence is one of the most common complications of craniopharyngiomas and usually occurs within the first 3 to 4 years following treatment.[12,15,17,21,30,32,33,35,36,53,55,56,68,72,77,87] In modern series, it occurs in roughly 20% of cases following imaging-confirmed complete resection and in 20 to 30% of cases following radiation therapy.[3,12,14,15,17,20,21,23,30–36,53, 55,56,66,72,75,76,87] These facts must be considered when assessing the efficacy and safety of any treatment algorithm. Thus, in addition to the commonly reported morbidity, one must consider the potentially deleterious effects of early irradiation on the safety and efficacy of subsequent treatments, which prove necessary in up to one third of children. In experienced hands, radical resection alone may afford a greater chance of upfront disease control and potential cure compared with planned limited resection plus radiation and provide more effective and safer treatment options should recurrence arise.

Craniopharyngiomas in Very Young Children

The aforementioned risks of radiation therapy are even more common and potentially detrimental in very young children (ages 5 and under).[22,42] Multiple centers have reported worse functional outcomes, higher rates of tumor recurrence, and decreased overall survival rates in younger children.[17,22,24,30,31,68,75,88–90] Importantly, one of the main treatment modalities following subtotal resection (STR) or recurrence—radiation therapy—is usually withheld in very young patients given the age-dependent cognitive morbidity, risk of secondary malignancy, visual deterioration, hypothalamic-pituitary-axis dysfunction, and cerebrovasculopathy, namely, moyamoya disease.[22,37–45] In accordance with other centers, we strongly advocate radical resection as the optimal treatment in very young children with craniopharyngiomas.[26,75,77,90]

A retrospective review of our entire series of 86 children revealed 19 children who were age 5 or younger at the time of surgery. GTR was achieved in all but one child, who had undergone numerous prior resections, radiation therapy, and cyst aspirations prior to referral to the senior author for salvage therapy. All remaining (18) patients (95%) were alive at a mean follow-up of 9.4 years. Six patients experienced a total of seven recurrences. Six of these were successfully cured with repeat resection, and the final child had radiosurgery, given the presence of a fusiform dilatation of the internal carotid artery. Four patients had transient cranial nerve palsies, but no permanent neurologic deficits occurred. New cases of diabetes insipidus occurred in 50% of these children, and only one child (6%) experienced visual deterioration. Mean body mass index (BMI) following resection was +1.4 standard deviations and within normal limits. New hypothalamic morbidity occurred in two children (short-term memory impairment and obesity, respectively), and two patients had worsening of their severe hypothalamic disturbance that was present preoperatively. Only 1 of 15 (6.7%) children with normal BMI prior to surgery experienced obesity, and a single patient experienced cognitive deterioration after radical resection. We found no differences in the rates of recurrence, recurrence-free, or overall survival between children ages 5 and younger and those who were older at the time of surgery. No child required conventional fractionated radiotherapy.

Given the increased risk of radiation therapy in young children, we agree with other centers[26,75,77,90] and strongly advocate radical resection as the optimal treatment in very young children with craniopharyngiomas. As our results demonstrate, in experienced hands, excellent oncological and functional outcomes can be obtained in this population with minimal morbidity—sparing this vulnerable population the inherent risks of cranial irradiation.

Conclusion

We continue to believe that children with craniopharyngiomas should be treated with curative intent at presentation, whether via radical surgery or limited surgery plus irradiation. In accordance with other authors,[14,30,32,74,77,91] however, we believe that in experienced hands radical resection of pediatric craniopharyngioma at both presentation and recurrence offers the best chance of a durable disease control and potential cure. Given that most recurrences happen in the first few years following resection and lower morbidity of reoperation on smaller tumors,[91] frequent surveillance imaging in the early postoperative period is necessary to identify recurrence early and immediately treat the tumor while small in size. Late recurrences, however, do occur and require continued long-term follow-up and imaging.

Nevertheless, the conclusions drawn from our experience may not be generalizable to all practices and patients. The success and safety of radical resection depend on surgical expertise,[26,34] postoperative endocrinologic support, and the familial and societal resources to cope with postoperative care and endocrine and hypothalamic deficits.[92] Educational assistance or tutoring may be required to maintain schooling at appropriate grade level. If family structure and socioeconomic conditions of an individual patient do not provide appropriate support for this chronic disease, the potential morbidity of radical resection may overshadow the merits of curative resection.[93]

♦ Subtotal Resection with Adjuvant Therapy

Frederick A. Boop, David A. Yam, and Thomas E. Merchant

History and Background

Early pioneers in neurologic surgery recognized that tumors in the suprasellar region were challenging to manage. Surgical outcomes were quite poor, and some experts concluded that the region was not to be disturbed by the surgeon.[94] Numerous attempts at both cranial and transsphenoidal approaches continued with occasional success, but for the most part, the results were generally unsatisfying. To make matters worse, these exceptionally rare tumors make up only ~0.8% of all brain tumors, which made experienced surgeons somewhat of a rarity. This problem persists today. Even in the most talented hands, surgical morbidity and mortality rates remain high.[95]

The introduction of corticosteroid therapy in the 1950s revolutionized postoperative management. This was followed by the introduction of desmopressin (trade name DDAVP), which allowed a means to control postoperative diabetes insipidus for the first time. The introduction of the operating microscope and better microsurgical instrumentation to neurosurgery in the 1970s was a milestone that markedly improved survival rates. Because craniopharyngiomas are benign tumors, it was once held that the primary goal of treatment should be a surgical cure by radical resection.[96,97] The use of adjuvant therapy such as radiation treatment or chemotherapy was eschewed and only offered to patients with recurrent disease or those too sick for a surgical procedure. After decades of reviewing the results of attempted GTR, several neurosurgeons expressed concerns about quality of life and mortality after radical resection. Thus began a small but growing trend of performing subtotal resection to decompress the optic apparatus and the hypothalamus followed by adjuvant radiotherapy. After over a century of improvements in radiographic imaging, pre- and postoperative care, microsurgical techniques, and the addition of adjuvant therapy, the controversies surrounding this rare disease still remain.

Clinical Case 1

A 7-year-old boy presented to his primary care physician offering a 19-week history of nausea, vomiting, and headache. He then developed facial drooping, which prompted evaluation in a local emergency department, where he was found to have a tumor and associated hydrocephalus. His review of systems was positive for decreased visual acuity without a recent change in vision and was negative for symptoms of neuroendocrine dysfunction. His physical exam was remarkable for anisocoria with a dilated but reactive left pupil, decreased acuity on the left eye of 20/200, and a field cut in the left eye. A mild facial droop was present on the left. His exam was otherwise unremarkable. Laboratory studies revealed normal cortisol, prolactin, testosterone, thyroid-stimulating hormone (TSH), free T4 (thyroxine), and antidiuretic hormone but decreased luteinizing hormone, follicle-stimulating hormone, and growth hormone (GH). His radiographic images are included (**Figs. 6.5** and **6.6**).

Diagnosis and Treatment Considerations

When a child such as this presents with a suspected craniopharyngioma, the neurosurgeon has two major obligations: to obtain a confirmed pathologic diagnosis and to initiate comprehensive treatment. Although radiographic imaging

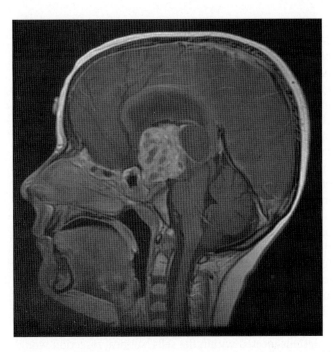

Fig. 6.5 Sagittal MRI T1-weighted image with contrast of a 7-year-old boy showing a large sellar and suprasellar mass with cystic regions and radiographic findings consistent with a craniopharyngioma.

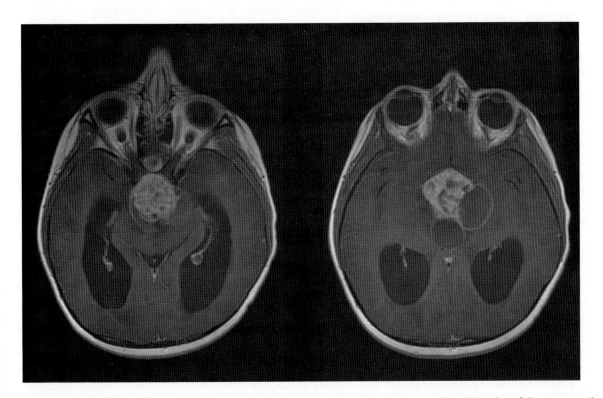

Fig. 6.6 Axial MRI T1-weighted images with contrast of the same 7-year-old boy showing the relationship of the tumor to the hypothalamus, the brainstem, and the ventricles.

has dramatically improved over the last few decades, a wide variety of lesions can occur in this region, including craniopharyngioma, pituitary adenoma, epidermoid tumors, optic pathway gliomas, meningiomas, colloid cysts, arachnoid cysts, and inflammatory lesions. For these reasons, biopsy of the mass is almost always indicated except in the most classic cases as confirmed by clinical presentation and radiographic imaging. If the child's tumor is discovered incidentally, stereotactic biopsy may be the quickest and least invasive method. If, however, there is concern regarding mass effect and neurologic change, open biopsy and resection may be indicated.

For each patient, the treatment should be individualized based on several factors. These include patient characteristics, tumor location, size, preoperative comorbidities, visual function, the presence of hydrocephalus, and hypothalamic/pituitary-axis integrity. Each and every issue must be addressed to the fullest extent possible, and the side effects of available treatments must be considered. For tumors with little to no involvement of the anterior hypothalamus such as lesions located within the sella, surgical resection would seem to be a reasonable approach if the surgeon and patient are willing to accept the risk of diabetes insipidus.[98–100] The more commonly encountered, more extensive tumors with hypothalamic involvement such as the case presented here, however, clearly represent a challenge for the surgeon. Although GTR of large tumors involving the hypothalamus has been performed with success, such success often comes at a high price, leading many to favor an equally effective use of limited surgery and adjuvant radiotherapy.

Radical Resection

Although craniopharyngiomas are histologically benign tumors, the risk of critical adjacent structures being damaged by either the tumor or the proposed treatment remains significant. The surgeon has two main options in the treatment of these tumors: either attempted total resection or subtotal resection supplemented by other therapies to keep the residual tumor from growing. The goal of the radical resection approach is to obtain a surgical cure of this benign disease, thus sparing the patient the risk of radiotherapy. Radical resection can be an effective treatment with excellent rates of long-term progression-free survival.[101] For the experienced craniopharyngioma surgeon, published risks may be acceptable; however, for the average neurosurgeon who has seen only a handful of these tumors in his or her professional lifetime, those statistics do not translate. For tumors involving the hypothalamus, surgical resection has met with severe cost to the patient with a wide range of neuroendocrine and cognitive dysfunction.[101,102] From the early days of craniopharyngioma surgery to the present, GTR even in highly experienced hands was achievable in only ~45 to 75% of cases.[103–105] As such, a

fairly large number of patients with residual disease go on to receive observation, additional surgery, and/or delayed salvage radiotherapy. Recurrence after reported GTR alone without radiotherapy is undeniably common and occurs in up to 53% of cases.[106,107] Death in patients who undergo attempted radical resection of craniopharyngioma is not uncommon, with a 4 to 9% mortality rate reported in the American Society of Pediatric Neurosurgeons' survey and higher rates in some series.[95,100] Morbidity following attempted GTR is an equally significant problem. Of patients with attempted radical resection, up to 96% have a wide range of permanent endocrinopathies related to the operative intervention[106] (**Table 6.2**).[98,102,106,108,109] Epilepsy is more frequent in patients managed by attempted radical resection, occurring in up to 40% of patients. Epilepsy is virtually nonexistent in those patients receiving limited surgery followed by adjuvant radiotherapy.[98] In addition, hypothalamic injury sufficient to alter the quality of life is reported in up to 86% of patients undergoing radical resection.[106,110,111] Considering these issues regarding mortality, morbidity, residual disease, frequency of recurrence, and quality of life, it is the authors' opinion that radical resection should be limited to small tumors that do not involve the hypothalamus. Furthermore, given the high recurrence rates in patients with proven GTRs, it behooves us that these patients be followed indefinitely.

Subtotal Resection and Adjuvant Therapy

In contrast to radical resection, the use of subtotal resection and adjuvant radiotherapy aims at maintaining the child's quality of life by surgically addressing mass effect, tumor volume, and hydrocephalus while halting tumor progression with radiotherapy or other modalities. This approach has been labeled palliative by advocates of radical resection; however, it is clear that this treatment does have proven long-term efficacy at the control of tumor progression equal to that of radical resection.[112] It is also a treatment strategy that is not as dependent upon the skill or experience of the neurosurgeon. Thus, limited surgery followed by focused radiotherapy is a treatment that can be widely applied, whereas radical resection, if it is to be done, should only be done in regional referral centers and by experienced microneurosurgeons with a proven track record. In terms of operative and perioperative mortality, several series have reported patients managed with subtotal resection and adjuvant therapy with no reported deaths.[98,113,114] Visual acuity is preserved or improved in the majority of patients using this treatment regimen.[98] In the GTR group, the vast majority of patients suffer from neuroendocrine disorders, whereas patients in the limited surgery and adjuvant treatment group have less early and lower overall neuroendocrinologic dysfunction. This is especially true in regards to cortisol function and diabetes insipidus (**Table 6.2**). Most

Table 6.2 Long-Term Endocrine Deficiencies Following Surgery or Limited Surgery with Radiation Therapy

Source	Modality (n)	Thyroid	Adrenal	GH	Gn	DI
Tomita (2005)[72]						
	Radical resection (n = 54)	50 (93%)	50 (93%)	50 (93%)	50 (93%)	47 (87%)
Poretti (2004)[89]						
	Radical resection (n = 25)	21 (84%)	19 (76%)	20 (80%)	21 (84%)	23/25 (92%)
Merchant (2002)[23]						
	Surgery (n = 15)	15 (100%)	14 (93%)	14 (93%)	4 (27%)	11 (73%)
	Limited surgery + RT (n = 14/15)	14 (93%)	10 (67%)	14 (93%)	8 (53%)	5 (33%)
Thompson (2005)[90]						
	Radical resection (25)	NA*	NA*	NA*	NA*	24 (96%)
	Subtotal Resection + RT (n = 23)	NA*	NA*	NA*	NA*	11 (47%)
Moon (2005)[109]						
	Limited surgery + RT (n = 25)	-*	-*	-*	-*	10 (38%)

* Data not provided in reference.

Abbreviations: DI, diabetes insipidus; GH, growth hormone; Gn, gonadotropins; RT, radiotherapy.

patients following attempted total resection require replacement of GH, TSH, cortisol, and vasopressin. With limited surgery and radiotherapy, hormone dysfunction will exist; however, the avoidance of diabetes insipidus prevents a major cause of death and morbidity in young children with craniopharyngioma.

Although no prospective randomized data are available, large cohort studies do exist looking at the quality of life of patients managed with limited surgery and adjuvant therapy. In these, combined treatment modalities with limited surgery have been shown to have better quality of life outcomes compared with those patients treated by radical resection.[106,107,109,111,114] In the Boston Children's series, major disability was found in 33% of radical surgery patients as compared with 15% in those treated with limited surgery and radiotherapy.[115,116] In the Royal Marsden series of 173 patients treated with limited surgery and radiotherapy, 52% of patients had no disability and lead active lives.[117] This is compared with studies involving radical resection, with up to 80% of survivors describing major disability and impairment.[101,106] Another cohort of 48 patients treated by either subtotal surgery followed by radiotherapy or radical resection showed that the 62% of patients treated by limited surgery were functional enough to attend normal school versus 37% of those receiving attempted radical resection.[123]

In summary, the use of limited surgery and adjuvant therapy has allowed for improved quality of life with a lower incidence of disability. This has led several regional referral centers to alter their treatment paradigms in favor of limited surgery and adjuvant therapy, including either

radiotherapy or chemotherapy.[118–120] In some centers, the use of intratumoral bleomycin or interferon-α has been advocated in younger children to delay more aggressive treatments, including the delaying of radiotherapy.[118,121]

The use of limited surgery and adjuvant therapy has been proven to prolong survival and control progression of disease. The 10- and 20-year progression-free survival rates reported are 83% and 79%, respectively, in one large series with extended postradiation follow-up.[117] Similar rates of tumor control have been reported at other centers.[98,114,122] Considering the improved quality of life, lower incidence of endocrinopathies, comparable rates of vision control, excellent rates of tumor control, and widespread applicability, subtotal resection with adjuvant radiotherapy clearly offers most neurosurgeons and patients a distinct advantage over radical resection.

When using radiation, there are known early and delayed risks that must be considered. Proponents of radical resection are quick to point these out. Earlier studies using conventional opposing beam fields exposed a significant normal brain volume to radiation and its side effects. Improvements in conformal and stereotactic radiosurgery have allowed reduction in these side effects with no diminution in rates of disease control.[114] Documented side effects of radiotherapy have included vasculopathy, cerebral infarction, visual loss, brain necrosis, secondary neoplasia, and neurocognitive sequelae. It should be noted that, although these effects do occur in patients undergoing limited surgery and radiation therapy, many of these side effects also occur in patients treated with radical surgery alone. A common argument against the use of radiation therapy in children is the development of neurocognitive sequelae. However, as was noted, patients who had had radical resection experience a greater decline in IQ than those managed with limited surgery and radiation.[98] In addition, the use of three-dimensional conformal radiation has reduced the number of complications and the drop-off in IQ.[114] With continued advancements in conformal radiotherapy and stereotactic radiosurgery, these side effects will likely continue to decrease.

Approach to Case 1

Given the patient's presentation and radiographic findings, this child is likely to have a craniopharyngioma. There is clear hypothalamic involvement, and the cystic regions of the tumor appear to be causing obstruction of CSF flow. The patient's premorbid conditions include endocrinologic dysfunction, although he does not currently have diabetes insipidus or hypocortisolism, loss of vision in the left eye, and hydrocephalus. Given the lack of acute visual change, this patient does not require emergent or urgent decompression of his optic nerves or chiasm. He does need decompression of his ventricles for treatment of his hydrocephalus, from which he is symptomatic. Because two cystic components are present and contributing to his hydrocephalus, the patient could reasonably be taken to surgery for stereotactic-guided insertion of an Ommaya reservoir, which can be used to aspirate the cyst. The cyst fluid should be sent for cytology, and biopsies can be obtained using framed stereotactic or endoscopic guidance. At the time of surgery, a septum pellucidotomy can be performed, and either a ventricular reservoir or shunt may be inserted for the treatment of hydrocephalus. In this case, the ventricular reservoir is particularly useful, as the CSF obstruction may resolve with the initiation of steroid therapy and adjuvant radiation. This may obviate the need for CSF diversion altogether. Within 24 to 48 hours after placement of the cyst Ommaya and the ventricular Ommaya reservoirs, the patient would likely be ready for discharge. A short time later he could begin adjuvant radiotherapy as an outpatient. Additionally, the use of intratumoral agents is feasible through the Ommaya reservoir. The child will need to be followed long term with serial imaging, neurocognitive assessments, endocrine laboratories, and visual field examinations. Should his tumor progress after treatment, surgical resection would still be a good option, given that all of the arachnoid planes are well preserved.

Clinical Case 2

A 14-year-old male patient presented in coma. He had shown deterioration of his school performance and personality change for 3 months prior to this, but his parents were afraid to question him about it because they were afraid he might be taking drugs. On the morning of presentation, they went to his room to awaken him for school but were unable to arouse him. On presentation he was purposeful to pain. He was in bigeminy with bradycardia and an elevated blood pressure. He had absent reflexes. Following an emergent CT scan, he was moved to the intensive care unit, where bifrontal ventricular catheters were placed. After ventricular drainage, the patient awakened and stabilized. An MRI was performed the next day showing a large cystic and solid suprasellar tumor. His cardiac arrhythmia was felt to be secondary to severe hypothyroidism, which was corrected over 3 to 4 days. He was subsequently taken to surgery.

Discussion of Case 2

This patient was managed with GTR alone. His initial postoperative course was unremarkable and uncomplicated aside from diabetes insipidus. He has panhypopituitarism requiring hormone replacement therapy, including vasopressin therapy to manage his diabetes insipidus. His Glasgow Outcome Scale was a 5, and eventually he was able to return to the public school system to attend classes. According to the Karnofsky Performance Scale, he was independent in his activities of daily living and would perform at nearly 100%. By all the usual measures this patient appeared to have an excellent outcome from his tumor resection. However, these measures do not account for the fact that the child had gone from being a straight A to a C student, with both attentional and behavioral problems. They do not account for the 150 lb weight gain over the next 12 months. They do not account for the fact that he had one useful quadrant of vision in each eye. They do not account for the fact that over the next 3 years a carotid artery pseudoaneurysm developed that necessitated arterial reconstruction. Despite postoperative scans showing a GTR, his tumor recurred in the posterior fossa 3 years later, necessitating a petrosal approach for reresection.

General Discussion

Craniopharyngioma was once treated solely with attempts at GTR, often with unsatisfactory outcomes. Because morbidity and mortality rates used to be unacceptably high, improvements in the management of these patients has focused on reducing these rates and not on true quality of life measures. More sensitive quality of life measures have pointed out major problems in patients managed with attempted radical resection alone. These include abulia, learning and memory impairment, hypothalamic obesity, and social dysfunction, which were not measured in earlier studies. Considering these realities, a treatment paradigm has evolved that not only focuses on mortality and survival rates but also stresses the importance of the child's quality of life. Due to the rarity and regional referral patterns surrounding the management of craniopharyngioma, it is unlikely that a prospective randomized trial comparing the two ideologies of treatment could ever be performed. It is likely that there are two subsets of patients with craniopharyngioma: the most common being those with a larger tumor with hypothalamic involvement and the rarer being those with a smaller sellar or suprasellar lesion without hypothalamic involvement. It has been well described that GTR can be performed for patients without hypothalamic involvement; this approach is still widely accepted at many centers, the trade-off being permanent, iatrogenic diabetes inspidus and a higher mortality rate.[95,112] In using this approach, however, it remains critical that these patients be followed closely for years, given the high rates of endocrinopathy and recurrence. In considering the more commonly encountered subset of patients with tumor that involves the hypothalamus, limited surgery and adjuvant therapy have produced equivalent rates of control with a better quality of life and less dependence on hormone replacement therapy.

It should be acknowledged that craniopharyngiomas occur so rarely that no class I evidence as to best management for all scenarios is available; hence, controversy as to optimal management is likely always to exist. We still do not know what the optimal treatment is for the very young child who presents with headaches, normal visual, and normal hormonal functions. We still do not understand the optimal timing of radiation and/or chemotherapeutic agents. We still do not know what the 20-year follow-up result is for a large cohort of patients who have undergone radiotherapy and limited surgery, although we have several patients who are approaching this duration who appear to be functioning well. We still do not know the long-term effect of growth hormone replacement therapy and its potential effect on regrowth of tumor. With many unanswered questions, it is understandable that craniopharyngioma management has remained controversial. Hopefully, future studies will seek to answer existing questions and many other questions that will lead to continued improvements in patient outcomes.

Conclusion

As medical technology advances, the treatment of benign intracranial tumors continues to evolve. The management approaches of cavernous sinus meningiomas and schwannomas are prime examples of how much change is occurring in the field of neurosurgery. The use of three-dimensional conformal and stereotactic radiotherapies has allowed the more precise delivery of radiation while limiting the toxicity to adjacent regions of the brain. Although radiation and chemotherapy have their own associated side effects, these treatments have shown promise in the management of benign disease while maintaining better outcomes than surgical management alone. The combined use of surgery and adjuvant therapy in the management of pediatric craniopharyngioma is a proven strategy that can be applied by neurosurgeons with limited surgical experience with this disease. Perhaps most importantly, this strategy allows for a higher quality of life for children with craniopharyngiomas than in the past when the goal of the surgeon was to resect all of the tumor at all costs. Because of its clear benefits for most patients and the fact that it can be safely instituted in centers with lower clinical volumes, subtotal resection with adjuvant radiation therapy should be considered the best initial treatment for the majority of childhood craniopharyngiomas.

◆ Lessons Learned

The philosophy of treatment of craniopharyngiomas has been a classic controversy in pediatric neurosurgery for two generations. It remains a debate as to what level of surgical aggressivity is appropriate and what degree of neurologic and endocrine morbidity is acceptable. As Dr. Wisoff, a proponent of the "aggressive school," wisely puts it, it is indeed a matter of treatment philosophy rather than the nuts and bolts of scientific evidence. The argument for aggressive surgical resection is best determined by experienced surgeons who serve as referral centers for these rare tumors. This approach which avoids the long term side effects of radiation therapy provides the best opportunity in a potential cure for these locally aggressive tumors. Both groups of authors admit that the role of the experienced surgeon is paramount in achieving a complete resection without a host of functional problems. But beyond the small number of surgeons experienced in resecting this rare tumor, how is experienced to be measured?

Dr. Boop's group strongly point toward the significant morbidity, even considerable mortality, of attempts to remove craniopharyngioma completely. The fact that we even must take mortality seriously into account is uncomfortable. Massive rates (up to 86%) of hypothalamic dysfunction affecting the quality of life lead them to advocate a more conservative philosophy. They argue that an attempt for radical resection should only be made if the hypothalamus is not significantly involved in the tumor growth. Those where the hypothalamus is infiltrated should be treated by debulking surgery alone with the explicit aim to maintain the child's quality of life. Adding radiotherapy to this conservative surgical approach maintains a sufficient tumor control comparable to that achieved by radical resection.

The long-term progression-free survival data are in fact impressive, with 83% in 10 years. This treatment approach calls for a reasonable resection of the tumor without injury to the hypothalamus or surrounding structures with hope of reducing the radiation field. These surgeons do not advocate simple biopsies but rather conservative tumor resections.

Dr. Boop and his colleagues also argue for a referral of the few craniopharyngioma patients to sufficiently experienced centers, at least those patients who have hypothalamic involvement.

Who is right? Restraint is certainly desirable. And as surgeons we are easier following our instinct to "get it all out" rather than our ability to consider advantages of "leaving something behind." Given the fact that not all patients will ever be treated by the handful of most experienced craniopharyngioma surgeons, and given the, in our view, very acceptable long-term survival rate of patients treated with conservative resection and radiotherapy, the latter approach will work well for more patients than will the radical surgery philosophy.

References

1. Burger P, Scheithauer B, Vogel F. Surgical Pathology of the Nervous System and Its Coverings. 3rd ed. New York: Wiley; 1991
2. Russell D, Rubinstein L. Pathology of Tumors of the Nervous System. 5th ed. Baltimore: Williams & Wilkins; 1989
3. Baskin DS, Wilson CB. Surgical management of craniopharyngiomas: a review of 74 cases. J Neurosurg 1986;65(1):22–27
4. Carmel PW, Antunes JL, Chang CH. Craniopharyngiomas in children. Neurosurgery 1982;11(3):382–389
5. Matson DD, Crigler JF Jr. Radical treatment of craniopharyngioma. Ann Surg 1960;152:699–704
6. Bunin GR, Surawicz TS, Witman PA, Preston-Martin S, Davis F, Bruner JM. The descriptive epidemiology of craniopharyngioma. J Neurosurg 1998;89(4):547–551
7. Weiner HL, Wisoff JH, Rosenberg ME, et al. Craniopharyngiomas: a clinicopathological analysis of factors predictive of recurrence and functional outcome. Neurosurgery 1994;35(6):1001–1010, discussion 1010–1011
8. Mollá E, Martí-Bonmatí L, Revert A, et al. Cranio-pharyngiomas: identification of different semiological patterns with MRI. Eur Radiol 2002;12(7):1829–1836
9. Prabhu VC, Brown HG. The pathogenesis of craniopharyngiomas. Childs Nerv Syst 2005;21(8–9):622–627
10. Pusey E, Kortman KE, Flannigan BD, Tsuruda J, Bradley WG. MR of craniopharyngiomas: tumor delineation and characterization. AJR Am J Roentgenol 1987;149(2):383–388
11. Wang KC, Hong SH, Kim SK, Cho BK. Origin of craniopharyngiomas: implication on the growth pattern. Childs Nerv Syst 2005;21(8–9):628–634
12. Wisoff JH. Surgical management of recurrent craniopharyngiomas. Pediatr Neurosurg 1994;21(Suppl 1):108–113
13. Cushing H. The craniopharyngiomas. In Thomas CC, ed. Intracranial Tumors: Notes upon a Series of Two Thousand Verified Cases with Surgical Mortality Percentages Thereto. Springfield, IL: Charles C Thomas; 1932
14. Caldarelli M, Massimi L, Tamburrini G, Cappa M, Di Rocco C. Long-term results of the surgical treatment of craniopharyngioma: the experience at the Policlinico Gemelli, Catholic University, Rome. Childs Nerv Syst 2005;21(8–9):747–757
15. Dhellemmes P, Vinchon M. Radical resection for craniopharyngiomas in children: surgical technique and clinical results. J Pediatr Endocrinol Metab 2006;19(Suppl 1):329–335
16. Di Rocco C, Caldarelli M, Tamburrini G, Massimi L. Surgical management of craniopharyngiomas—experience with a pediatric series. J Pediatr Endocrinol Metab 2006;19(Suppl 1):355–366
17. Erçahin Y, Yurtseven T, Ozgiray E, Mutluer S. Craniopharyngiomas in children: Turkey experience. Childs Nerv Syst 2005;21(8–9):766–772
18. Habrand JL, Ganry O, Couanet D, et al. The role of radiation therapy in the management of craniopharyngioma: a 25-year experience and review of the literature. Int J Radiat Oncol Biol Phys 1999;44(2):255–263
19. Hetelekidis S, Barnes PD, Tao ML, et al. Twenty-year experience in childhood craniopharyngioma. Int J Radiat Oncol Biol Phys 1993;27(2):189–195
20. Kalapurakal JA, Goldman S, Hsieh YC, Tomita T, Marymont MH. Clinical outcome in children with craniopharyngioma treated with primary surgery and radiotherapy deferred until relapse. Med Pediatr Oncol 2003;40(4):214–218
21. Karavitaki N, Brufani C, Warner JT, et al. Craniopharyngiomas in children and adults: systematic analysis of 121 cases with long-term follow-up. Clin Endocrinol (Oxf) 2005;62(4):397–409
22. Merchant TE, Kiehna EN, Kun LE, et al. Phase II trial of conformal radiation therapy for pediatric patients with craniopharyngioma and correlation of surgical factors and radiation dosimetry with change in cognitive function. J Neurosurg 2006;104(2, Suppl):94–102
23. Merchant TE, Kiehna EN, Sanford RA, et al. Craniopharyngioma: the St. Jude Children's Research Hospital experience 1984–2001. Int J Radiat Oncol Biol Phys 2002;53(3):533–542
24. Rajan B, Ashley S, Gorman C, et al. Craniopharyngioma—a long-term results following limited surgery and radiotherapy. Radiother Oncol 1993;26(1):1–10
25. Regine WF, Kramer S. Pediatric craniopharyngiomas: long-term results of combined treatment with surgery and radiation. Int J Radiat Oncol Biol Phys 1992;24(4):611–617
26. Sanford RA. Craniopharyngioma: results of survey of the American Society of Pediatric Neurosurgery. Pediatr Neurosurg 1994;21(Suppl 1):39–43
27. Scott RM, Hetelekidis S, Barnes PD, Goumnerova L, Tarbell NJ. Surgery, radiation, and combination therapy in the treatment of childhood craniopharyngioma—a 20-year experience. Pediatr Neurosurg 1994;21(Suppl 1):75–81
28. Tomita T. Management of craniopharyngiomas in children. Pediatr Neurosci 1988;14(4):204–211
29. Wen BC, Hussey DH, Staples J, et al. A comparison of the roles of surgery and radiation therapy in the management of craniopharyngiomas. Int J Radiat Oncol Biol Phys 1989;16(1):17–24
30. Zuccaro G. Radical resection of craniopharyngioma. Childs Nerv Syst 2005;21(8–9):679–690

31. De Vile CJ, Grant DB, Kendall BE, et al. Management of childhood craniopharyngioma: can the morbidity of radical surgery be predicted? J Neurosurg 1996;85(1):73–81

32. Kim SK, Wang KC, Shin SH, Choe G, Chi JG, Cho BK. Radical excision of pediatric craniopharyngioma: recurrence pattern and prognostic factors. Childs Nerv Syst 2001;17(9):531–536, discussion 537

33. Lena G, Paz Paredes A, Scavarda D, Giusiano B. Craniopharyngioma in children: Marseille experience. Childs Nerv Syst 2005;21(8–9): 778–784

34. Puget S, Garnett M, Wray A, et al. Pediatric craniopharyngiomas: classification and treatment according to the degree of hypothalamic involvement. J Neurosurg 2007;106(1, Suppl):3–12

35. Sosa IJ, Krieger MD, McComb JG. Craniopharyngiomas of childhood: the CHLA experience. Childs Nerv Syst 2005;21(8–9): 785–789

36. Yaşargil MG, Curcic M, Kis M, Siegenthaler G, Teddy PJ, Roth P. Total removal of craniopharyngiomas: approaches and long-term results in 144 patients. J Neurosurg 1990;73(1):3–11

37. Anderson V, Godber T, Smibert E, Ekert H. Neurobehavioural sequelae following cranial irradiation and chemotherapy in children: an analysis of risk factors. Pediatr Rehabil 1997;1(2):63–76

38. Anderson VA, Godber T, Smibert E, Weiskop S, Ekert H. Cognitive and academic outcome following cranial irradiation and chemotherapy in children: a longitudinal study. Br J Cancer 2000; 82(2):255–262

39. Keene DL, Johnston DL, Grimard L, Michaud J, Vassilyadi M, Ventureyra E. Vascular complications of cranial radiation. Childs Nerv Syst 2006;22(6):547–555

40. Mabbott DJ, Spiegler BJ, Greenberg ML, Rutka JT, Hyder DJ, Bouffet E. Serial evaluation of academic and behavioral outcome after treatment with cranial radiation in childhood. J Clin Oncol 2005;23(10):2256–2263

41. Mulhern RK, Merchant TE, Gajjar A, Reddick WE, Kun LE. Late neurocognitive sequelae in survivors of brain tumours in childhood. Lancet Oncol 2004;5(7):399–408

42. Neglia JP, Robison LL, Stovall M, et al. New primary neoplasms of the central nervous system in survivors of childhood cancer: a report from the Childhood Cancer Survivor Study. J Natl Cancer Inst 2006;98(21):1528–1537

43. Ron E, Modan B, Boice JD Jr, et al. Tumors of the brain and nervous system after radiotherapy in childhood. N Engl J Med 1988; 319(16):1033–1039

44. Schmiegelow M, Feldt-Rasmussen U, Rasmussen AK, Lange M, Poulsen HS, Müller J. Assessment of the hypothalamo-pituitary-adrenal axis in patients treated with radiotherapy and chemotherapy for childhood brain tumor. J Clin Endocrinol Metab 2003;88(7):3149–3154

45. Spiegler BJ, Bouffet E, Greenberg ML, Rutka JT, Mabbott DJ. Change in neurocognitive functioning after treatment with cranial radiation in childhood. J Clin Oncol 2004;22(4):706–713

46. Carpentieri SC, Waber DP, Scott RM, et al. Memory deficits among children with craniopharyngiomas. Neurosurgery 2001;49(5): 1053–1057, discussion 1057–1058

47. Cavazzuti V, Fischer EG, Welch K, Belli JA, Winston KR. Neurological and psychophysiological sequelae following different treatments of craniopharyngioma in children. J Neurosurg 1983;59(3): 409–417

48. Müller HL, Bueb K, Bartels U, et al. Obesity after childhood craniopharyngioma—German multicenter study on pre-operative risk factors and quality of life. Klin Padiatr 2001;213(4):244–249

49. Riva D, Pantaleoni C, Devoti M, Saletti V, Nichelli F, Giorgi C. Late neuropsychological and behavioural outcome of children surgically treated for craniopharyngioma. Childs Nerv Syst 1998;14(4–5):179–184

50. Sands SA, Milner JS, Goldberg J, et al. Quality of life and behavioral follow-up study of pediatric survivors of craniopharyngioma. J Neurosurg 2005;103(4, Suppl):302–311

51. Al-Mefty O, Hassounah M, Weaver P, Sakati N, Jinkins JR, Fox JL. Microsurgery for giant craniopharyngiomas in children. Neurosurgery 1985;17(4):585–595

52. Colangelo M, Ambrosio A, Ambrosio C. Neurological and behavioral sequelae following different approaches to craniopharyngioma: long-term follow-up review and therapeutic guidelines. Childs Nerv Syst 1990;6(7):379–382

53. Hoffman HJ, De Silva M, Humphreys RP, Drake JM, Smith ML, Blaser SI. Aggressive surgical management of craniopharyngiomas in children. J Neurosurg 1992;76(1):47–52

54. Sweet WH. Radical surgical treatment of craniopharyngioma. Clin Neurosurg 1976;23:52–79

55. Fahlbusch R, Honegger J, Paulus W, Huk W, Buchfelder M. Surgical treatment of craniopharyngiomas: experience with 168 patients. J Neurosurg 1999;90(2):237–250

56. Van Effenterre R, Boch AL. Craniopharyngioma in adults and children: a study of 122 surgical cases. J Neurosurg 2002;97(1):3–11

57. Samii M, Bini W. Surgical treatment of craniopharyngiomas. Zentralbl Neurochir 1991;52(1):17–23

58. Shibuya M, Takayasu M, Suzuki Y, Saito K, Sugita K. Bifrontal basal interhemispheric approach to craniopharyngioma resection with or without division of the anterior communicating artery. J Neurosurg 1996;84(6):951–956

59. Zhang YQ, Ma ZY, Wu ZB, Luo SQ, Wang ZC. Radical resection of 202 pediatric craniopharyngiomas with special reference to the surgical approaches and hypothalamic protection. Pediatr Neurosurg 2008;44(6):435–443

60. Symon L, Sprich W. Radical excision of craniopharyngioma: results in 20 patients. J Neurosurg 1985;62(2):174–181

61. Al-Mefty O, Ayoubi S, Kadri PA. The petrosal approach for the resection of retrochiasmatic craniopharyngiomas. Neurosurgery 2008; 62(5, Suppl 2):ONS331–ONS335, discussion ONS335–ONS336

62. Chakrabarti I, Amar AP, Couldwell W, Weiss MH. Long-term neurological, visual, and endocrine outcomes following transnasal resection of craniopharyngioma. J Neurosurg 2005;102(4): 650–657

63. Gardner PA, Kassam AB, Snyderman CH, et al. Outcomes following endoscopic, expanded endonasal resection of suprasellar craniopharyngiomas: a case series. J Neurosurg 2008;109(1):6–16

64. Laws ER Jr. Transsphenoidal removal of craniopharyngioma. Pediatr Neurosurg 1994;21(Suppl 1):57–63

65. Maira G, Anile C, Albanese A, Cabezas D, Pardi F, Vignati A. The role of transsphenoidal surgery in the treatment of craniopharyngiomas. J Neurosurg 2004;100(3):445–451

66. Albright AL, Hadjipanayis CG, Lunsford LD, Kondziolka D, Pollack IF, Adelson PD. Individualized treatment of pediatric craniopharyngiomas. Childs Nerv Syst 2005;21(8–9):649–654

67. Fischer EG, Welch K, Shillito J Jr, Winston KR, Tarbell NJ. Craniopharyngiomas in children: long-term effects of conservative surgical procedures combined with radiation therapy. J Neurosurg 1990;73(4):534–540

68. Fisher PG, Jenab J, Gopldthwaite PT, et al. Outcomes and failure patterns in childhood craniopharyngiomas. Childs Nerv Syst 1998;14(10):558–563

69. Mottolese C, Szathmari A, Berlier P, Hermier M. Craniop-haryngiomas: our experience in Lyon. Childs Nerv Syst 2005;21(8–9): 790–798

70. Ohmori K, Collins J, Fukushima T. Craniopharyngiomas in children. Pediatr Neurosurg 2007;43(4):265–278

71. Stripp DC, Maity A, Janss AJ, et al. Surgery with or without radiation therapy in the management of craniopharyngiomas in children and young adults. Int J Radiat Oncol Biol Phys 2004; 58(3):714–720

72. Tomita T, Bowman RM. Craniopharyngiomas in children: surgical experience at Children's Memorial Hospital. Childs Nerv Syst 2005;21(8–9):729–746

73. Barua KK, Ehara K, Kohmura E, Tamaki N. Treatment of recurrent craniopharyngiomas. Kobe J Med Sci 2003;49(5–6):123–132

74. Caldarelli M, di Rocco C, Papacci F, Colosimo C Jr. Management of recurrent craniopharyngioma. Acta Neurochir (Wien) 1998; 140(5):447–454

75. Choux M, Lena G. [Craniopharyngioma in children: 41st Annual Congress of the French Society of Neurosurgery. Lisbon, Portugal, 4–7 June 1991.] Neurochirurgie 1991;37(Suppl 1):1–174

76. Duff J, Meyer F, Ilstrup D, Laws E, Schleck C, Scheithauer B. Long-term outcomes for surgically resected craniopharyngiomas. Neurosurgery 2000;46(2):291–302, discussion 302–305

77. Vinchon M, Dhellemmes P. Craniopharyngiomas in children: recurrence, reoperation and outcome. Childs Nerv Syst 2008; 24(2):211–217

78. Djordjević M, Djordjević Z, Janićijević M, Nestorović B, Stefanović B, Ivkov M. Surgical treatment of craniopharyngiomas in children. Acta Neurochir Suppl (Wien) 1979;28(2):344–347

79. Gordy PD, Peet MM, Kahn EA. The surgery of the craniopharyngiomas. J Neurosurg 1949;6(6):503–517

80. Guidetti B, Fraioli B. Craniopharyngiomas: results of surgical treatment. Acta Neurochir Suppl (Wien) 1979;28(2):349–351

81. Kahn EA, Gosch HH, Seeger JF, Hicks SP. Forty-five years experience with the craniopharyngiomas. Surg Neurol 1973;1(1):5–12

82. Rougerie J. What can be expected from the surgical treatment of craniopharyngiomas in children: report of 92 cases. Childs Brain 1979;5(5):433–449

83. Shapiro K, Till K, Grant DN. Craniopharyngiomas in childhood: a rational approach to treatment. J Neurosurg 1979;50(5):617–623

84. Trippi AC, Garner JT, Kassabian JT, Shelden CH. A new approach to inoperable craniopharyngiomas. Am J Surg 1969;118(2):307–310

85. Ammirati M, Samii M, Sephernia A. Surgery of large retrochiasmatic craniopharyngiomas in children. Childs Nerv Syst 1990;6(1):13–17

86. Katz EL. Late results of radical excision of craniopharyngiomas in children. J Neurosurg 1975;42(1):86–93

87. Tomita T, McLone DG. Radical resections of childhood craniopharyngiomas. Pediatr Neurosurg 1993;19(1):6–14

88. Hayward R. The present and future management of childhood craniopharyngioma. Childs Nerv Syst 1999;15(11–12):764–769

89. Poretti A, Grotzer MA, Ribi K, Schönle E, Boltshauser E. Outcome of craniopharyngioma in children: long-term complications and quality of life. Dev Med Child Neurol 2004;46(4):220–229

90. Thompson D, Phipps K, Hayward R. Craniopharyngioma in childhood: our evidence-based approach to management. Childs Nerv Syst 2005;21(8–9):660–668

91. Minamida Y, Mikami T, Hashi K, Houkin K. Surgical management of the recurrence and regrowth of craniopharyngiomas. J Neurosurg 2005;103(2):224–232

92. Shiminski-Maher T, Rosenberg M. Late effects associated with treatment of craniopharyngiomas in childhood. J Neurosci Nurs 1990;22(4):220–226

93. Wisoff J, Donahue B. Management of craniopharyngiomas. In: Pollack I, Adelson P, Albright L, eds. Principles and Practice of Pediatric Neurosurgery. 2nd ed. Stuttgart: Thieme Medical Publishers; 2008:560–577

94. Frazier CH. The achievements and limitations of neurologic surgery. Arch Surg 1921;3:543–559

95. Yaşargil MG, Curcic M, Kis M, Siegenthaler G, Teddy PJ, Roth P. Total removal of craniopharyngiomas: approaches and long-term results in 144 patients. J Neurosurg 1990;73(1):3–11

96. Sweet WH. Radical surgical treatment of craniopharyngioma. Clin Neurosurg 1976;23:52–79

97. Hoffman HJ, Hendrick EB, Humphreys RP, Buncic JR, Armstrong DL, Jenkin RD. Management of craniopharyngioma in children. J Neurosurg 1977;47(2):218–227

98. Merchant TE, Kiehna EN, Sanford RA, et al. Craniopharyngioma: the St. Jude Children's Research Hospital experience, 1984–2001. Int J Radiat Oncol Biol Phys 2002;53(3):533–542

99. Sanford RA. Craniopharyngioma: results of survey of the American Society of Pediatric Neurosurgery. Pediatr Neurosurg 1994; 21(Suppl 1):39–43

100. Sanford RA, Muhlbauer MS. Craniopharyngioma in children. Neurol Clin 1991;9(2):453–465

101. Hoffman HJ, De Silva M, Humphreys RP, Drake JM, Smith ML, Blaser SI. Aggressive surgical management of craniopharyngiomas in children. J Neurosurg 1992;76(1):47–52

102. Tomita T, Bowman RM. Craniopharyngiomas in children: surgical experience at Children's Memorial Hospital. Childs Nerv Syst 2005;21(8–9):729–746

103. Dhellemmes P, Vinchon M. Radical resection for craniopharyngiomas in children: surgical technique and clinical results. J Pediatr Endocrinol Metab 2006;19(Suppl 1):329–335

104. Zuccaro G. Radical resection of craniopharyngioma. Childs Nerv Syst 2005;21(8–9):679–690

105. Fahlbusch R, Honegger J, Paulus W, Huk W, Buchfelder M. Surgical treatment of craniopharyngiomas: experience with 168 patients. J Neurosurg 1999;90(2):237–250

106. Poretti A, Grotzer MA, Ribi K, Schönle E, Boltshauser E. Outcome of craniopharyngioma in children: long-term complications and quality of life. Dev Med Child Neurol 2004;46(4):220–229

107. Puget S, Garnett M, Wray A, et al. Pediatric craniopharyngiomas: classification and treatment according to the degree of hypothalamic involvement. J Neurosurg 2007;106(1, Suppl):3–12

108. Thompson D, Phipps K, Hayward R. Craniopharyngioma in childhood: our evidence-based approach to management. Childs Nerv Syst 2005;21(8–9):660–668

109. Moon SH, Kim IH, Park SW, et al. Early adjuvant radiotherapy toward long-term survival and better quality of life for craniopharyngiomas—a study in single institute. Childs Nerv Syst 2005;21(8–9):799–807

110. Pierre-Kahn A, Recassens C, Pinto G, et al. Social and psycho-intellectual outcome following radical removal of craniopharyngiomas in childhood: a prospective series. Childs Nerv Syst 2005; 21(8–9):817–824

111. Sands SA, Milner JS, Goldberg J, et al. Quality of life and behavioral follow-up study of pediatric survivors of craniopharyngioma. J Neurosurg 2005;103(4, Suppl):302–311

112. Hoffman HJ. Aggressive treatment of craniopharyngiomas. In: Al-Metfy O, Origitano TC, and Harkey HL, eds. Controversies in Neurosurgery. New York: Thieme Medical Publishers; 1996: 25–27

113. Stripp DCH, Maity A, Janss AJ, et al. Surgery with or without radiation therapy in the management of craniopharyngiomas in children and young adults. Int J Radiat Oncol Biol Phys 2004; 58(3):714–720

114. Merchant TE, Kiehna EN, Kun LE, et al. Phase II trial of conformal radiation therapy for pediatric patients with craniopharyngioma and correlation of surgical factors and radiation dosimetry with change in cognitive function. J Neurosurg 2006;104(2, Suppl): 94–102

115. Fischer EG, Welch K, Shillito J, et al. Long-term effects of conservative surgical procedures combined with radiation therapy. J Neurosurg 1998;73:534–540

116. Hetelekidis S, Barnes PD, Tao ML, et al. Twenty-year experience in childhood craniopharyngioma. Int J Radiat Oncol Biol Phys 1993;27(2):189–195

117. Rajan B, Ashley S, Gorman C, et al. Craniopharyngioma—a long-term results following limited surgery and radiotherapy. Radiother Oncol 1993;26(1):1–10

118. Hukin J, Visser J, Sargent M, Goddard K, Fryer C, Steinbok P. Childhood craniopharyngioma: Vancouver experience. Childs Nerv Syst 2005;21(8–9):758–765

119. Mottolese C, Szathmari A, Berlier P, Hermier M. Craniop-haryngiomas: our experience in Lyon. Childs Nerv Syst 2005;21(8–9): 790–798

120. Scott RM. Craniopharyngioma: a personal (Boston) experience. Childs Nerv Syst 2005;21(8–9):773–777

121. Cavalheiro S, Dastoli PA, Silva NS, Toledo S, Lederman H, da Silva MC. Use of interferon alpha in intratumoral chemotherapy for cystic craniopharyngioma. Childs Nerv Syst 2005;21(8–9): 719–724

122. Ohmori K, Collins J, Fukushima T. Craniopharyngiomas in children. Pediatr Neurosurg 2007;43(4):265–278

123. Zuccaro G, Jaimovich R, Mantes B, Monges J. Complications in pediatric craniopharyngioma treatment. Childs Nerv System 1996;12(7): 385–391

7 Optic Pathway/Hypothalamic Gliomas

♦ Management

Charles Teo

Optic pathway/hypothalamic gliomas (OPHGs) present a management dilemma. They represent < 1% of brain tumors seen in all age groups and 3 to 5% of all brain tumors in the pediatric age group.[1] Patients may present with very subtle or devastating symptoms, have widely diverse imaging, and run either an extremely benign course that may never require intervention or a rapidly progressive course that may result in early death. Predicting the biological nature of these tumors is difficult; therefore, treatment paradigms are poorly defined. It would be wrong to discuss the surgical management of these tumors without first reviewing the different classifications.

Classification

A review of the recent literature is at best confusing. These tumors have been classified according to clinical presentation, radiologic imaging, histologic subtype, anatomical location, and the presence or absence of neurofibromatosis (NF).[2–4] Although each system has certain merits, they result in considerable overlap; subsequently, treatment paradigms are poorly defined. Clearly, if we could predict the biological activity of the tumor, then surgical intervention could be reserved for those aggressive types that result in early visual loss, hydrocephalus, and hypothalamic disturbance. Those with predictable biological inertia could be followed with serial imaging or clinical assessment.

Prognosis by Location

1. Optic nerve involvement only (prechiasmatic): best
2. Optic nerves and chiasm (sparing the hypothalamus): fair
3. Hypothalamic involvement: poor

Prognosis by Age

1. 0 to 5 years of age: poor
2. 5 to 20 years of age: best
3. 20+ years: fair

Prognosis by Histology

1. Juvenile pilocytic astrocytoma: best
2. Fibrillary astrocytoma: fair
3. Pilomyxoid variant: poor

Prognosis by Presentation

1. Unilateral visual loss: best
2. Bilateral visual loss: fair
3. Mostly hypothalamic dysfunction: poor

After a review of the literature, it is clear that there is a consensus that those "anterior" tumors confined to the optic nerve should be discussed separately from true optic chiasmatic-hypothalamic gliomas (OCHGs). The prechiasmatic, optic pathway tumor is usually found in children with neurofibromatosis type 1 (NF1), rarely spreads to the contralateral nerve or chiasm, runs a very indolent course, is mostly of the pilocytic variety and invariably does not progress, and therefore rarely requires treatment. The "posterior" tumors that affect the chiasm and hypothalamus are sometimes classified separately as primarily chiasmatic or primarily hypothalamic, have often been called exophytic, and, most would concede, are hard to distinguish from one another on imaging.

Natural History

The growth rates of optic pathway tumors can vary dramatically. Some are so indolent that they have been called hamartomas. Indeed, spontaneous regression has been seen with the "anterior" located tumors in NF1 patients.[5] Others are so aggressive that they run a malignant course with rapid recurrence and early death. Rarely, they may even disseminate along the neuraxis.[6] This is a phenomenon of low-grade gliomas seen in only 5% of all cases, but when present, more than half the cases are the "posterior" located tumors.[7] Along with the recognized prognosticators listed above, other factors that may play a role in the natural history of optic pathway tumors are the gender of the patient and whether there is a background of NF1. In the surgical series of Ahn et al, only 21% of boys showed tumor progression compared with 71% of girls.[6] Listernick et al found progression of tumor in only 2 of 17 patients with NF1 versus 12 of 19 children with glioma not associated with NF1.[8]

Undoubtedly, the worst prognosis is with those patients who present at a very young age with hypothalamic dysfunction. These tumors are often large with secondary hydrocephalus and intracranial hypertension. Untreated, virtually all of these patients die before 1 year of age.[9]

Pathology

The most common histologic type is the pilocytic astrocytoma (PA). Prechiasmatic tumors are mostly of this type. Other types are low-grade fibrillary astrocytomas, gangliogliomas, and, rarely, malignant gliomas.

Burger's group[10] described a disturbing variety of astrocytoma that was monomorphous and myxoid in appearance and associated with a more aggressive course (**Fig. 7.1**). They called this the pilomyxoid astrocytoma (PMA). Other features of this subtype resembled the PA, but there was a clear absence of Rosenthal fibers and very few eosinophilic granular bodies (**Fig. 7.2**). Those patients with the pilomyxoid variety had a progression-free survival (PFS) rate at 1 year of 38.7% compared with those patients with pilocytic tumors whose PFS rate was 69.2%.[11]

Microvessel density may be another method of prognosticating. This can be determined by immunostaining with factor VIII. A higher density may be associated with reduced PFS.[12]

Clinical Manifestation

The clinical presentation varies according to the age of the patient and the anatomical location of the tumor. Visual disturbance is common and can be prechiasmatic, chiasmatic, or postchiasmatic. If the patient is younger than 3 years old, visual disturbance is subtle and so insidious that the patient may be near blind at presentation and not have any visual complaints. Of course, if the tumor is prechiasmatic, involving the optic nerve alone, visual disturbance will be confined to the one eye, and examination may demonstrate proptosis. If the tumor is chiasmatic, examination may demonstrate a pendular-type nystagmus and asymmetrical and patchy visual field loss due to confrontation. Fundoscopy often shows optic atrophy, although papilledema may be seen with large tumors or secondary hydrocephalus. If the hypothalamus is affected, patients may present with precocious puberty, short stature, gelastic seizures, and/or the diencephalic syndrome of Russell. This syndrome is found in children younger than 3 years of age and is characterized by emaciation without gastrointestinal abnormalities, euphoria, and a hyperkinetic state. The

older child and adult with hypothalamic involvement may present with obesity, diabetes insipidus, hypogonadism, hypopituitarism, headache from secondary hydrocephalus, memory disturbance, and emotional lability. Hypothalamic disturbance is less common in adults than in children.

Management

The imaging study of choice is magnetic resonance imaging (MRI) with and without gadolinium. The entire neuraxis should be imaged to determine if dissemination has occurred. Patchy or uniform enhancement is common and does not indicate malignancy. Delineating the margins of tumor from the optic chiasm and hypothalamus is difficult. The prechiasmatic type shows fusiform enlargement of the optic nerve and other features of neurofibromatosis. The differential diagnosis of suprasellar tumors in childhood includes craniopharyngioma (more often cystic and calcified), germ cell tumors (more homogeneous in enhancement and less cystic), dermoid cyst, and sarcoidosis. MR spectroscopy may help assess biological activity, as some have found elevated choline-to-creatine ratios in the peritumoral tissue of patients with OPHGs.[13] All patients should be evaluated by the ophthalmology and endocrinology teams. Particular emphasis should be placed on the preoperative visual fields, as objective loss of vision can be severe without patients complaining of visual disturbance.

Treatment

Observation

Observation is recommended for those patients in whom the tumor is found incidentally. These patients usually have NF1 and have had an MRI to stage their disease. Even in patients with minor symptoms, one tries not to treat in the absence of clinical or radiologic progression.

Surgery

Surgery is recommended in very special circumstances:

1. Those patients with tumors confined to the optic nerve who are showing radiologic and/or clinical progression and in whom vision is severely compromised or indeed who are blind should have curative tumor resection. The cure rate with surgery is 100%. The surgical approach is through a frontal craniotomy and entrance through the orbital roof.
2. Patients with hydrocephalus secondary to third ventricular obstruction are candidates for surgery. The aim of surgery is threefold: tissue diagnosis, reestablishment of cerebrospinal fluid (CSF) pathways, and preservation of neurologic function. There is no evidence to date to show a relationship between the degree of resection and either overall survival or PFS.[6,14]

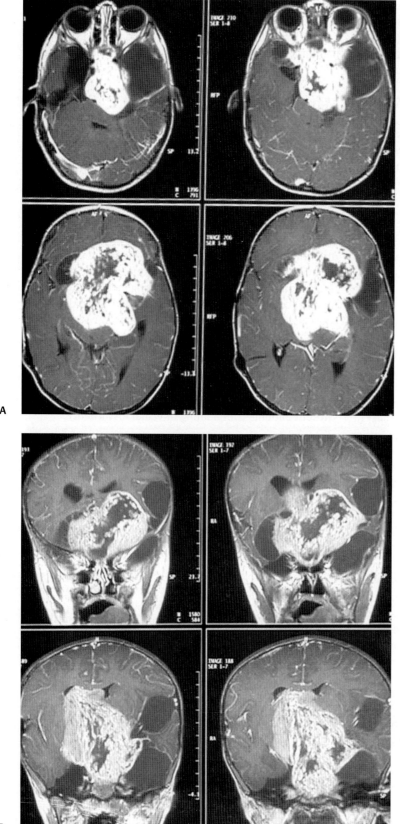

Fig. 7.1 (A–C) Magnetic resonance imaging (MRI) of a 3-year-old boy with a rapidly progressive optic chiasmatic-hypothalamic glioma (OCHG). He presented with the diencephalic syndrome.

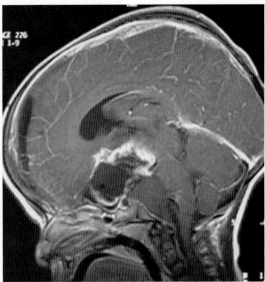

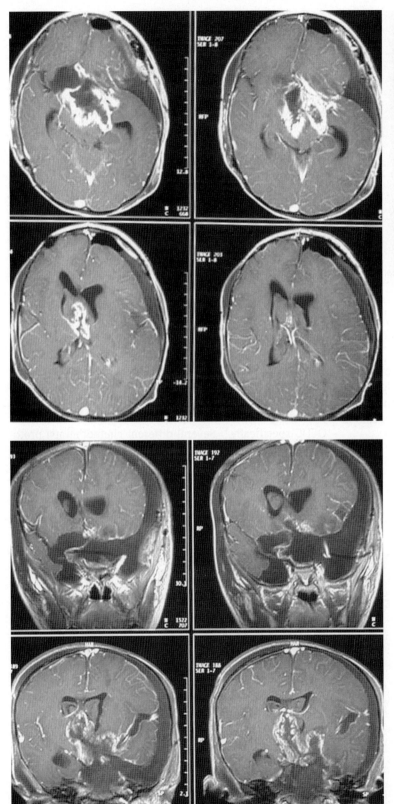

Fig. 7.1 (*Continued*) **(D–F)** Immediate postoperative MRI showing a radical but subtotal resection. His vision deteriorated after surgery, but all other hypothalamic problems improved. The histology of the tumor is shown in **Fig. 7.2.**

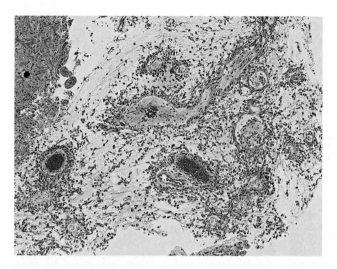

Fig. 7.2 Hematoxylin-eosin stain showing the typical appearance of a pilomyxoid astrocytoma.

Therefore, it is imperative to remove as much tumor as is necessary to open the third ventricle but not to damage the hypothalamus and chiasm (**Fig. 7.3**).

3. If patients have failed chemotherapy and radiotherapy, and the tumor continues to progress clinically and/or radiologically, then subtotal resection is indicated. Surprisingly, progression of residual tumor appears to be halted or at least slowed by surgery (**Fig. 7.1**).

Radiotherapy

Radiotherapy is reserved for those patients who present over 5 years of age with progressive disease but without hydrocephalus. Because many of these tumors are large, it is difficult not to include the temporal lobes and pituitary fossa in the radiation fields. Conformal fractionated stereotactic radiotherapy may reduce the number of short- and long-term side effects.[15] Preradiotherapy surgery may reduce the dose of radiotherapy, but no studies have shown a survival advantage from this protocol. Radiotherapy after subtotal surgical resection is delayed until there is progression of the residual tumor. The rationale for this is the phenomenon of growth retardation after surgical intervention. Furthermore, the older the patient is before radiotherapy is given, the less chance there is of negative cognitive sequelae.

Chemotherapy

Chemotherapy is recommended in patients who present younger than 5 years of age with progressive disease and no hydrocephalus. There is an argument to try chemotherapy in all patients who present with progressive disease despite their age.[16] An interesting study looking at patients who were diagnosed with high-grade gliomas by inexperienced pathologists and treated with combination chemotherapy/radiotherapy but were subsequently felt to have low-grade gliomas by a central registry found no survival advantage to combined treatment compared with chemotherapy alone. This study looked at all pediatric low-grade tumors, not OCHG specifically.[17] Several different chemotherapy protocols have been used, including vincristine, actinomycin D, carboplatin, and etoposide. Although initial disease control is seen in ~90% of patients, very few have significant reduction in tumor volume.[18] Intratumoral injection of I-125 iododeoxyuridine has been used with limited success.[19]

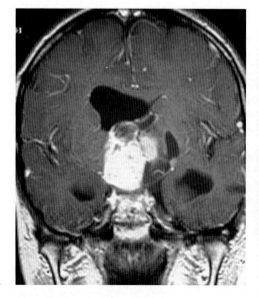

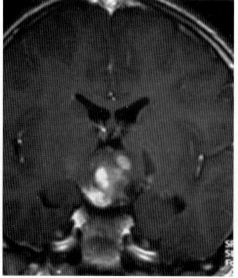

A

B

Fig. 7.3 (A) This 9-year-old boy presented with symptoms and signs of intracranial hypertension. His OCHG had been followed for many years. **(B)** This postoperative MRI demonstrates a subtotal resection but sufficient enough to decompress the third ventricle and reestablish normal cerebrospinal fluid pathways. His postoperative course was uneventful with no worsening of hypothalamic or visual function.

Prognosis

Unfortunately, the literature has many inconsistencies. First, very few studies have separated the "anterior" optic nerve tumors from the true OCHGs.[14] Second, the histologic subtype of PMA has only recently been described and may account for the wide spectrum of survival rates.

Komotar et al[20] showed that the PMA group of patients were clearly disparate from the PA group. The mean ages at diagnosis for the PMA and PA groups were 18 months and 58 months, respectively. The mean PFS times for the PMA and PA groups were 26 and 147 months, respectively. The mean overall survival times for the PMA and PA groups were 63 and 213 months, respectively. CSF dissemination of disease was seen in the PMA group only. Within the follow-up period, seven patients with PMAs (33%) and seven patients with PAs (17%) died as a result of their disease. In an age-matched set, the mean PFS times for the PMA and PA groups were 25 and 163 months, respectively, and the mean overall survival times for the PMA and PA groups were 60 and 233 months, respectively.

If one disregards the various subtypes, then the overall actuarial survival is over 85%.[21] In older children or adults with PA of the chiasm/hypothalamus, surgery alone may offer excellent outcomes[22] (**Fig. 7.4**). Of course, one should expect at least minimal neuroendocrinologic complications, such as diabetes insipidus and visual deterioration. However, the prognosis is almost diametrically opposite in younger children, who often harbor the more sinister PMA variety. Recurrence rates are high, and

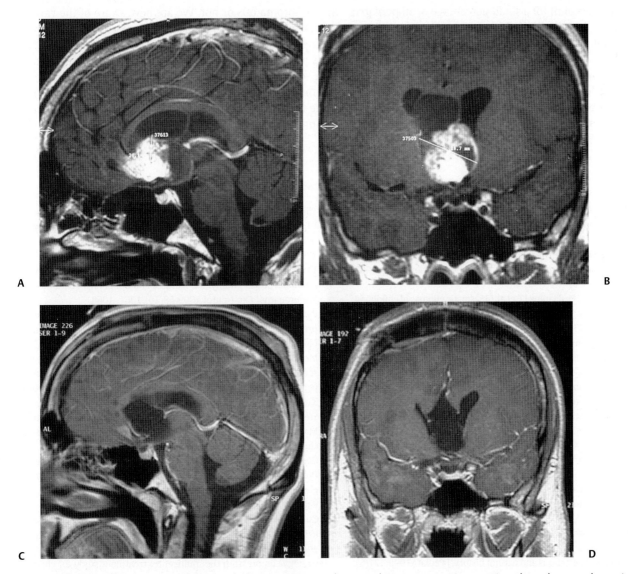

Fig. 7.4 (A,B) MRI of a 17-year-old boy with deteriorating visual function and clear radiologic progression. He had minimal hypothalamic symptoms of poor temperature control and short-term memory disturbance. **(C,D)** Immediate postoperative MRI shows a complete macroscopic resection through an endoscopic-assisted interhemispheric/transforaminal approach. The patient was discharged from the hospital on day 1 in excellent neurologic condition and is currently attending college.

almost all of these infants will succumb to their disease within 5 years.

Conclusion

The term *optic pathway glioma* encompasses a wide variety of tumors. They can be extremely benign in patients with NF1, especially when they involve the optic nerve alone, and hence never require surgical intervention. Conversely, they can be extremely malignant when they occur in infants with mostly hypothalamic dysfunction and are of the PMA variety. Despite all treatment options, these patients progress rapidly and often have a fatal outcome.

Contemporary operative techniques, such as endoscopy and frameless stereotactic guidance, have improved surgical results but have failed to produce long-term benefits or cure except in a small subset of patients. In the future, we look to our oncological colleagues for novel treatment options against one of pediatric neurosurgery's most challenging tumors.

◆ Lessons Learned

These tumors account for a small percentage of all pediatric brain tumors but are probably the most heterogeneous entity. Although the majority of these tumors are low-grade gliomas, there are subsets with different predilections based on location, age, and prognosis. This chapter does an excellent job of presenting the various options for the treatment of these rare tumors. The natural history is mainly determined by the genetic predisposition, that is, neurofibromatous or not. We are now aware of the various histologic types in this location, in particular, the more aggressive PA, which is more common in young children. This particular histology has a significantly worse PFS rate. The discussion concerning adjuvant radiotherapy or chemotherapy is clear and concise. The figures clearly illustrate the growth potential of these tumors and the results of surgery.

References

1. Duffner PK, Cohen ME. Isolated optic nerve gliomas in children with and without neurofibromatosis. Neurofibromatosis 1988;1(4):201–211
2. Tenny RT, Laws ER Jr, Younge BR, Rush JA. The neurosurgical management of optic glioma: results in 104 patients. J Neurosurg 1982;57(4):452–458
3. Packer RJ, Savino PJ, Bilaniuk LT, et al. Chiasmatic gliomas of childhood: a reappraisal of natural history and effectiveness of cranial irradiation. Childs Brain 1983;10(6):393–403
4. Hoffman HJ, Humphreys RP, Drake JM, et al. Optic pathway/hypothalamic gliomas: a dilemma in management. Pediatr Neurosurg 1993;19(4):186–195
5. Piccirilli M, Lenzi J, Delfinis C, Trasimeni G, Salvati M, Raco A. Spontaneous regression of optic pathways gliomas in three patients with neurofibromatosis type I and critical review of the literature. Childs Nerv Syst 2006;22(10):1332–1337
6. Ahn Y, Cho BK, Kim SK, et al. Optic pathway glioma: outcome and prognostic factors in a surgical series. Childs Nerv Syst 2006;22(9):1136–1142
7. Gajjar A, Bhargava R, Jenkins JJ, et al. Low-grade astrocytoma with neuraxis dissemination at diagnosis. J Neurosurg 1995;83(1):67–71
8. Listernick R, Darling C, Greenwald M, Strauss L, Charrow J. Optic pathway tumors in children: the effect of neurofibromatosis type 1 on clinical manifestations and natural history. J Pediatr 1995;127(5):718–722
9. Burr IM, Slonim AE, Danish RK, Gadoth N, Butler IJ. Diencephalic syndrome revisited. J Pediatr 1976;88(3):439–444
10. Tihan T, Fisher PG, Kepner JL, Godfraind C, McComb RD, Goldwaithe PT, Burger PC. Pediatric astrocytomas with monomorphous pilomyxoid features and a less favorable outcome. J Neuropathol Exp Neurol 1999;58(10):1061–1068
11. Tihan T, Fisher PG, Kepner JL, et al. Pediatric astrocytomas with monomorphous pilomyxoid features and a less favorable outcome. J Neuropathol Exp Neurol 1999;58(10):1061–1068
12. Bartels U, Hawkins C, Jing M, et al. Vascularity and angiogenesis as predictors of growth in optic pathway/hypothalamic gliomas. J Neurosurg 2006;104(5, Suppl):314–320
13. Morales H, Kwock L, Castillo M. Magnetic resonance imaging and spectroscopy of pilomyxoid astrocytomas: case reports and comparison with pilocytic astrocytomas. J Comput Assist Tomogr 2007;31(5):682–687
14. Steinbok P, Hentschel S, Almqvist P, Cochrane DD, Poskitt K. Management of optic chiasmatic/hypothalamic astrocytomas in children. Can J Neurol Sci 2002;29(2):132–138
15. Combs SE, Schulz-Ertner D, Moschos D, Thilmann C, Huber PE, Debus J. Fractionated stereotactic radiotherapy of optic pathway gliomas: tolerance and long-term outcome. Int J Radiat Oncol Biol Phys 2005;62(3):814–819
16. Gnekow AK, Kortmann RD, Pietsch T, Emser A. Low-grade chiasmatic-hypothalamic glioma-carboplatin and vincristin chemotherapy effectively defers radiotherapy within a comprehensive treatment strategy: report from the multicenter treatment study for children and adolescents with a low grade glioma—HIT-LGG 1996—of the Society of Pediatric Oncology and Hematology (GPOH). Klin Padiatr 2004;216(6):331–342

17. Fouladi M, Hunt DL, Pollack IF, et al. Outcome of children with centrally reviewed low-grade gliomas treated with chemotherapy with or without radiotherapy on Children's Cancer Group high-grade glioma study CCG-945. Cancer 2003;98(6):1243–1252

18. Mahoney DH Jr, Cohen ME, Friedman HS, et al. Carboplatin is effective therapy for young children with progressive optic pathway tumors: a Pediatric Oncology Group phase II study. Neuro-oncol 2000;2(4):213–220

19. Suárez JC, Viano JC, Zunino S, et al. Management of child optic pathway gliomas: new therapeutical option. Childs Nerv Syst 2006; 22(7):679–684

20. Komotar RJ, Burger PC, Carson BS, et al. Pilocytic and pilomyxoid hypothalamic/chiasmatic astrocytomas. Neurosurgery 2004;54(1):72–79, discussion 79–80

21. Sutton LN, Molloy PT, Sernyak H, et al. Long-term outcome of hypothalamic/chiasmatic astrocytomas in children treated with conservative surgery. J Neurosurg 1995;83(4):583–589

22. Wisoff JH, Abbott R, Epstein F. Surgical management of exophytic chiasmatic-hypothalamic tumors of childhood. J Neurosurg 1990; 73(5):661–667

8 Ependymomas

◆ Surgical Resection

M. Memet Özek and Su Gülsün Berrak

Ependymoma arises from the ependymal cells that line the cerebral ventricles and central canal of the spinal cord. It is the third most common brain tumor in children,[1] with ~70 to 80% of the cases presenting in children younger than 8 years of age.[2-4] Two thirds of patients with intracranial ependymomas present with posterior fossa tumors, and 7 to 15% present with disseminated disease at diagnosis[5,6] (**Fig. 8.1**).

Prognosis and Treatment

Surgery

The optimal treatment of these tumors is surgical resection.[6-11] The most significant prognostic factor predicting survival in children with ependymomas is the extent of surgical resection.[7,8,11-18] Location, histology, and other prognostic

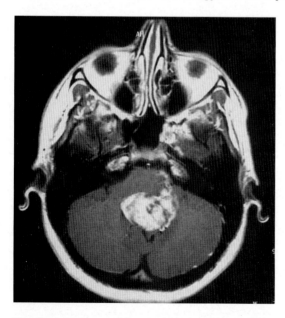

Fig. 8.1 A fourth ventricle ependymoma with peripontine infiltration and two seeding lesions on the right cerebellar cortex.

variables appear to have a minor impact on long-term survival rates in comparison to the extent of surgical resection.[6,9,18-20] The 5-year survival rate for ependymomas has been found to be between 60 and 89% after gross total resection (GTR), but this decreases to 21 to 46% in incompletely resected tumors.[2,7,15,21-24] The frequency of complete resections ranges from 25 to 93% for supratentorial ependymomas and from 5 to 72% for infratentorial ependymomas despite the presence of novel surgical techniques.[6,18,25-29] However, in some instances, a preoperative plan for a subtotal resection in ependymoma is the rule: on imaging studies, the presence of a lesion that involves the pontocerebellar angle refers to infiltration of most cranial nerves and diffuse infiltration of the floor of the fourth ventricle, indicating a preoperative subtotal removal plan for the neurosurgeon (**Figs. 8.2** and **8.3**). Similarly, GTR of a tumor infiltrating the pons usually would be extremely difficult and morbid for the patient, if not impossible and lethal. The presence of a distant metastasis on full neuraxis imaging should also have a major impact on the goals of surgery, such as planning subtotal removal rather than GTR preoperatively. It has been established that the rate of GTR is dependent on location, being up to 100% in the roof of the fourth ventricle, 86% in midfloor tumors, and 54% in the lateral recesses.[18] It is well known that the extent of resection is the strongest prognostic factor for survival rates. Subtotal resection is sometimes preoperatively planned by the neurosurgeon; sometimes the presence of a subtotal resection is reported postoperatively either by the neurosurgeon or by the imaging studies performed in the early postoperative days. Even in patients for whom complete resection cannot be obtained, the Children's Cancer Group (CCG) 921 trial suggests that a residual tumor measuring < 1.5 cm² predicts improved survival.[6] Reoperation with attempted complete resection, when safe and feasible after initial resection, allows proven survival benefits in children with ependymoma and residual bulky disease.[12,30-32] But the role of second surgery is still debated, and the Children's Oncology Group (COG) has developed a

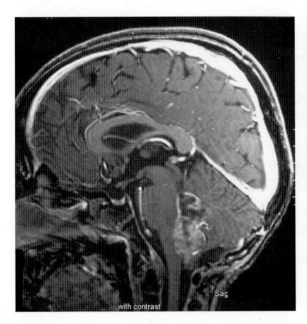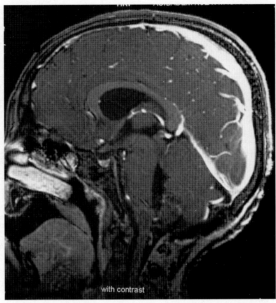

Fig. 8.2 (A) Enhancement of the wide infiltration of the fourth ventricle floor. **(B)** Early postoperative magnetic resonance imaging (MRI) of the patient.

study in which second-look surgery is being performed in patients with residual local disease, following adjuvant chemotherapy before definitive radiation (COG ACNS0121).

Radiotherapy

For many years radiotherapy has been established as an important modality in the subsequent treatment of intracranial ependymoma. Although local field radiation was used in the 1960s and 1970s, in 1975 extending the radiation field to include the whole brain was recommended based on the theoretical shedding of tumor cells into the cerebrospinal fluid (CSF). Reports of similar failure rates in localized versus craniospinal radiation by the late 1980s led to the recommendation of a local radiation dose > 4500 cGy (in 1.5–1.8 Gy fractions) for better local control.[23,24,33–35]

The method of increasing the chances of local tumor control in ependymoma using hyperfractionated radiotherapy (HFRT) has been adopted.[12] In the Pediatric Oncology Group (POG) 9132 study, in 15 patients who had subtotal resection, a HFRT dose of 69.6 Gy given in 58 twice-daily fractions resulted in a 3-year event-free survival (EFS) rate of 52%.[36] This result compared favorably with a similar historic group of patients treated with conventional fractionation that had a 5-year EFS rate of 27%.[36] But this study was not able to demonstrate any clear benefit of HFRT in patients with GTR.[36] Massimino et al[12] reported on a series of 63 patients with ependymoma who were given HFRT for GTR or four courses of chemotherapy followed by HFRT for subtotal resection. However, they were not able to demonstrate a dramatically improved local control rate compared

with the historical series, especially in patients with residual disease and anaplastic histology. New radiotherapy treatment techniques, such as conformal or stereotactic radiotherapy (SRT), have been developed to minimize the acute and long-term toxicities of radiotherapy. SRT uses highly focal, precise radiotherapy with the biologic advantages of fractionation.[37–39] There are several reports with promising 3- to 5-year local control rates[40] using SRT as a boost after conventional radiation therapy or for the treatment of recurrent ependymoma.[40–46] It must be acknowledged, however, that there is no long-term follow-up on patients treated using this method, so that efficacy has not yet been determined. Conformal radiotherapy has also been used in 88 localized 1- to 21-year-old patients with ependymomas.[47] The 3-year EFS rate was found to be ~75% in one series.[47] Of note, 74 of 88 children in this preliminary report had GTRs.[47] Twenty-four months after the initiation of conformal radiotherapy, no statistically significant change in the measures of neurocognitive effects (i.e., no more than +10 points from the normative mean for the appropriate age group) could be demonstrated.[47] Current studies have also adopted a conformal approach for all patients older than 12 months of age. The American Pediatric Brain Tumor Consortium study of children younger than 3 years of age uses intrathecal chemotherapy, or systemic chemotherapy, as the first-line treatment option and saves conformal radiotherapy for patients with higher-risk disease. COG also suggests conformal radiotherapy as a treatment option in a subgroup of patients older than 1 year of age with higher-risk localized ependymomas. With the help of ongoing trials, the benefits of conformal radiotherapy will be appreciated only

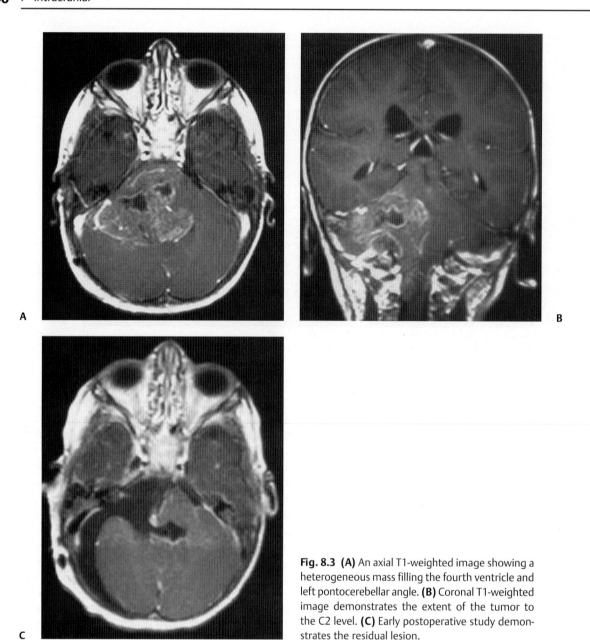

Fig. 8.3 **(A)** An axial T1-weighted image showing a heterogeneous mass filling the fourth ventricle and left pontocerebellar angle. **(B)** Coronal T1-weighted image demonstrates the extent of the tumor to the C2 level. **(C)** Early postoperative study demonstrates the residual lesion.

if there is no increase in the rate of failure. Because acute and late toxicities should be within the predicted limits, these toxicity assessments need to be very carefully performed.

There are other studies reporting on EFS rates following GTRs suggesting that a subgroup of patients may benefit from deferral strategies, thus avoiding immediate postoperative radiotherapy.[9,10,27,48–50] In these studies, 3 to 6 patients out of 6 to 20 patients[9,10,27,51] have been reported to be long-term survivors who did not receive postoperative radiotherapy. These authors concluded that surgery alone was a reasonable option for totally resected, low-grade ependymomas. However, in a retrospective review with 45 patients, Rogers et al[22] demonstrated that GTR and observation had an inferior 10-year overall survival rate when compared with GTR and irradiation (67% vs 83%, respectively; $p > .05$).

Chemotherapy

Radiotherapy deferral strategies are also a part of the therapy plan for infants and young children. Earlier studies from the POG and CCG planned to use delayed irradiation in their infant protocols. In a later study by the Societé Française d'Oncologie Pédiatrique (SFOP) on infants and young children with ependymoma, the main aim was to avoid radiotherapy as first-line treatment. According to the updated results of the Baby POG I study, the 5-year survival rate was

25.7% in patients who had radiotherapy deferred for 2 years, and the 5-year survival rate was 63.3% in patients with 1-year radiotherapy deferral.[16] The aforementioned difference in survival, as a result of deferred radiation, persisted even in children with a GTR and no metastases at diagnosis.[16] These data suggest the sensitivity of ependymomas to chemotherapy while indicating the fact that radiation cannot be totally eliminated from treatment options. In the French Society of Pediatric Oncology Baby Protocol 90, infants were planned to be given radiotherapy only in case of progression under a multiagent chemotherapy regimen.[52] With this strategy, radiation could be avoided in 23% of patients in this study.[52] Additionally, the 5-year overall survival rate (52%) was found to be similar to that found in the Baby POG I study (63.3%).[16] This finding demonstrates that some children with ependymoma can be cured without radiotherapy. CCG 9921,[53] German Pediatric Brain Tumor Study clinical trials HIT-SKK 87 and 92,[54] and the United Kingdom Children's Study Group/International Society of Pediatric Oncology (UKCCSG/SIOP)[55] prospective studies also deferred radiotherapy to progression/relapse with similar overall survival results: 59.0%, (5-year), 55.9% (3-year), and 60.0% (5-year), respectively. Nevertheless, the Headstart I and II studies with myeloablative chemotherapy and autologous hematopoietic stem cell rescue revealed an inferior 5-year survival rate of 38%,[56] in comparison to the approach of multiagent chemotherapy with deferral of radiation to progression or relapse.[52-55]

In light of these studies, the deferral of irradiation to the time of first relapse could be recommended in children younger than 3 years old with radiologically proven GTR. However, because most patients with radiologically proven tumor residuum would show tumor progression in 1 year, such deferral of radiation might be lethal. Therefore, in children younger than 3 years old with residual tumor, conformal irradiation is strongly recommended with minimal deferral.

Including the above-mentioned studies, there are several reviews that considered the role of chemotherapy in the management of ependymoma in children.[52-55,57-59] However, all retrospective studies in the early 1980s failed to show a survival advantage.[2,5,7,8,24,31] The only study using radiotherapy and chemotherapy with vincristine and lomustine versus radiotherapy in a randomized prospective manner was not able to demonstrate an improvement in the outcome of children with ependymoma.[60] It could well be argued that the chemotherapy drugs used in this randomized study were not optimal. Needle et al[61] reported a 5-year progression-free survival rate of 80% for patients older than 36 months of age with incompletely resected ependymoma who were treated with irradiation followed by carboplatin and vincristine alternating with ifosfamide and etoposide. Another CCG study (CCG 921), a prospective randomized trial that investigates the effect of lomustine, vincristine, and prednisone versus "eight in one" chemotherapy after radiotherapy in

ependymoma patients older than 3 years of age, demonstrated similar survival rates (50%) for both chemotherapy arms.[6] Multimodal treatment regimens used in the HIT 88/89/91 trial, consisting of adjuvant combined irradiation and chemotherapy (either ifosfamide, etoposide, methotrexate, cisplatin, or cytarabine and radiotherapy vs radiotherapy and methotrexate, cisplatin, or vincristine), were found to have increased 3-year survival rates to 75% in the treatment of anaplastic ependymomas in childhood.[14] In some other reports, the 5-year survival rates for anaplastic versus nonanaplastic ependymomas have been found to range between 10 and 47% versus 45 and 87%, respectively.[26,62-65]

The current policy for children newly diagnosed with ependymoma is maximally feasible resection followed by local irradiation. Chemotherapy in the upfront setting is recommended in all patients younger than 3 years to delay or avoid radiotherapy. Chemotherapy is also recommended to decrease the rate of relapse in patients with GTR and increase survival rates in patients known to have a poor prognosis at the time of diagnosis. Thus, chemotherapy in the adjuvant setting is an option for patients in whom GTR could not be achieved and/or who have anaplastic ependymoma.

Recurrent Ependymoma

In the recurrence setting, chemotherapy options are very limited, and they are palliative rather than curative. Reoperation of tumors that are surgically accessible, irradiation if not previously given, and salvage chemotherapy are the recommended management options in recurrent ependymomas.[8,57,66] The role of STR for recurrence is under investigation.[40,43,45] Because salvage chemotherapy is not curative, a variety of agents and schedules are also still under investigation.[8,30,67-70] The agents to show mildly promising results have been cisplatin and etoposide.[68-71] High-dose intensive chemotherapy with autologous bone marrow transplant rescue has also been investigated in the setting of recurrent ependymoma. Unfortunately, there was very little clinical response with a very high incidence of fatal toxicity.[57,66] In conclusion, chemotherapy has very little effect in the setting of recurrent intracranial ependymoma.

Conclusion

Ependymomas account for 8 to 14% of brain tumors in children. Approximately 85% of ependymomas present with localized disease. Gross total resection is the most important predictor of outcome. Conformal field radiotherapy is recommended as adjuvant therapy in most patients, especially in infants. Chemotherapy in the upfront setting is recommended in all infants to delay or avoid radiotherapy. The role of chemotherapy in achieving the optimal surgical outcome and/or rendering the patient free of visible residual disease is still under investigation. Chemotherapy is also recommended to decrease the rate of relapse in patients with GTR and increase survival rates in patients who are known to have poor prognosis at diagnosis. Thus, chemotherapy in the adjuvant setting is an option in patients in whom GTR could not be achieved or who have anaplastic ependymoma. Currently, the overall survival rate of all children with ependymoma is in the range of 39 to 69%. With approximately half of the patients eventually succumbing to disease, therapies aimed at improving survival are needed. Frequently, children who underwent posterior fossa irradiation for this tumor have relatively low intelligence quotients (IQs); therapeutic modifications such as conformal radiotherapy are aimed at decreasing the long-term neurologic morbidity. The development of new strategies to improve survival with minimum toxicity is the main focus of current studies.

◆ Surgical Resection with Adjuvant Therapy

Ali Shirzadi and Moise Danielpour

Intracranial ependymomas are the second most common malignant tumor of childhood. Despite a seemingly benign pathology and slow growth, their 5-year survival rates and long-term prognosis remain poor.[72–79] Surgical resection is the initial treatment goal for these tumors.[79–81] The majority of these tumors arise in the posterior fossa and are intimately associated with vital structures, making it difficult to attain a complete resection without significant morbidity. Even in the face of a GTR, the recurrence rate is significant, with various studies illustrating the need for adjuvant therapy.[80,82,83] The decision of how to approach these tumors is currently controversial; radiotherapy is effective but not without risk of significant adverse effects. Chemotherapy has shown some promise in children who are too young for radiotherapy, but it is not curative.[82,84] Therefore, treating physicians are left with the dilemma of deciding the use and timing of adjuvant therapy. Based on the current literature, we discuss the role and timing of adjuvant radiation and chemotherapy for children with intracranial ependymoma, as well as potential new targets for treatment of this disease.

Epidemiology

Brain tumors are the most common solid pediatric malignancy, with equal distribution in children up to 14 years of age. Intracranial ependymomas comprise ~2 to 14% of all pediatric brain tumors,[81,85–87] with 60% diagnosed in children younger than 16 years.[85,88] They are known to be the second most malignant tumor of children younger than 2 years of age, following medulloblastomas.[84] Their presentation is mostly at a very young age, with a mean age of 24 to 72 months.[89,90] They are equally distributed among boys and girls[91] or with slight male predominance.[90,92] A majority of these tumors are located infratentorially[89–91] and can be intimately involved with the lower cranial nerves and vascular structures (**Figs. 8.4, 8.5** and **8.6**).

Radiation versus Chemotherapy

Radiotherapy has been used as an adjunct for treatment of ependymomas for decades. However, there is an ongoing debate on the impact of radiotherapy, recommended dose, and timing of radiation. Radiotherapy can have adverse effects on a young child's developing nervous system, significantly affecting cognition (IQ) and memory.[93–96] Additionally, neuroendocrine and second cancers are known to be delayed effects of radiotherapy.[97] Suc et al[98] reported on more than 5-year follow-up of 20 long-term brain tumor survivors younger than 3 years of age at diagnosis. In this study, 85% had impaired cognition, with 55% requiring special education. Similarly, in the study by Ater et al,[99] infants treated with postoperative Mustargen, vincristine, procarbazine, and

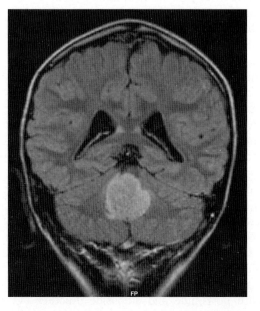

Fig. 8.4 A 9-year-old boy presents with 2-month complaints of nausea and daytime headaches. His brain MRI revealed an irregular enhancing mass in the fourth ventricle. A flair coronal image is presented here.

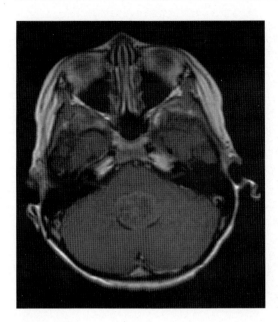

Fig. 8.5 Axial contrast image showing an irregular enhancing fourth ventricle mass.

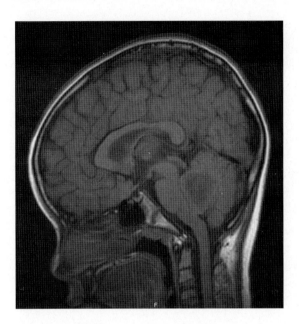

Fig. 8.6 Sagittal T1 noncontrast image showing a fourth ventricle mass with slight dilatation of the lateral ventricles.

prednisone (MOPP) chemotherapy without radiation had a normal IQ (101) in comparison with the declining IQ of children requiring radiotherapy (85 at 5.8-year and 63 at 10-year follow-up). Over the past decades, there has been a growing interest in delaying radiotherapy and initiating treatment with chemotherapy, especially in the subgroup of children younger than 3 years.[82,84,100] Therefore, with the intention of avoiding or delaying radiotherapy, the Pediatric Oncology Group study was conducted.[84]

In the POG study, 48 children younger than 3 years with intracranial ependymomas were treated with a combination of surgical resection and chemotherapy in an effort to delay radiation. Thirty-one were younger than 2 years at the time of diagnosis and received 2 years of chemotherapy followed by radiation, whereas 17 were 24 to 36 months old at the time of diagnosis and received chemotherapy for 1 year followed by radiation. Of the children who had residual disease after surgery, there was 48% complete or partial response to two cycles of cyclophosphamide and vincristine, with 61.8% survival at 3 years. Unfortunately, these optimistic results did not persist. A significant divergence in survival and prognosis appeared as a result of a delay in radiation. Children in which radiation therapy had been delayed for 2 years while they received chemotherapy had only a 25.7% survival rate compared with 63.3% for children who had received 1 year of chemotherapy followed by radiation. This divergence was also noted in children with GTR and no metastases at diagnosis. The survival rate for the 16 children in this subgroup was 62.5%. The eight children who were 24 to 36 months years old had a 5-year survival rate of 87.5%, whereas the eight who were younger than 24 months had a

5-year survival rate of only 37.5%. The survival difference among these subgroups led to the conclusion that delay of radiation of more than 1 year adversely affected survival. The authors of the POG study concluded that, although ependymomas may be chemosensitive, they are not chemocurative.

The UKCCSG/SIOP study[82] followed children who were 3 years old or younger with ependymoma who where treated primarily with chemotherapy to avoid or delay radiotherapy. Eighty-nine children with intracranial ependymomas were studied over an 11-year period. Of these patients, nine had metastatic disease at the time of diagnosis. GTR was documented by surgeons at the end of the operations. After maximal resection, the children had alternating cycles of myelosuppresive and nonmyelosuppresive chemotherapy blocks of 14 days for 1 year. Radiotherapy was avoided until there was radiographic evidence of disease progression or tumor recurrence. Chemotherapy was started at an average of 23 days following surgery. It was terminated in 27 patients prior to receiving maximal myeloablative dosing due to disease progression (11 patients), unacceptable toxicity (10 patients), residual disease (1 patient), without tumor on imaging (1 patient), and without clear reason for the remaining 4 patients. The investigators used relative dose intensity (RDIChemo) to adjust for the cumulative dose of the chemotherapy regimen and the time it took to administer the medication to that defined by the protocol. RDIChemo resulted in a mean of 0.87 (0.53–1.41) equivalent of 90% of that intention. One third of patients had an RDIChemo < 0.78 and one third > 0.93. Comparing the postchemotherapy 5-year survival rate among these different RDIChemo subgroups, those achieving optimum RDIChemo (> 0.93) had a 76%

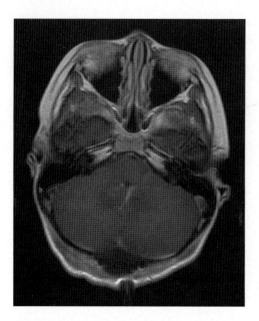

Fig. 8.7 Immediate postoperative contrast axial image reveals complete resection of a grade II ependymoma.

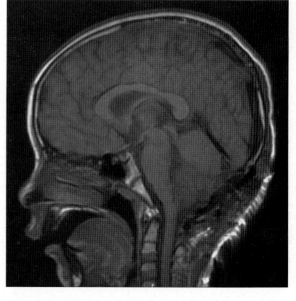

Fig. 8.8 Sagittal T1 noncontrast image showing the reduction in the size of the lateral ventricle.

survival rate in comparison with 52% survival in the nonoptimum (< 0.78) RDIChemo subgroup. Therefore, patients with higher "dose intensity chemotherapy" tended to have an increased survival rate. Of the nonmetastatic patients, 50 had disease progression, and 36 of them underwent radiotherapy in addition to 6 of the 9 metastatic patients, all of whom had progression of their tumor. The mean time from surgery to radiotherapy was 20.3 months, with a mean age of 3.6 at the time of radiation. In patients with disease progression, those who underwent radiotherapy had an EFS rate of > 40% compared with < 20% among patients with no radiotherapy. Comparing different prognostic values, supratentorial tumors had a better survival rate, although the findings were not statistically significant. Also, neurosurgical resection based on the surgeon's intraoperative review was viewed as a powerful predictor of outcome (**Figs. 8.7** and **8.8**), and metastatic disease suggested a poor survival rate. The investigators concluded that chemotherapy with the highest achieved dose intensity in children younger than age 3 with ependymoma is effective but not curative.

The study by the French Society of Pediatric Oncology[100] evaluated the benefits of postoperative chemotherapy and additional surgery at the completion of chemotherapy or tumor progression to avoid or delay radiotherapy in 73 children 5 years or younger. In the study, the progression-free survival (PFS) rate was estimated as 33% and 22% at the 2nd and 4th year, respectively, of tumor diagnosis. During the intended chemotherapy period, 50% of patients experienced relapse, and 72% required further surgery and radiation. The investigators concluded that the decreased PFS as well as

the high risk of progression in their patients further illustrated the requirement for radiotherapy and the lack of strong evidence for chemotherapy as the primary adjuvant treatment.

Similarly, in a study by Shu and associates at the Children's Hospital of Philadelphia (CHOP)/Hospital of the University of Pennsylvania (HUP),[81] patients treated immediately with radiotherapy postoperatively ($N = 34$) were compared with patients with delayed radiotherapy ($N = 13$) due to chemotherapy ($N = 10$) or no immediate treatment ($N = 3$). This study found a worse outcome for patients with delayed treatment. However, this finding was not statistically significant and had a small sample size. These studies and other cooperative group studies[100,101] have reported limited success with trials using chemotherapy to delay radiotherapy and favored immediate postoperative radiation therapy in these patients. Additionally, the studies' authors concluded that an age older than 3 years, a dose > 54 Gy, GTR, no cord extension, and a histologically low grade of tumor were associated with a better prognosis (**Figs. 8.9, 8.10,** and **8.11**). Therefore, radiation may be able to be differed temporally but could not be completely eliminated, even in children with a GTR.

Many questions remain in the use of adjuvant therapy for ependymoma following surgical resection. One of the most significant is the dosage of radiotherapy that is the most effective in preventing recurrence with the least risk of neurocognitive decline. Shu and associates at CHOP/HUP[81] radiated 39 patients with doses > 54 Gy and 8 patients with doses < 54 Gy. They concluded that statistically significant improved overall survival ($p < .0005$) and PFS ($p = .35$) rates

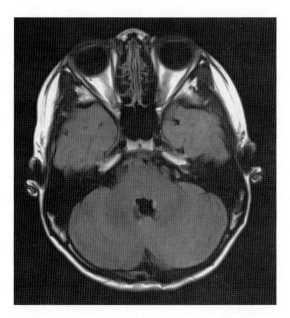

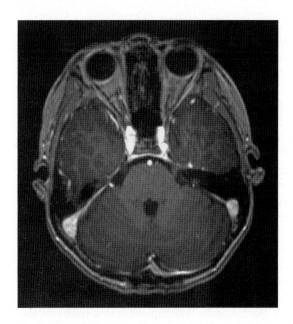

Fig. 8.9 Flair image showing stable MRI without recurrence taken 2 years after resection and a dose of 59.4 Gy at standard fractionation of 1.8 Gy to the posterior fossa.

Fig. 8.10 Axial T1 contrast image taken after resection and radiation shows no enhancement in the posterior fossa.

were observed in higher doses of radiation. Therefore, radiation doses ≥ 54 Gy were correlated with a better prognosis.

Merchant at el[83] conducted a study to determine whether the irradiated volume could be reduced to decrease central nervous system–related side effects without diminishing the rate of disease control. They followed 88 patients with a median age of 2.85 who received conformal radiation therapy

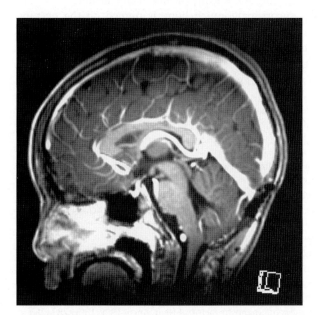

Fig. 8.11 Sagittal contrast image showing no tumor recurrence to the posterior fossa and lateral ventricles that have decreased to their normal size. The patient is doing well and is back to normal daily activities.

(CRT) following surgical resection. CRT was defined as a spectrum of radiation and techniques to deliver the highest dose of radiation to the volume at risk of recurrence to spare the normal tissue. Seventy-three of these children were given a radiation dose of 59.4 Gy, and the rest (11 younger than 18 months) received 54 Gy to their gross tumor volume (tumor bed, residual tumor, or both) with a margin of 1 cm. Neurocognitive testing was performed at baseline at 6, 12, 24, 36, 48, and 60 months following CRT. The PFS rate was measured from radiation to neuroimaging documentation of tumor recurrence. The 3-year PFS rate was estimated to be 74.7% +/− 5.7% in comparison with the previously reported 2- to 5-year PFS rates of 50 to 67% by other studies.[77,102-105] Investigators attributed part of their success to the high proportion of cases in which GTR was achieved, 84% compared with the national average of 40 to 60%.[105] In their study, high-grade tumor (differentiated 90.3 +/− 4.6% vs anaplastic 43.7% +/− 14.3% ; $p < .0001$) and less than GTR (77.6 +/− 5.8% vs near total/STR 42.9 +/−16.2%; $p = .0031$) adversely affected outcome and the hazard ratio for PFS. Additionally, preirradiation chemotherapy marginally affected PFS by univariate statistic ($p = .0446$). In regards to the neurocognitive effects, patients underwent 316 examinations to evaluate changes in IQ, memory, academic achievement, adaptive behavior, and visual-auditory learning. In their conclusion, Merchant and associates found no statistical significance in these measurements 2 years after CRT among children either younger or older than 3 years. Even though younger age at the time of diagnosis is traditionally associated with a poor prognosis, the authors attributed this poor prognosis to hesitancy in giving radiation, lower dose of radiation, or more aggressive behavior of the tumor. Based on these findings, it can be stated that age is not a factor in PFS, and focal conformal radiation therapy with doses as high as 59 Gy can be applied safely, even to children younger than 3 years.

Central to discussions on the treatment of pediatric brain tumors and translational studies is the increasing awareness that only a few atypical cells within a brain tumor may be responsible for the growth and recurrence of some brain tumors.[105-107] Ependymomas may represent clinically[108] and genetically[109] different diseases with a common cell of origin that has gone awry, requiring a better knowledge of these so-called cancer stem cells that could function as a therapeutic target. The bulk of the cells of most cancers are generated by a rare fraction of "stem cell–like" cancer cells,[107,110-118] which are responsible for growth and recurrence of these tumors, and may be resistant to current treatments, including classic chemotherapy and surgical regimens. With this in mind, it is likely that future advances in the treatment of ependymomas and other pediatric tumors will come from targeted molecular therapies using cell cycle and differentiation pathways in stem cells.

Conclusion

Although there are various trials being conducted in regards to the most effective treatment with the fewest side effects for intracranial ependymomas, the current literature strongly supports the concept of GTR of this tumor as the initial treatment. Additionally, the chemotherapy-first approach may be used as an initial adjuvant therapy, but evidence heavily calls for treating infants with postoperative conformational radiotherapy. Reoperation for tumor progression should be evaluated on a case-by-case basis dependent on the advice of the treating team of physicians and the desires of the patients' family. It is likely that future advances in the treatment of pediatric brain tumors will come with better characterization of stem cell–like tumor cells and targeted molecular therapies.

♦ Lessons Learned

Ependymomas apparently still pose the management dilemmas they did over the past 2 decades. GTR is the best indicator for long survival, but it often cannot be achieved because of the anatomical constraints of infiltration of cranial nerves and brainstem, which would cause unacceptable and debilitating morbidity. Radiation is effective in delaying tumor recurrence but causes tremendous morbidity in young children, particularly as only higher doses (> 54 Gy) appear to be sufficient. Chemotherapy has an effect, but a limited one. Trials have shown that delaying radiation more than 1 year has resulted in a significant deterioration of survival. None of the newer "tricks" of radiation oncologists, such as HFRT and CRT, appear to resolve this issue in any meaningful way that would be generally accepted.

What we can learn about the treatment of this obstinate tumor continues to be further complicated by its relative rarity and the inevitably small numbers of all studies that are hampering statistically profound conclusions.

Not surprisingly, much hope is pinned on the ongoing research in molecular biology. After going two steps forward and one step back with ependymomas for a generation, it is hoped that the understanding about tumor stem cells will open a window for substantial progress.

References

1. Kun LEHJ, Rorke-Adams LB, Lau C, Strother D, Pollack IF. Tumors of the central nervous system. In: Pizzo PA, ed. Principles and Practice of Pediatric Oncology. Philadelphia: Lippincott Williams & Wilkins; 2006:786–864
2. Goldwein JW, Leahy JM, Packer RJ, et al. Intracranial ependymomas in children. Int J Radiat Oncol Biol Phys 1990;19(6):1497–1502
3. Gilles FH, Sobel EL, Tavaré CJ, Leviton A, Hedley-Whyte ET; The Childhood Brain Tumor Consortium. Age-related changes in diagnoses, histological features, and survival in children with brain tumors: 1930–1979. Neurosurgery 1995;37(6):1056–1068
4. Polednak AP, Flannery JT. Brain, other central nervous system, and eye cancer. Cancer 1995;75(1, Suppl):330–337
5. Perilongo G, Massimino M, Sotti G, et al. Analyses of prognostic factors in a retrospective review of 92 children with ependymoma: Italian Pediatric Neuro-oncology Group. Med Pediatr Oncol 1997; 29(2):79–85
6. Robertson PL, Zeltzer PM, Boyett JM, et al. Survival and prognostic factors following radiation therapy and chemotherapy for ependymomas in children: a report of the Children's Cancer Group. J Neurosurg 1998;88(4):695–703
7. Pollack IF, Gerszten PC, Martinez AJ, et al. Intracranial ependymomas of childhood: long-term outcome and prognostic factors. Neurosurgery 1995;37(4):655–666, discussion 666–667
8. Chiu JK, Woo SY, Ater J, et al. Intracranial ependymoma in children: analysis of prognostic factors. J Neurooncol 1992;13(3):283–290
9. Nazar GB, Hoffman HJ, Becker LE, Jenkin D, Humphreys RP, Hendrick EB. Infratentorial ependymomas in childhood: prognostic factors and treatment. J Neurosurg 1990;72(3):408–417

10. Awaad YM, Allen JC, Miller DC, Schneider SJ, Wisoff J, Epstein FJ. Deferring adjuvant therapy for totally resected intracranial ependymoma. Pediatr Neurol 1996;14(3):216–219

11. Geyer JR, Zeltzer PM, Boyett JM, et al. Survival of infants with primitive neuroectodermal tumors or malignant ependymomas of the CNS treated with eight drugs in 1 day: a report from the Children's Cancer Group. J Clin Oncol 1994;12(8):1607–1615

12. Massimino M, Gandola L, Giangaspero F, et al; AIEOP Pediatric Neuro-Oncology Group. Hyperfractionated radiotherapy and chemotherapy for childhood ependymoma: final results of the first prospective AIEOP (Associazione Italiana di Ematologia-Oncologia Pediatrica) study. Int J Radiat Oncol Biol Phys 2004;58(5):1336–1345

13. Korshunov A, Golanov A, Sycheva R, Timirgaz V. The histologic grade is a main prognostic factor for patients with intracranial ependymomas treated in the microneurosurgical era: an analysis of 258 patients. Cancer 2004;100(6):1230–1237

14. Timmermann B, Kortmann RD, Kühl J, et al. Combined postoperative irradiation and chemotherapy for anaplastic ependymomas in childhood: results of the German prospective trials HIT 88/89 and HIT 91. Int J Radiat Oncol Biol Phys 2000;46(2):287–295

15. Paulino AC, Wen BC, Buatti JM, et al. Intracranial ependymomas: an analysis of prognostic factors and patterns of failure. Am J Clin Oncol 2002;25(2):117–122

16. Duffner PK, Krischer JP, Sanford RA, et al. Prognostic factors in infants and very young children with intracranial ependymomas. Pediatr Neurosurg 1998;28(4):215–222

17. Agaoglu FY, Ayan I, Dizdar Y, Kebudi R, Gorgun O, Darendeliler E. Ependymal tumors in childhood. Pediatr Blood Cancer 2005;45(3):298–303

18. Spagnoli D, Tomei G, Ceccarelli G, et al. Combined treatment of fourth ventricle ependymomas: report of 26 cases. Surg Neurol 2000;54(1):19–26, discussion 26

19. Ross GW, Rubinstein LJ. Lack of histopathological correlation of malignant ependymomas with postoperative survival. J Neurosurg 1989;70(1):31–36

20. Merchant TE, Haida T, Wang MH, Finlay JL, Leibel SA. Anaplastic ependymoma: treatment of pediatric patients with or without craniospinal radiation therapy. J Neurosurg 1997;86(6):943–949

21. Oya N, Shibamoto Y, Nagata Y, Negoro Y, Hiraoka M. Postoperative radiotherapy for intracranial ependymoma: analysis of prognostic factors and patterns of failure. J Neurooncol 2002;56(1):87–94

22. Rogers L, Pueschel J, Spetzler R, et al. Is gross-total resection sufficient treatment for posterior fossa ependymomas? J Neurosurg 2005;102(4):629–636

23. Rousseau P, Habrand JL, Sarrazin D, et al. Treatment of intracranial ependymomas of children: review of a 15-year experience. Int J Radiat Oncol Biol Phys 1994;28(2):381–386

24. Carrie C, Mottolese C, Bouffet E, et al. Non-metastatic childhood ependymomas. Radiother Oncol 1995;36(2):101–106

25. McLaughlin MP, Marcus RB Jr, Buatti JM, et al. Ependymoma: results, prognostic factors and treatment recommendations. Int J Radiat Oncol Biol Phys 1998;40(4):845–850

26. Stüben G, Stuschke M, Kroll M, Havers W, Sack H. Postoperative radiotherapy of spinal and intracranial ependymomas: analysis of prognostic factors. Radiother Oncol 1997;45(1):3–10

27. Hukin J, Epstein F, Lefton D, Allen J. Treatment of intracranial ependymoma by surgery alone. Pediatr Neurosurg 1998;29(1):40–45

28. Imhof HG, Hany M, Wiestler OD, Glanzmann C. Long-term follow-up in 39 patients with an ependymoma after surgery and irradiation. Strahlenther Onkol 1992;168(9):513–519

29. Robertson PL, Zeltzer PM, Boyett JM, et al. Survival and prognostic factors following radiation therapy and chemotherapy for ependymomas in children: a report of the Children's Cancer Group. J Neurosurg 1998;88(4):695–703

30. Goldwein JW, Glauser TA, Packer RJ, et al. Recurrent intracranial ependymomas in children: survival, patterns of failure, and prognostic factors. Cancer 1990;66(3):557–563

31. Foreman NK, Love S, Thorne R. Intracranial ependymomas: analysis of prognostic factors in a population-based series. Pediatr Neurosurg 1996;24(3):119–125

32. Foreman NK, Love S, Gill SS, Coakham HB. Second-look surgery for incompletely resected fourth ventricle ependymomas: technical case report. Neurosurgery 1997;40(4):856–860, discussion 860

33. Vanuytsel L, Brada M. The role of prophylactic spinal irradiation in localized intracranial ependymoma. Int J Radiat Oncol Biol Phys 1991;21(3):825–830

34. Shaw EG, Evans RG, Scheithauer BW, Ilstrup DM, Earle JD. Postoperative radiotherapy of intracranial ependymoma in pediatric and adult patients. Int J Radiat Oncol Biol Phys 1987;13(10):1457–1462

35. Goldwein JW, Corn BW, Finlay JL, Packer RJ, Rorke LB, Schut L. Is craniospinal irradiation required to cure children with malignant (anaplastic) intracranial ependymomas? Cancer 1991;67(11):2766–2771

36. Kovnar EH, Curran W, Tomita T, et al. Hyperfractionated irradiation for childhood ependymoma: early results of a phase III Pediatric Oncology Group study. J Neurooncol 1997;33:268

37. Merchant TE, Zhu Y, Thompson SJ, Sontag MR, Heideman RL, Kun LE. Preliminary results from a Phase II trial of conformal radiation therapy for pediatric patients with localised low-grade astrocytoma and ependymoma. Int J Radiat Oncol Biol Phys 2002;52(2):325–332

38. Tarbell NJ, Loeffler JS. Recent trends in the radiotherapy of pediatric gliomas. J Neurooncol 1996;28(2–3):233–244

39. Plathow C, Schulz-Ertner D, Thilman C, et al. Fractionated stereotactic radiotherapy in low-grade astrocytomas: long-term outcome and prognostic factors. Int J Radiat Oncol Biol Phys 2003;57(4):996–1003

40. Jawahar A, Kondziolka D, Flickinger JC, Lunsford LD. Adjuvant stereotactic radiosurgery for anaplastic ependymoma. Stereotact Funct Neurosurg 1999;73(1–4):23–30

41. Aggarwal R, Yeung D, Kumar P, Muhlbauer M, Kun LE. Efficacy and feasibility of stereotactic radiosurgery in the primary management of unfavorable pediatric ependymoma. Radiother Oncol 1997;43(3):269–273

42. Hirato M, Nakamura M, Inoue HK, et al. Gamma Knife radiosurgery for the treatment of brainstem tumors. Stereotact Funct Neurosurg 1995;64(Suppl 1):32–41

43. Stafford SL, Pollock BE, Foote RL, Gorman DA, Nelson DF, Schomberg PJ. Stereotactic radiosurgery for recurrent ependymoma. Cancer 2000;88(4):870–875

44. Endo H, Kumabe T, Jokura H, Shirane R, Tominaga T. Stereotactic radiosurgery for nodular dissemination of anaplastic ependymoma. Acta Neurochir (Wien) 2004;146(3):291–298, discussion 298

45. Kinoshita M, Izumoto S, Kagawa N, Hashimoto N, Maruno M, Yoshimine T. Long-term control of recurrent anaplastic ependymoma with extracranial metastasis: importance of multiple surgery and stereotactic radiosurgery procedures—case report. Neurol Med Chir (Tokyo) 2004;44(12):669–673

46. Hodgson DC, Goumnerova LC, Loeffler JS, et al. Radiosurgery in the management of pediatric brain tumors. Int J Radiat Oncol Biol Phys 2001;50(4):929–935

47. Merchant TE, Mulhern RK, Krasin MJ, et al. Preliminary results from a phase II trial of conformal radiation therapy and evaluation of radiation-related CNS effects for pediatric patients with localized ependymoma. J Clin Oncol 2004;22(15):3156–3162

48. Ernestus RI, Schröder R, Stützer H, Klug N. Prognostic relevance of localization and grading in intracranial ependymomas of childhood. Childs Nerv Syst 1996;12(9):522–526

49. Palma L, Celli P, Cantore G. Supratentorial ependymomas of the first two decades of life: long-term follow-up of 20 cases (including two subependymomas). Neurosurgery 1993;32(2):169–175

50. Papadopoulos DP, Giri S, Evans RG. Prognostic factors and management of intracranial ependymomas. Anticancer Res 1990;10(3):689–692

51. Ernestus RI, Wilcke O, Schröder R. Supratentorial ependymomas in childhood: clinicopathological findings and prognosis. Acta Neurochir (Wien) 1991;111(3–4):96–102

52. Grill J, Le Deley MC, Gambarelli D, et al; French Society of Pediatric Oncology. Postoperative chemotherapy without irradiation for ependymoma in children under 5 years of age: a multicenter trial of the French Society of Pediatric Oncology. J Clin Oncol 2001;19(5):1288–1296

53. Geyer JR, Sposto R, Jennings M, et al; Children's Cancer Group. Multiagent chemotherapy and deferred radiotherapy in infants with malignant brain tumors: a report from the Children's Cancer Group. J Clin Oncol 2005;23(30):7621–7631

54. Timmermann B, Kortmann RD, Kühl J, et al. Role of radiotherapy in anaplastic ependymoma in children under age of 3 years: results of the prospective German brain tumor trials HIT-SKK 87 and 92. Radiother Oncol 2005;77(3):278–285

55. Grundy RG, Wilne SA, Weston CL, et al; Children's Cancer and Leukaemia Group (formerly UKCCSG) Brain Tumour Committee. Primary postoperative chemotherapy without radiotherapy for intracranial ependymoma in children: the UKCCSG/SIOP prospective study. Lancet Oncol 2007;8(8):696–705

56. Zacharoulis S, Levy A, Chi SN, et al. Outcome for young children newly diagnosed with ependymoma, treated with intensive induction chemotherapy followed by myeloablative chemotherapy and autologous stem cell rescue. Pediatr Blood Cancer 2007;49(1):34–40

57. Grill J, Kalifa C, Doz F, et al. A high-dose busulfan-thiotepa combination followed by autologous bone marrow transplantation in childhood recurrent ependymoma: a phase II study. Pediatr Neurosurg 1996;25(1):7–12

58. Souweidane MM, Bouffet E, Finlay J. The role of chemotherapy in newly diagnosed ependymoma of childhood. Pediatr Neurosurg 1998;28(5):273–278

59. Siffert J, Allen JC. Chemotherapy in recurrent ependymoma. Pediatr Neurosurg 1998;28(6):314–319

60. Evans AE, Anderson JR, Lefkowitz-Boudreaux IB, Finlay JL. Adjuvant chemotherapy of childhood posterior fossa ependymoma: craniospinal irradiation with or without adjuvant CCNU, vincristine, and prednisone—a Children's Cancer Group study. Med Pediatr Oncol 1996;27(1):8–14

61. Needle MN, Goldwein JW, Grass J, et al. Adjuvant chemotherapy for the treatment of intracranial ependymoma of childhood. Cancer 1997;80(2):341–347

62. Tihan T, Zhou T, Holmes E, Burger PC, Ozuysal S, Rushing EJ. The prognostic value of histological grading of posterior fossa ependymomas in children: a Children's Oncology Group study and a review of prognostic factors. Mod Pathol 2008;21(2):165–177

63. Schild SE, Nisi K, Scheithauer BW, et al. The results of radiotherapy for ependymomas: the Mayo Clinic experience. Int J Radiat Oncol Biol Phys 1998;42(5):953–958

64. Di Marco A, Campostrini F, Pradella R, et al. Postoperative irradiation of brain ependymomas. Analysis of 33 cases. Acta Oncol 1988;27(3):261–267

65. Kovalic JJ, Flaris N, Grigsby PW, Pirkowski M, Simpson JR, Roth KA. Intracranial ependymoma long-term outcome, patterns of failure. J Neurooncol 1993;15(2):125–131

66. Mason WP, Goldman S, Yates AJ, Boyett J, Li H, Finlay JL. Survival following intensive chemotherapy with bone marrow reconstitution for children with recurrent intracranial ependymoma—a report of the Children's Cancer Group. J Neurooncol 1998;37(2):135–143

67. Friedman HS, Krischer JP, Burger P, et al. Treatment of children with progressive or recurrent brain tumors with carboplatin or iproplatin: a Pediatric Oncology Group randomized phase II study. J Clin Oncol 1992;10(2):249–256

68. Chamberlain MC. Recurrent intracranial ependymoma in children: salvage therapy with oral etoposide. Pediatr Neurol 2001;24(2):117–121

69. Bertolone SJ, Baum ES, Krivit W, Hammond GD. A phase II study of cisplatin therapy in recurrent childhood brain tumors: a report from the Children's Cancer Study Group. J Neurooncol 1989;7(1):5–11

70. Sexauer CL, Khan A, Burger PC, et al. Cisplatin in recurrent pediatric brain tumors: a POG Phase II study. Cancer 1985;56(7):1497–1501

71. Khan AB, D'Souza BJ, Wharam MD, et al. Cisplatin therapy in recurrent childhood brain tumors. Cancer Treat Rep 1982;66(12):2013–2020

72. Duffner PK, Krischer JP, Sanford RA, et al. Prognostic factors in infants and very young children with intracranial ependymomas. Pediatr Neurosurg 1998;28(4):215–222

73. Garrett PG, Simpson WJ. Ependymomas: results of radiation treatment. Int J Radiat Oncol Biol Phys 1983;9(8):1121–1124

74. Gornet MK, Buckner JC, Marks RS, Scheithauer BW, Erickson BJ. Chemotherapy for advanced CNS ependymoma. J Neurooncol 1999;45(1):61–67

75. McCormick PC, Stein BM. Intramedullary tumors in adults. Neurosurg Clin N Am 1990;1(3):609–630

76. Pollack IF, Gerszten PC, Martinez AJ, et al. Intracranial ependymomas of childhood: long-term outcome and prognostic factors. Neurosurgery 1995;37(4):655–666, discussion 666–667

77. Rousseau P, Habrand JL, Sarrazin D, et al. Treatment of intracranial ependymomas of children: review of a 15-year experience. Int J Radiat Oncol Biol Phys 1994;28(2):381–386

78. Stüben G, Stuschke M, Kroll M, Havers W, Sack H. Postoperative radiotherapy of spinal and intracranial ependymomas: analysis of prognostic factors. Radiother Oncol 1997;45(1):3–10

79. Metellus P, Barrie M, Figarella-Branger D, et al. Multicentric French study on adult intracranial ependymomas: prognostic factors analysis and therapeutic considerations from a cohort of 152 patients. Brain 2007;130(Pt 5):1338–1349

80. Rogers L, Pueschel J, Spetzler R, et al. Is gross-total resection sufficient treatment for posterior fossa ependymomas? J Neurosurg 2005;102(4):629–636

81. Shu HK, Sall WF, Maity A, et al. Childhood intracranial ependymoma: twenty-year experience from a single institution. Cancer 2007;110(2):432–441

82. Grundy RG, Wilne SA, Weston CL, et al; Children's Cancer and Leukaemia Group (formerly UKCCSG) Brain Tumour Committee.

Primary postoperative chemotherapy without radiotherapy for intracranial ependymoma in children: the UKCCSG/SIOP prospective study. Lancet Oncol 2007;8(8):696–705

83. Merchant TE, Mulhern RK, Krasin MJ, et al. Preliminary results from a phase II trial of conformal radiation therapy and evaluation of radiation-related CNS effects for pediatric patients with localized ependymoma. J Clin Oncol 2004;22(15):3156–3162

84. Duffner PK, Horowitz ME, Krischer JP, et al. The treatment of malignant brain tumors in infants and very young children: an update of the Pediatric Oncology Group experience. Neuro-oncol 1999;1(2):152–161

85. Brandes AA, Cavallo G, Reni M, et al. A multicenter retrospective study of chemotherapy for recurrent intracranial ependymal tumors in adults by the Gruppo Italiano Cooperativo di Neuro-Oncologia. Cancer 2005;104(1):143–148

86. Gurney JG, Smith MA, Bunin GR. CNS and Miscellaneous Intracranial and Intraspinal Neoplasm. Bethesda, MD: National Cancer Institute, SEER Program; 1999

87. Tomita T. Neurosurgical perspectives in pediatric neurooncology. Childs Nerv Syst 1998;14(3):94–96

88. Reni M, Brandes AA. Current management and prognostic factors for adult ependymoma. Expert Rev Anticancer Ther 2002;2(5):537–545

89. Foreman NK, Love S, Thorne R. Intracranial ependymomas: analysis of prognostic factors in a population-based series. Pediatr Neurosurg 1996;24(3):119–125

90. Perilongo G, Massimino M, Sotti G, et al. Analyses of prognostic factors in a retrospective review of 92 children with ependymoma: Italian Pediatric Neuro-oncology Group. Med Pediatr Oncol 1997;29(2):79–85

91. Robertson PL, Zeltzer PM, Boyett JM, et al. Survival and prognostic factors following radiation therapy and chemotherapy for ependymomas in children: a report of the Children's Cancer Group. J Neurosurg 1998;88(4):695–703

92. Central Brain Tumor Registry of United States. Statistical Report: Primary Brain Tumors in the United States, 1995–1999. Hinsdale, IL: Author; 2002

93. Copeland DR, deMoor C, Moore BD III, Ater JL. Neurocognitive development of children after a cerebellar tumor in infancy: a longitudinal study. J Clin Oncol 1999;17(11):3476–3486

94. Mulhern RK, Merchant TE, Gajjar A, Reddick WE, Kun LE. Late neurocognitive sequelae in survivors of brain tumours in childhood. Lancet Oncol 2004;5(7):399–408

95. Riva D, Giorgi C. The neurodevelopmental price of survival in children with malignant brain tumours. Childs Nerv Syst 2000;16(10–11):751–754

96. Spiegler BJ, Bouffet E, Greenberg ML, Rutka JT, Mabbott DJ. Change in neurocognitive functioning after treatment with cranial radiation in childhood. J Clin Oncol 2004;22(4):706–713

97. Duffner PK, Krischer JP, Horowitz ME, et al. Second malignancies in young children with primary brain tumors following treatment with prolonged postoperative chemotherapy and delayed irradiation: a Pediatric Oncology Group study. Ann Neurol 1998;44(3):313–316

98. Suc E, Kalifa C, Brauner R, et al. Brain tumours under the age of 3: the price of survival—a retrospective study of 20 long-term survivors. Acta Neurochir (Wien) 1990;106(3-4):93–98

99. Ater JL, van Eys J, Woo SY, Moore B III, Copeland DR, Bruner J. MOPP chemotherapy without irradiation as primary postsurgical therapy for brain tumors in infants and young children. J Neurooncol 1997;32(3):243–252

100. Grill J, Le Deley MC, Gambarelli D, et al; French Society of Pediatric Oncology. Postoperative chemotherapy without irradiation for ependymoma in children under 5 years of age: a multicenter trial of the French Society of Pediatric Oncology. J Clin Oncol 2001;19(5):1288–1296

101. Duffner PK, Horowitz ME, Krischer JP, et al. Postoperative chemotherapy and delayed radiation in children less than 3 years of age with malignant brain tumors. N Engl J Med 1993;328(24):1725–1731

102. Horn B, Heideman R, Geyer R, et al. A multi-institutional retrospective study of intracranial ependymoma in children: identification of risk factors. J Pediatr Hematol Oncol 1999;21(3):203–211

103. Kovalic JJ, Flaris N, Grigsby PW, Pirkowski M, Simpson JR, Roth KA. Intracranial ependymoma long-term outcome, patterns of failure. J Neurooncol 1993;15(2):125–131

104. Massimino M, Gandola L, Giangaspero F, et al. Hyperfractionated radiotherapy and chemotherapy for childhood ependymoma: final results of the first prospective AIEOP (Associazione Italiana di Ematologia-Oncologia Pediatrica) study. Int J Radiat Oncol Biol Phys 2004;58:1336–1345

105. Poppleton H, Gilbertson RJ. Stem cells of ependymoma. Br J Cancer 2007;96(1):6–10

106. Gilbertson RJ. Brain tumors provide new clues to the source of cancer stem cells: does oncology recapitulate ontogeny? Cell Cycle 2006;5(2):135–137

107. Vescovi AL, Galli R, Reynolds BA. Brain tumour stem cells. Nat Rev Cancer 2006;6(6):425–436

108. Moynihan TJ. Ependymal tumors. Curr Treat Options Oncol 2003;4(6):517–523

109. Ebert C, von Haken M, Meyer-Puttlitz B, et al. Molecular genetic analysis of ependymal tumors. NF2 mutations and chromosome 22q loss occur preferentially in intramedullary spinal ependymomas. Am J Pathol 1999;155(2):627–632

110. Pardal R, Clarke MF, Morrison SJ. Applying the principles of stem-cell biology to cancer. Nat Rev Cancer 2003;3(12):895–902

111. Al-Hajj M, Clarke MF. Self-renewal and solid tumor stem cells. Oncogene 2004;23(43):7274–7282

112. Bonnet D, Dick JE. Human acute myeloid leukemia is organized as a hierarchy that originates from a primitive hematopoietic cell. Nat Med 1997;3(7):730–737

113. Lapidot T, Sirard C, Vormoor J, et al. A cell initiating human acute myeloid leukaemia after transplantation into SCID mice. Nature 1994;367(6464):645–648

114. Hemmati HD, Nakano I, Lazareff JA, et al. Cancerous stem cells can arise from pediatric brain tumors. Proc Natl Acad Sci U S A 2003;100(25):15178–15183

115. Ignatova TN, Kukekov VG, Laywell ED, Suslov ON, Vrionis FD, Steindler DA. Human cortical glial tumors contain neural stem-like cells expressing astroglial and neuronal markers in vitro. Glia 2002;39(3):193–206

116. Singh SK, Hawkins C, Clarke ID, et al. Identification of human brain tumour initiating cells. Nature 2004;432(7015):396–401

117. Al-Hajj M, Wicha MS, Benito-Hernandez A, Morrison SJ, Clarke MF. Prospective identification of tumorigenic breast cancer cells. Proc Natl Acad Sci U S A 2003;100(7):3983–3988

118. Taylor MD, Poppleton H, Fuller C, et al. Radial glia cells are candidate stem cells of ependymoma. Cancer Cell 2005;8(4):323–335

9 Scaphocephaly/Sagittal Synostosis

◆ Early Strip Craniectomy

Erin N. Kiehna and John A. Jane Jr.

Since Lane performed the first sagittal synostectomy in 1892, surgeons have sought to correct the cosmetic deformity caused by sagittal synostosis and prevent any of its possible deleterious effects.[1] Efforts have ranged from a simple strip craniectomy advocated by Shillito and Matson[2] and Hunter and Rudd,[3] to the more extensive procedure pioneered by Jane,[4] to extensive cranial vault remodeling popularized in the 1990s by Marsh et al,[5] Boop et al,[6] Penslar et al,[7] Maugans et al,[8] and others with varying degrees of success.[9] After decades of research, it is now apparent that there may not be a single "gold standard" for sagittal synostosis. Rather, different procedures are indicated based on the age of presentation and the degree of scaphocephaly.

Although scaphocephaly is present in ~2 of every 10,000 live births,[10] most infants do not present for neurosurgical evaluation until they are an average of 5 months, which may exclude simple suturectomies as they often do not address the long-term scaphocephalic shape and suture recrudescence.[6] However, as the awareness of craniosynostosis increases in the community, the average age at presentation may decrease. Younger age at presentation may allow for less invasive procedures on relatively younger infants, thereby lowering intraoperative blood loss and potential morbidity while still improving aesthetics.

Cranial vault remodeling (CVR) has several disadvantages when compared with a simple strip suturectomy. It is associated with more extensive blood loss and exposes a much larger surface area of the brain over a longer period of time, raising the risk of morbidity and mortality.[11,12] In addition, CVR requires a joint effort between neurosurgeons and plastic surgeons, the use of absorbable plates, and a longer hospital stay, which drastically raises the expense of the procedure.[13] Given these disadvantages, it would be beneficial for a select group of infants younger than 3 months of age with minimal deformity to undergo a less invasive approach.

Diagnosis

The diagnosis of scaphocephaly is generally made from the physical examination. According to Virchow's law, bony direction ceases in the direction perpendicular to the sagittal suture and compensates in the opposite direction. As a result, these infants usually have a long, narrow head with a prominent bony ridge along the sagittal suture. Predictable compensatory growth occurs at adjacent sutures and can affect the shape of the entire skull.[4] As a result, frontal bossing or an occipital prominence may also be noted. Plain radiographs are useful for demonstrating fused sutures. In addition, a three-dimensional computed tomography (CT) scan can provide further proof of suture fusion and can also identify any underlying brain abnormalities.[14]

Operative Technique

Patient Selection

Surgical treatment for craniosynostosis is generally preferred within the first year of life, when the infant's skull is malleable and the nonpathologic sutures have not yet fused.[15] Although craniosynostosis may be detected by the third trimester on fetal ultrasound,[16] most patients do not typically present for evaluation until they are several months old. Typically, the first 2 months of life involve rapid growth of the cranial vault, accompanied by nearly doubling of brain mass by the first 6 months of life.[17] Surgery during this period has many challenges, but it also may benefit from the intracranial dynamics. Although a simple strip craniectomy poses a risk of rapid suture recrudescence, early suture release within the first few months of life can take advantage of rapid brain growth and development to aid in natural CVR with or without the aid of external devices.[18] Surgeons therefore must weigh the ability of the infant to tolerate the surgery, which increases with age, against the changing malleability of the skull, which favors early surgery. As such, a simple strip craniectomy is ideally performed in infants younger than 3 months with mild scaphocephaly without significant frontal bossing or occipital knobs.[19] For older infants between 6 and 12 months of age or those with more significant deformities, cranial vault reconstruction may be more appropriate. In addition, infants who have undergone a simple strip suturectomy should be followed with serial exams and head circumferences to assess whether they will need further CVR in the future.[20]

Operative Procedure

The patient is placed in the supine position with the head resting in a padded suboccipital support (**Fig. 9.1**). The infant is then prepped and draped widely. Local anesthetic with epinephrine is used to decrease postoperative pain and minimize incisional bleeding from the scalp. A midline skin incision is made from 1 to 2 cm anterior to the anterior fontanelle to 1 to 2 cm posterior to the lambda (**Fig. 9.2A**). This incision may be elongated for patients with occipital prominence. Skin clips are used to reduce bleeding from the scalp edges. The scalp is then reflected bilaterally, dissecting through the loose areolar plane of the scalp, above the pericranium, as its preservation reduces blood loss. When the anterior fontanelle is open, a curet is used to separate the dura underlying the fontanelle from the overlying pericranium. Two bur holes are then made on either side of the sagittal suture just anterior to the lambdoid sutures. A craniotome is used to connect these bur holes to the edges of the anterior

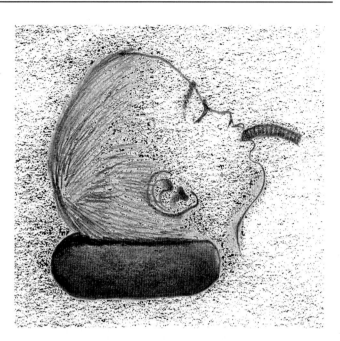

Fig. 9.1 Positioning of the patient with sagittal synostosis.

fontanelle (**Fig. 9.2B**). Great care is taken when removing the bone overlying the sagittal sinus, with either Kerrison punches or rongeurs. The width of the suturectomy is based on surgeon preference, weighing the risk of suture recrudescence against the need for future cranioplasty if significant bony regrowth does not occur. Venous bleeding is controlled with the use of cottonoid patties, bipolar electrocautery, and

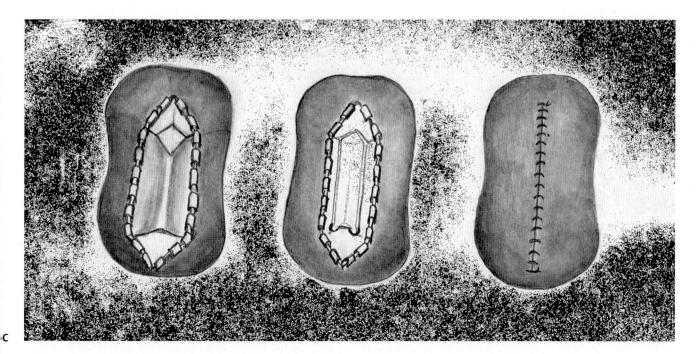

C

Fig. 9.2 Operative technique for early strip craniectomy. **(A)** Exposure of the sagittal suture. **(B)** Craniotomy. **(C)** Closure.

surgical hemostatic matrix. Following copious irrigation, the incision is then closed with resorbable sutures in the galea and a running resorbable suture through the scalp (**Fig. 9.2C**). We have not endorsed the use of drains.

Morbidity and mortality of craniosynostosis repair often have as much to do with anesthetic considerations as they do with surgical considerations. Armored endotracheal tubes are typically used to minimize potential compromise of the tube and ensure adequate ventilation throughout the operative case. Arterial lines are needed to maintain continuous blood pressure monitoring and blood sampling during the case and the immediate postoperative period. Central venous lines may also be inserted to allow for rapid transfusion of blood products and fluids as needed. The infant's core body temperature must be closely monitored, even in suturectomies, which expose less surface area than CVR. The surgeon must maintain meticulous hemostasis throughout the case, and the anesthesia team must closely monitor blood loss (often hidden in lap pads) and replace blood products early. Positioning the infant in the supine position with modest head elevation (< 30 degrees) reduces venous bleeding without significantly increasing the risk of venous air embolism.

Postoperative Treatment

Patients are generally extubated immediately following the case and cared for in the pediatric intensive care unit until they have achieved hemodynamic stabilization. We transfuse for hematocrits < 22, platelets < 100, or an international normalized ratio (INR) > 1.3. Scheduled alternating ibuprofen and Tylenol is used for pain control. The entire hospital stay rarely exceeds 4 days.

Adjuvant Treatment

In addition to a simple strip craniectomy, many devices exist on the market today to prevent restenosis of the excised sutures and aid in correction of the scaphocephalic shape. Although the strip craniectomy alone often corrects the biparietal dimension, it can fail in the correction of the anteroposterior elongation. This is where additional operative techniques and external devices may play a critical role.

Bone Growth Inhibitors

Silastic and other plastic strips have been used to impede regrowth of bone at the suture site. Although effective at preventing suture recrudescence, their use has fallen out of favor in an effort to avoid permanent implants. Another effort to reduce bony regrowth involved applying Zecker solution to the underlying dura. However, its predisposition to lowering the seizure threshold has reduced its usage. New research has focused on the use of Noggin, a bone morphogenetic protein (BMP) inhibitor, to prevent postoperative resynostosis in infants with craniosynostosis.[21] Preliminary data on rabbits are promising, but further clinical correlates are needed.

Helmets

For centuries, various civilizations have demonstrated the effectiveness of external pressure on molding cranial shape. Skull-molding caps were originally designed over 30 years ago to provide additional cranial molding after surgery. These devices have been demonstrated to result in greatly improved cranial shapes than those created by surgery alone.[22] Although surgical correction is still the mainstay of treatment for craniosynostosis, modern molding helmet therapy continues to be a valuable tool in promoting normal growth patterns postoperatively, even after a helmeting course is completed.[23,24] Patients typically wear a series of two helmets over the course of 1 to 2 years to promote gradual remodeling over time. It is unknown whether helmeting alone would be effective for sagittal synostosis, as this has not been studied secondary to the lack of funding for correction of scaphocephaly in the absence of surgical repair.

Springs

Since the late 1990's, Lauritzen has pioneered the use of internal springs to correct nonsyndromic sagittal suture synostosis. His studies of strip craniectomy combined with placement of internal springs at an average age of 3 to 4 months resulted in efficacious treatment of sagittal synostosis.[25] Further studies comparing spring-assisted cranial remodeling with external helmeting would be advantageous.

Outcomes

Although substantial research has been conducted to elucidate any impact of craniosynostosis on long-term cognitive development, no clear association has been made. Certainly, learning disabilities do exist in this population of patients; however, the frequency does not seem to be affected by surgical intervention.[26,27] The more commonly reported measure of surgical outcomes for sagittal synostosis is the cephalic index (CI), an easily calculated ratio of width to length based on CT scans. However, this is an imperfect grading scale, as it may fail to account for "hourglass" bitemporal distortion of severe frontal or occipital bossing. This leaves us with a photographic aesthetics end point, which is more or less subjective, often based on the child's and the parents' perspective as they age.[28,29]

Conclusion

A simple strip craniectomy with or without an external molding device is an option for the correction of nonsyndromic, isolated sagittal synostosis without frontal bossing or an occipital prominence in infants younger than 3 months of age. Newer techniques involving retrievable springs may provide a reasonable alternative to helmeting. For older infants or those exhibiting signs of more extensive suture fusion, CVR would be indicated.

♦ Late Craniofacial Reconstruction

Oliver Simmons

Sagittal synostosis, the premature fusion of the sagittal suture, is the most common form of craniosynostosis. It is generally not recognized until scaphocephaly becomes clinically observable. Sagittal synostosis accounts for 40 to 60% of single-suture synostoses. It is generally accepted that the incidence of scaphocephaly ranges from 1 in 2000 to 1 in 5000 live births.[30] The skull deformity resulting from premature closure of the sagittal suture is predictable. Transverse growth of the skull will be restricted, and the calvarium will be long anteroposteriorly and narrow in the temporoparietal region with ridges at the site of the fused suture (**Fig. 9.3**). Schmelzer et al[31] identified four predictable patterns of calvarial dysmorphology in patients with scaphocephaly: bifrontal bossing, bitemporal retrusion, coronal constriction, and occipital protuberance (**Fig. 9.4**).

The etymology of the word *scaphocephaly* indicates this clinical appearance (from the Greek *scaphos*, meaning "boat," and *kephaly*, meaning "head"). Additional changes such as frontal and occipital bossing will vary among individuals. Signs of scaphocephaly will usually present between 1 and 4 months of age and should be identified by an astute pediatrician.

The etiopathogenesis of primary scaphocephaly remains mainly unknown. Multiple theories have been offered. Virchow, in 1851, initially proposed that the suture was the primary abnormality and was translated to the cranial base. More than 100 years later, Moss, in 1955, theorized that tension at the cranial base was translated to the cranial vault suture. It is now relatively well accepted that misregulation in apoptosis might be related to early maturation of cranial sutures.[32] Furthermore, environmental and genetic factors play a role in the pathogenesis of scaphocephaly. As shown by the work of Lajeunie et al,[33] a genetic component is supported by the higher risk in monozygotic twins, whereas the presence of an environmental component is reinforced by the high rate of twinning, normal monozygotic/dizygotic twin ratio, and a < 100% concordance rate in monozygotic twins.

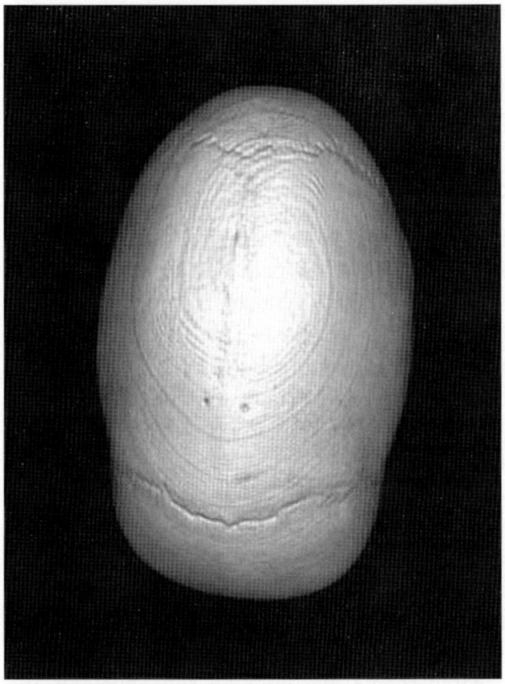

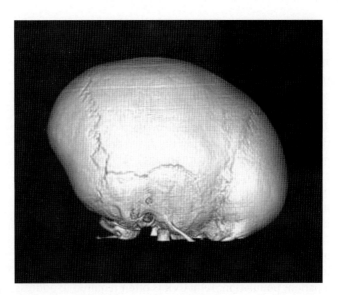

Fig. 9.3 Three-dimensional computed tomography (CT) scan showing the fused sagittal suture and increased length-to-width ratio of the calvarium.

Fig. 9.4 Three-dimensional CT scan of a patient with scaphocephaly showing the prominent occipital protuberance.

Diagnosis

Clinical examination will often be sufficient to develop suspicion of isolated sagittal synostosis. Some centers routinely request CT scans to confirm their clinical diagnosis. Such studies not only allow confirmation of a clinical diagnosis but can also be used for presurgical planning and will provide another tool to follow these patients and objectively evaluate outcomes. Nevertheless, this represents radiation that might be construed as unnecessary by some. In fact, the work of Agrawal et al[34] elegantly showed that diagnosis and treatment planning of isolated sagittal synostosis can be reliably made clinically.

The CI represented by the maximal transverse width (euryon–euryon) divided by the maximum anteroposterior length (glabella–opisthocranium) is reduced.[35] It is usually calculated using a digital caliper from a CT study of the patient's calvarium. Normal head shape has an average CI of 76 to 78%. Classically, infants with isolated sagittal craniosynostosis will have a CI from 60 to 67%. These measurements can also be performed clinically, but the soft tissue envelope must be taken into consideration.

Radiology

In the past, several radiologic examinations were used to diagnose and treat the synostosis. Plain radiographs are used to show sclerosis and occasionally show "thumb printing" as a sign of increased intracranial pressure (ICP). These are also of historic significance, because of the widespread and easy access to CT scans. Magnetic resonance imaging (MRI) is of limited use in the bony anatomy and is mostly used to evaluate for subtle posterior fossa brain parenchyma deformities, such as Chiari malformations.

Treatment Planning

Treatment goals of scaphocephaly are to increase the potential space and reorient the vectors of cerebral growths, restore the cerebrospinal fluid dynamics, and improve the cosmetic appearance of the skull by reshaping the cranial vault. The latter is performed by correcting the deformational changes and excising the fused suture. When diagnosed early (before 6 months of age), this can be done using sagittal strip craniectomy and outfracture of the parietal bone. In cases where the patient presents between 6 and 12 months of age, subtotal calvarectomy with vault remodeling is typically performed and will be discussed here.

Late presentation (age 12 months and older) represents a more complex problem, as represented by more severe clinical findings. Weinzweig et al[36] reviewed their experience in a patient population. Total CVR is often required to address the fronto-orbital deformity. This can be performed in a single- or two-stage approach. When a staged procedure is planned, the fronto-orbital deformity is addressed at the same time as the anterior two thirds of the calvarium in the initial stage. Staging a procedure will decrease the operative time and the blood loss. Despite refinements in the management of delayed presentation, early diagnosis remains the best way of simplifying and directing the management of isolated sagittal suture synostosis.

Surgical Management

Preoperative Management

General guidelines for safe management of the craniofacial patient rely heavily on communication among all parties involved. The anesthesiologist sees the patient preoperatively and assesses the overall health of the child and his or her fitness to receive the operation outlined. Risks of large volumes of blood loss as well as the potential for air emboli make it necessary in all but the most minor intracranial procedure to establish arterial lines and central venous access and to place a precordial Doppler, as well as an end-tidal CO_2 monitor.

Surgical teams place a Foley catheter for urine measurement. The patient is positioned to pad all bony prominences. Typically, patients are positioned supine for a suturectomy. The patient who needs a posterior expansion is placed in a Mayfield horseshoe that has been triple padded with cotton to prevent facial pressure sores. Because the eyes are the most sensitive structure on the face, both the anesthesiologist and the surgeon must confirm that they are covered or have no pressure on them. Prior to this, the eyes are lubricated and covered in Tegaderm mesh dressing. Anterior advancements are done in the supine position, on a Mayfield horseshoe headrest.

Surgical Techniques

Since the earliest days of treatment, surgical techniques have been described to correct this pediatric deformity. They were first described for sagittal synostosis mainly because it is the most often detected synostosis. These techniques were aimed at correcting the deformity by re-creating what was not present in nature, the sagittal suture. These techniques were mainly employed when the surgery was felt to be safe and have been used on younger and younger patients to yield better results.

Although suturectomy is the mainstay in early treatment, it relies totally on the growth of the head to correct the deformity. These techniques have been augmented by the use of helmet therapy that had traditionally been used with nonsynosotic plagiocephalic children. Newer techniques, such as endoscopic repair, are pushing the envelope and allowing more osteotomies for reshaping that were not previously possible. They all, however, rely on the growth of the head and the helmet to reshape the patient postoperatively.

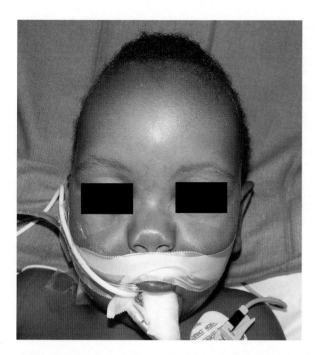

Fig. 9.5 Narrow biparietal distance with pseudoturricephaly.

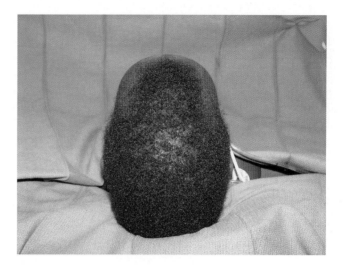

Fig. 9.6 Narrow biparietal distance.

Because the main risks of mortality in surgery are related to sagittal sinus injury, I do not believe that closed/endoscopic repairs are necessarily safer than other repairs as has been reported.[37] The main advantage I see to endoscopic repair is the fact that blood transfusions are not needed. Because of this, I am an advocate for earlier surgery whenever possible and minimal surgery when there is significant growth left and the family is committed to using a helmet to recontour the head. However, I treat most of my cases as standard open approaches, mainly because parents are not always willing to commit to the use of a helmet. It is inconvenient, time-consuming, and cannot be used to overcompensate the head to take into account future growth.

The majority of my patients are therefore not candidates for endoscopic techniques. The greatest advantage of the open approach is what I call the "what you see is what you get" result. Patients seem to come in two distinct groups: early presenters, who are treated without plastic surgery, and later presenters, who already have secondary deformations that I feel are not addressed with suturectomy techniques.

Preferred Technique

My technique is based on a modification of the "Pi" technique.[38] Typically, patients are photographed in the supine position before being turned prone (**Figs. 9.3, 9.4,** and **9.5**). Most first surgeries are posterior expansions. This provides the clear advantage in sagittal synostosis, as the main defect is the biparietal narrowness (**Fig. 9.6**). These patients if

caught early enough have only mild amounts of frontal bossing that does not typically require anterior remodeling (**Fig. 9.7**). A strip of bone left over the sagittal sinus is maintained, and instead of single larger osteotomies in the front, we perform multiple shorter osteotomies throughout the length of the bar (**Fig. 9.8**). This accomplishes two things. First, multiple short osteotomies allow for the necessary 1.5 cm or more of head shortening that is necessary for the remodeling, as well as for a gentler contour of the upper skull. A single osteotomy allows the bone to shift but not to round out in direction. Second, multiple osteotomies limit the amount of torque or tension on the dura in the region of the sagittal sinus.

Next, the deformed and overly flattened (**Figs. 9.9** and **9.10**) lateral "clam shells" of bone are reshaped by closing

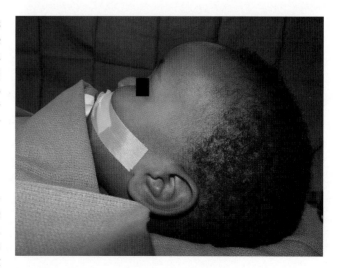

Fig. 9.7 Mild anterior bossing and posterior bossing.

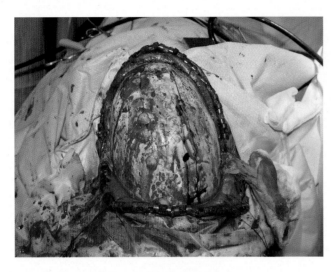

Fig. 9.8 Prone with bicoronal flaps and bur holes.

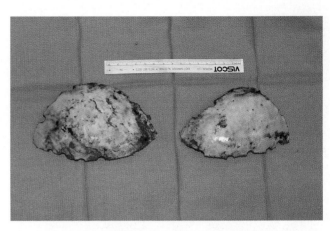

Fig. 9.9 Overly narrow "clam shells" with severe narrowed biparietal distance.

wedge osteotomies and switching from one side to the other, then performing closing wedge osteotomies on the flattened side and opening osteotomies on the overly rounded top portion (**Figs. 9.11, 9.12,** and **9.13**). The switching of the sides makes it easier to obtain the bilateral 1 to 2 cm of expansion needed for the midvault.

Lateral "barrel stave" osteotomies, as described by Persing et al,[39] are made down the remaining portion of the lateral skull to the skull base to allow for expansion of the noncraniectomized portion of the skull (**Fig. 9.14**). Finally, the posterior occipital bulge is infractured and plated in place (**Fig. 9.15**). The bone gaps are filled in with a mixture of bone paste and cut bones, as well as a sandwich of Surgicel (**Fig. 9.16**). This results in a normal head shape (**Fig. 9.17**).

Postoperative Outcomes

Fearon et al reviewed their experience in the surgical management of scaphocephaly of 89 patients treated predominantly with posterior cranial vault expansion.[40] They found a statistically significant decrease in cranial vault growth both in breadth and length, with expected growth in width being more affected. The poor growth observed may be related to an intrinsic problem that led to sagittal synostosis in the first place. Nevertheless, a trend toward normalization of the CI was noted. None of the patients in their series required or elected to undergo frontal remodeling after follow-up of up to 14 years. Given these findings, the goal of scaphocephaly correction should aim at overcorrection of the presenting deformity.[40]

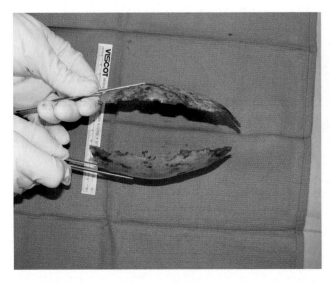

Fig. 9.10 Severely flattened "clam shells."

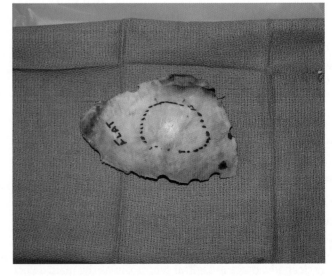

Fig. 9.11 Marked for flat and rounded areas.

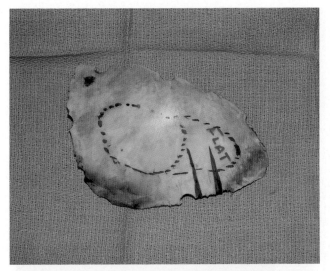

A

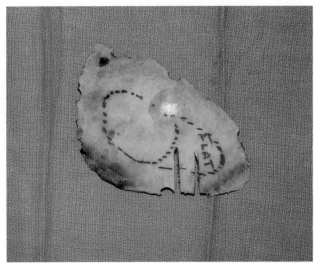

B

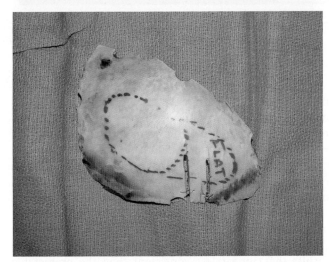

C

Fig. 9.12 (A–C) Plan for closing wedge osteotomy to round out the flat portions of the bone.

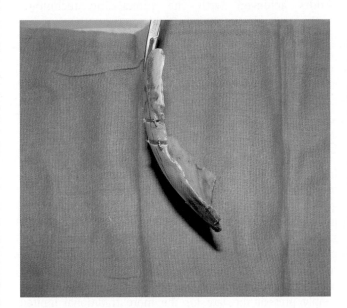

Fig. 9.13 Rounded out lateral "clams shells."

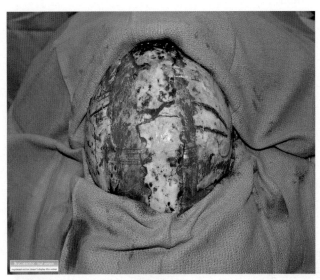

Fig. 9.14 Bones expanded and lateral "barrel staves" on the base of the skull, with transverse osteotomies to shorten the front-to-back distance.

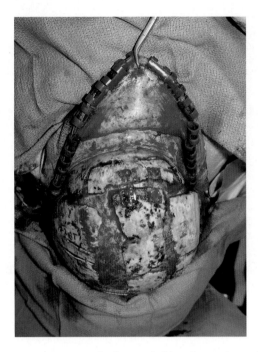

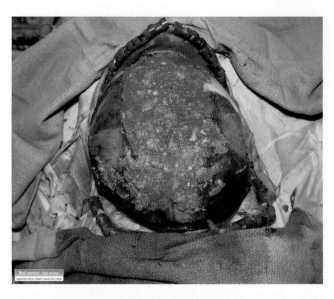

Fig. 9.16 DBX and bone chips fill in the gaps.

Fig. 9.15 Occipital infracture held in place with resorbable plates.

The reoperation rate in patients with single-suture sagittal synostosis has been reported to be 4.35% in patients who underwent strip craniectomy and 6.45% in patients who underwent CVR.[41] This difference may be explained by more severe deformation that requires more extensive initial surgery, leading to a higher risk of a secondary procedure. McCarthy et al[42] designed the "hung span" technique to address patients with scaphocephaly and persistent increase in ICP, which is unusual. It not only allows increasing the intracranial volume but also restores cranial vault harmony.

Arnaud et al[43] investigated the cognitive development of patients with nonsyndromic isolated sagittal suture synostosis. No statistically significant difference was noted in cognitive development of patients who were treated surgically versus patients who did not undergo surgery. There is a general consensus, though, that further investigation is required to elucidate the impact of isolated sagittal synostosis on neurodevelopment.[44]

Since the early 1990s, the minimally invasive philosophy has been applied to the management of scaphocephaly. Drawbacks of the endoscopic approach include results that appear less consistent than the predictable results achieved with the remodeling technique. Furthermore, the results rely highly on the patient's wearing a custom-made helmet for up to 1 year. Finally, performing a craniectomy with such a limited exposure potentially places the patient at greater risk for serious complications compared with an open procedure, especially if bleeding is encountered.

Discussion

Initial techniques of surgery for synostosis were geared toward simply removing the fused suture and allowing for growth to fix the problem. The initial approach to surgery just re-created what was there in nature and allowed for growth; the ensuing repair of the deformity relied on a complete intraoperative treatment that allowed for immediate reshaping of the skull. Although there are many treatment options for children with this condition, frequently patients simply present too late for the more traditional limited approach. In these cases, I feel that endoscopic treatment is

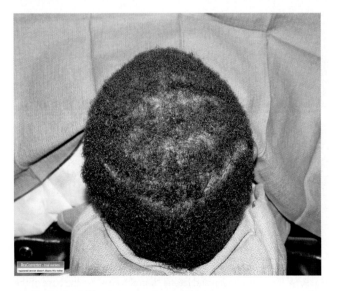

Fig. 9.17 On-table postoperative result.

too limited and unpredictable. The posterior expansion followed by an anterior reconstruction if needed allows for safe and easy increase in volume and shape of the skull. This is the tried-and-true method that allows on-the-table reliable change and does not require prolonged helmet wear and additional growth for reconstruction.

♦ Endoscopic Wide Vertex Craniectomy

David F. Jimenez, Constance M. Barone, and James N. Rogers

Sagittal synostosis, along with the scaphocephaly with which it typically presents, remains the most common type of craniosynostosis and the one most likely to be seen at a neurosurgical or craniofacial practice. Many surgical approaches have been developed to treat this condition, and favorable results are often obtained. However, excellent long-lasting results are difficult to obtain consistently regardless of the type of procedure done. A major contributor to this problem is the intrinsic, genetically driven dural forces that revert the operated cranium back to the presurgical scaphocephalic shape. Consequently, long-term follow-up of these patients commonly reveals suboptimal results in patients treated either with strip craniectomies or extensive calvarial remodeling techniques. During the last 10 years, we have been advocating the use of minimally invasive endoscopic techniques to perform endoscope-assisted wide vertex craniectomies and bilateral temporal and parietal wedge osteotomies, along with postoperative cranial orthotic treatment, to achieve excellent long-term results. We present our experience with this approach and strongly advocate its use.

Clinical Materials

Patient Demographics

A total of 185 patients presenting with the diagnosis of sagittal synostosis were treated with an endoscope-assisted wide vertex craniectomy and bilateral temporal and parietal wedge osteotomies, as well as postoperative helmet molding, between May 1997 and August 2007. There were 136 male patients (73.5%) and 49 female patients (26.5%). Following surgery, all patients were treated with custom-made Surlyn (Dupont, Wilmington, Delaware) helmets for up to 12 months. The patients were closely followed during the 12 months and then yearly thereafter.

Anesthesia

Craniosynostosis repair in infants is usually seen as one of the more critical anesthetic challenges for an anesthesiologist. Pediatric anesthesia textbooks describe at length the challenges to be faced during surgery, with a major concern being the extreme blood loss associated with these procedures. In fact, the recommendation is to have blood available immediately at the beginning of the surgery and to replace the blood lost, milliliter for milliliter, as the case begins. Venous air emboli and ventilation difficulties are other serious concerns. The usual long duration of the surgery often leads to significant heat loss and major fluid shifts that require aggressive monitoring, such as arterial lines and central venous catheters.

Endoscopic strip craniectomy for sagittal synostosis, with its minimal blood loss and short duration, significantly reduces the risks of surgery. Blood loss is typically minimal, making the need for blood transfusion unlikely. Major fluid shifts are minimized, necessitating only maintenance fluids for the duration of the case. Arterial lines and central venous catheters are unnecessary because hemodynamic stability is easily maintained. Preoperative laboratories are dictated by the patient's medical history. A minimum of a preoperative hematocrit is obtained for later comparison postoperatively.

Induction of anesthesia is accomplished with mask inhalation of sevoflurane in the operative suite after placement of two pulse oximeters, electrocardiogram, and non-invasive blood pressure monitors. Preoperative sedation with midazolam is usually not needed because the patients are too young to have separation anxiety issues. After induction, a peripheral intravenous (IV) line is placed in an extremity, and muscle relaxant is administered prior to intubation. After induction and securing the endotracheal tube, the patient is placed in the "sphinx" position, 180 degrees away from the anesthesia machine and the anesthesiologist. Close attention to padding of pressure points is important, even in short cases, to reduce the risk of nerve or skin injury. A preoperative hematocrit is obtained and sent to the laboratory. Prior to incision, antibiotics are administered, and 1 to 2 μg/kg of fentanyl are given. Maintenance of anesthesia is maintained with inhalation agents and muscle relaxants as needed.

Airway stability is always of critical importance, especially in infants. The sphinx position, with the patient prone, neck extended, and head elevated, can easily dislodge the endotracheal tube. Close attention to breath sounds with the change in position will allow immediate correction, before the patient is prepped and draped. Once the proper position is obtained, the tube should be well secured and a throat pack inserted to minimize leakage. The airway circuit is secured with tape to the operating room table to keep tension off the endotracheal tube. Eye care is provided with corneal shields or pads. We monitor all patients for possible venous air embolism with the placement of an appropriately padded precordial Doppler. Normothermia is maintained throughout the case with the use of a standard pediatric air flow body warmer.

Because the head is elevated above the heart in the sphinx position, air embolism is a concern but is typically not clinically significant. However, because infants are likely to have a patent ductus, the possibility of a right-to-left shunt, with the risk of a cerebral air embolism, is still a concern. A precordial Doppler monitor should be positioned over the heart to identify an air embolism quickly. It should be carefully padded to minimize pressure on the chest, as the patient will be in the prone sphinx position. IV lines should be flushed of all air. Close attention to hemostasis and adequate hydration of the patient significantly reduces the incidence of embolism. End-tidal CO_2 monitoring can also aid in identifying an embolism. If an air embolism is detected, the surgeons are immediately notified and the head lowered and the field flooded until control can be established.

As in all pediatric cases, maintenance of temperature is critical. A warm operating room, warming lights, and air blankets are used as indicated to maintain patient temperature. Muscle relaxation is important to make sure there is no patient movement during the surgical procedure. Rectal acetaminophen and local anesthesia when closing are helpful in minimizing postoperative pain.

After completion of the surgery, the anesthetic agents are discontinued, and muscle relaxant reversal agents are administered. A postoperative hematocrit is obtained and sent to the laboratory for comparison. The patient is placed again in the supine position, suctioned, and extubated when responsive and breathing spontaneously. The patient is then transported to the postoperative care unit with supplemental oxygen and pulse oximetry monitoring. Additional fentanyl may be needed if discomfort is evident.

Surgical Procedure

Positioning

The patient is placed in a modified prone (sphinx) position on a viscoelastic mat. The table is turned 180 degrees from the anesthesia team, and the surgeons work at the head of the infant with full access to the frontal and occipital areas. The scalp is minimally shaved, and the head is prepped with povidone–iodine solution.

Surgical Technique

To gain access to the subgaleal space, two incisions (2–3 cm in length) are made, with the epicenter over the sagittal suture. The anterior incision is made ~2 cm behind the anterior fontanelle, and the posterior incision is made immediately in front of the lambda. Using a monopolar (needle-tip) handpiece set at 15 W, a bloodless dissection plane is developed between the galea and pericranium. The plane of dissection is extended from the anterior fontanelle to the lambda and ~3 cm from the midline bilaterally.

A pediatric craniotome (7 mm) is used to make a bur hole on the lateral edge (on one side) of each incision. Osteotomies are created across the midline with Kerrison rongeurs (6 mm). After developing an epidural plane toward the anterior fontanelle, a wedge of bone is removed extending from the anterior ostectomy to the anterior fontanelle. A 30-degree rigid endoscope is inserted under the cranial bone and used to visualize the undersurface of the cranium and the posterior edge of the fontanelle.

The endoscope is held with the nondominant hand. A suction tip is handled with the dominant hand, which is used as an aspirating dissector. A plane is developed between the dura and the overlying bone by advancing the endoscope and suction tip in unison. Developing this plane is fairly easy, given the fact that stenosis of the suture frees the dural attachment fibers from the overlying bone. By gently pushing down on the dura with these instruments, the plane can be rapidly developed between the anterior and posterior osteotomies and several centimeters bilaterally from the midline (**Figs. 9.18** and **9.19**). Once the bone has been isolated from the overlying scalp and underlying dura, a pair of Mayo scissors are used to cut ostectomies on the lateral edges of the anterior and posterior osteotomies. The cut piece of bone can be sectioned or folded in two and removed from one of the scalp incisions. A large piece of Gelfoam is then placed over the dura, and light pressure is applied to the overlying scalp to obtain hemostasis. Wedge osteotomies are

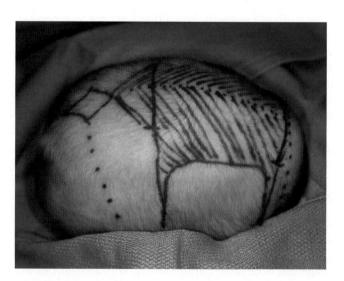

Fig. 9.18 Lateral view of the scalp showing the wedge-shaped osteotomies of the temporal (behind the coronal suture) and parietal (in front of the lambdoid suture) areas.

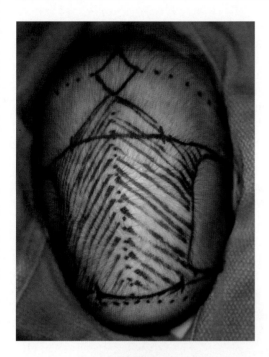

Fig. 9.19 Top view of the scalp demonstrates markings of the vertex craniectomy. The frontal incision is placed 2 to 3 cm behind the anterior fontanelle (AF); a wedge craniectomy is directed anteriorly to the AF and connected to the lateral wedge osteotomies.

made bilaterally posterior to each coronal suture and anterior to each lambdoid suture. Hemostasis from the diploic space is achieved by using suction–electrocautery (60 W) and cauterizing all edges of the calvaria that have been osteotomized. The scalp incisions are closed with absorbable Vicryl sutures and the skin with Steri-Strips and Mastisol.

Postoperative Care

The patient is observed overnight and discharged the following morning. Most commonly, some discomfort will be experienced for about 8 hours following surgery; then the patient returns to baseline. Pain is managed by treating the patient with alternating doses of acetaminophen and ibuprofen augmented with nalbuphine hydrochloride and morphine as needed for adequate pain control. Unlike traditional vault remodeling procedures, there is virtually no facial or cranial soft tissue swelling, and the patient does not experience pyrexia. On the fourth postoperative day, the head is scanned, and on the sixth day a custom-made helmet is delivered and properly fitted. The helmet is worn for ~6 to 8 weeks, then new ones are resized and worn for up to 10 to 12 months.

Results

Using CI measurements and standard anteroposterior, lateral, and top photographs, as well as selective occasional CT scans and plain radiographs, the patient is followed up at 6 weeks,

3 months, 6 months, 9 months, 12 months, 18 months, and yearly thereafter. Most patients we have treated have been closely followed up to the present time. One hundred and eighty-five patients were consecutively treated during a 10-year period. Seventy-three percent were male, and 26% were female. The mean age at the time of surgery was 3.7 months, with a median of 3.0 months. The mean width of the craniectomy size was 5.5 cm and mean length 10.5 cm. The mean estimated blood loss was 27 cc. The mean percent of estimated blood volume loss was 5.5%. The mean surgical time was 62 minutes. The mean length of hospitalization was 1.1 day, with 177 patients staying only 1 night (96%) and discharged the morning following surgery. Blood transfusions were required in 15 patients (8%), and only 2 patients (1%) were transfused intraoperatively. Complications included two postoperative deaths (1% mortality rate). In both cases, the surgeries were performed without technical problems. One patient developed systemic and massive hemolysis, and the second developed arterial and venous thromboses. In both cases the patient's parents requested removal of life support. Other complications included five superficial scalp irritations (early in the series) that healed with helmet removal for several days and local therapy. There was a minor sagittal sinus injury (cautery related) that was easily treated with a single suture. There were three dural tears with no intraparenchymal injuries that were primarily repaired with no untoward effects. Using CI as an outcome measure, results were rated as excellent: CI > 75, good: CI 81–75, and poor: CI < 70. The mean preoperative CI was 67. Using these criteria, we obtained 87.0% excellent, 8.7% good, and 4.3% poor results. These results were extensively correlated with standard photographic documentation.

Discussion

Our experience treating patients with sagittal craniosynostosis over a 20-year period includes the use of many surgical techniques, which include simple strip craniectomies, Pi procedures, reverse Pi, bifrontal craniotomies, biparietal craniotomies, vertex craniotomies, and various calvarial vault (CVR) techniques (e.g., Marchac transposition).[45-52] Our results with these techniques have been mixed. Early results in most cases are very good (6–12 months), but when followed long term, there is significant deterioration and return to baseline scaphocephalic shapes.[53] Additionally, the use of titanium plates and screws have been associated with several complications, which include dural and cortical penetration, as well as extrusion and skin breakdown and pseudocapsule formation.

Another concern has been the significant trauma and stress associated with extensive calvarial remodeling techniques. Large blood losses and voluminous blood transfusions are the norm.[54] Marked facial and cranial bruising and swelling are the rule. Consequently, we have attempted to obtain consistently superior results while minimizing the trauma and blood transfusion rates associated with traditional procedures. The basic concept is to operate on a very young infant,[55–58] minimizing blood loss, tissue damage, and injury while using the rapid brain growth phase to restore normalcy to the cranial base and vault. As such, we introduced the concept of minimizing the scalp incision with the use of endoscopes to achieve the necessary dissection planes below the galea and above the dura. Once the bone is fully exposed, the major osteotomies can be safely made in a circumferential fashion. A very important step in minimizing blood loss has

been the use of the suction–electrocautery unit (Valley Laboratory, Valley Forge, Pennsylvania) set at 60 W, blend 1. The diploic space can be substantially cauterized until it is blackened and no longer bleeding. This maneuver prevents postoperative hematomas and negates the need for subgaleal drains.

We have been working over the past decade with Orthomerica (Orlando, Florida) and developed a protocol for producing consistently well-fitting helmets at reasonable prices. As the brain rapidly grows and the head changes in shape, most patients have to wear up to three helmets. The helmet therapy can be divided into three phases. Phase 1 aims

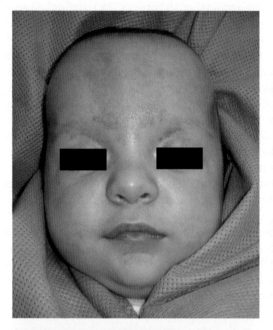

A

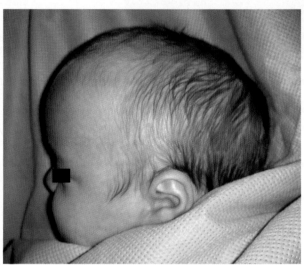

B

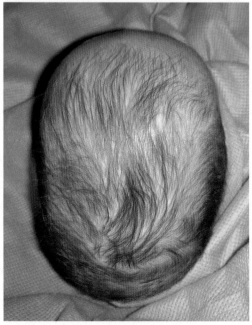

C

Fig. 9.20 (A) Four-month-old boy with sagittal synostosis and early and marked frontal bossing and bitemporal narrowing. **(B)** Side view of the same patient demonstrates significant frontal bossing. **(C)** Scaphocephalic shape is seen on the top view of the patient's head.

to correct the scaphocephalic into a normocephalic shape. Phase 2 aims to overcorrect and achieve a very round head with a CI > 80. Phase 3 is designed to keep the normal head shape and counteract the natural forces and tendency toward reverting to scaphocephaly. We consistently have noticed that whatever shape and CI a patient has at age 18 months, he or she will keep the same CI over the years to come. (The longest follow-up of 10 years corroborates this concept well.) We think that the failure of simple strip craniectomies has to do with the unopposed natural forces during the postoperative period, which can lead to unacceptable results.

We believe that we have achieved our goals given the high percentage of excellent results (87%) at the same time that we have had a very low transfusion rate (8%), low length of hospitalization (1 day), and short surgical times (1 hour). A commonly heard complaint from colleagues is in regards to the use of helmets following the surgery. It is our belief that the helmets play a crucial and essential role in the achievement of our final results. Skepticism about our approach to treating sagittal synostosis with endoscopic techniques has been repeatedly expressed by our colleagues since our first publication.[59] However, our short-term follow-up (**Figs. 9.18, 9.19, 9.20, 9.21,** and **9.22**) and

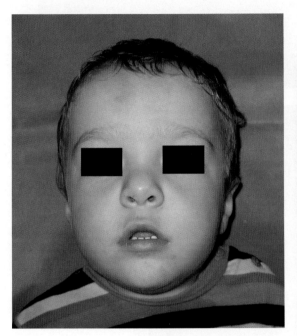

A

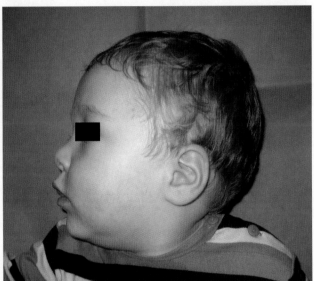

B

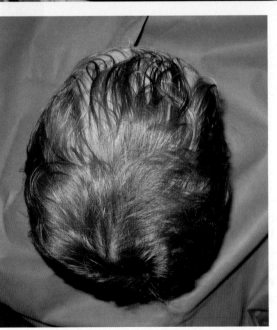

C

Fig. 9.21 (A) Frontal view 18 months after surgery shows lateral expansion of the temporal areas. **(B)** Correction of frontal bossing and recession of the forehead. **(C)** Correction of scaphocephaly and expansion of the parietal areas with rounding and normalization of the head.

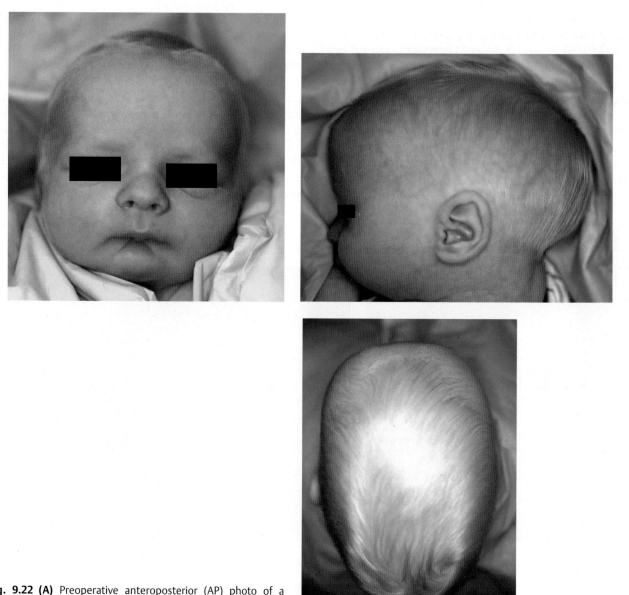

Fig. 9.22 (A) Preoperative anteroposterior (AP) photo of a 1-month-old boy with sagittal synostosis. **(B)** Lateral view shows prominent occipital protrusion and frontal bossing. **(C)** Top view demonstrates bifrontal enlargement and marked scaphocephaly.

long-term follow-up (**Figs. 9.23, 9.24, 9.25,** and **9.26**) demonstrate early and persistent correction of marked preoperative deformities. Furthermore, in most cases the scalp incisions are barely, if at all, visible, and the cranium and forehead exhibit no bumps, lumps, indentations, or prominent hardware. Anthropometric measurements (CI) collaborates long-standing correction of the patients' scaphocephaly. We attributed these results to early surgery and helmet therapy.

In summary, endoscope-assisted craniectomy, followed by well-tailored helmet therapy, is an excellent way to treat sagittal synostosis in an infant. It is associated with significantly less blood loss, lower transfusion rates, and shorter hospital stays. In the age of informed consent, this surgical alternative should be given to parents as a viable, safe, and effective option for treating this condition. Our 10-year data support the aforementioned conclusions.

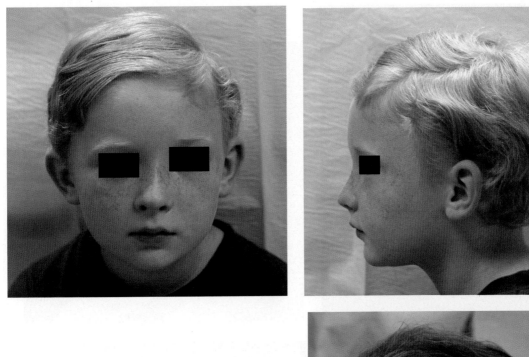

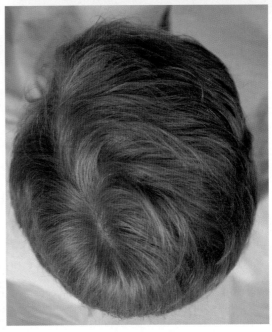

Fig. 9.23 (A) Long-term 9.5-year follow-up AP view demonstrates forehead normalization. **(B)** Lateral view reveals normocephaly with complete and sustained correction of the frontal and occipital abnormalities. **(C)** Top view displays a round and fully corrected scaphocephalic preoperative shape.

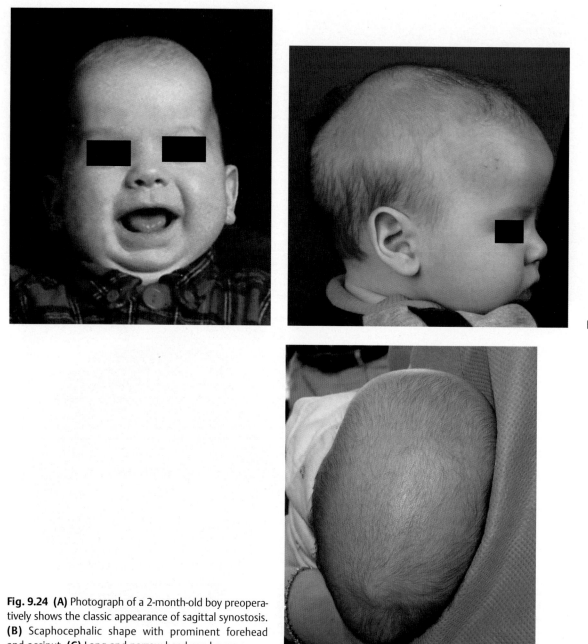

Fig. 9.24 **(A)** Photograph of a 2-month-old boy preoperatively shows the classic appearance of sagittal synostosis. **(B)** Scaphocephalic shape with prominent forehead and occiput. **(C)** Long and narrow head can be seen on a preoperative view from the top.

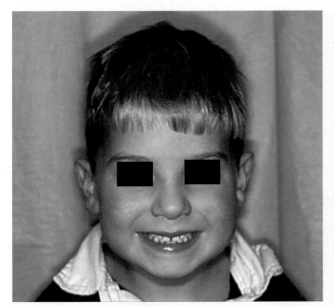

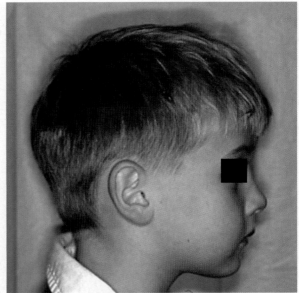

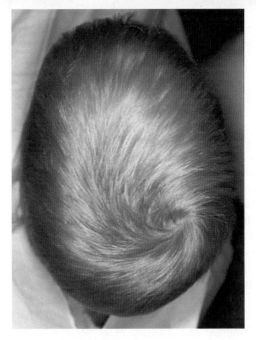

Fig. 9.25 **(A)** Four and a half years after surgery, normalization of the cranial vault can be appreciated. **(B)** Lateral view shows excellent forehead correction. **(C)** No longer scaphocephalic, biparietal expansion of the cranium can be noticed.

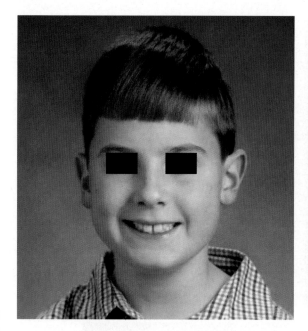 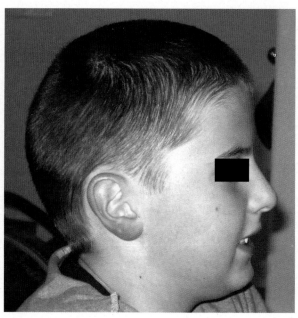

A   B

Fig. 9.26 (A) Photograph of the child 10.5 years after surgery demonstrates persistent correction of preoperative deformities. **(B)** Lateral view reveals continued improvement of the patient's forehead and occiput. The patient has no symptoms and is excelling at school.

♦ Lessons Learned

There has been considerable controversy about the optimal management of sagittal synostosis. The timing of surgery was disputed, but there is a reasonable consensus now that early surgery, preferably in the first 3 months of life, yields results similar to late reconstruction in terms of long-term correction of cranial deformity. Surely the question of optimal timing is determined by the time children are brought to the attention of the pediatric neurosurgeon. Surgical correction beyond the age of 6 months most certainly will require much more complex intervention than the issue discussed here. The authors are in agreement about the timing of surgery. Kiehna and Jane emphasize the open strip craniectomy technique, and Jimenez et al present their endoscope-assisted minimally invasive surgical technique. It all amounts to the same thing: operate early (i.e., around age 3 months), remove the synostotic sagittal suture, and provide the opening for growth of the brain on all sides. The open technique is indeed a rather easy standard. It is used by many pediatric neurosurgeons, probably with some technical variations, such as positioning and the use of lateral bone cuts ("barrel stave" osteotomies) to provide increased lateral diameter. The endoscope-assisted technique of Jimenez et al essentially employs a general and well-recognized surgical principle: minimize the size of the exposure and the size of the wound, and consequently the blood loss and the exposure of critical structures, such as the sagittal sinus. Given the flexibility of the infant's cranial

tissues and the malleability of the skull bone at this age, this technique continues to be intriguing, and the data appear to provide evidence for the notion of minimal invasiveness: smaller incisions, smaller blood loss, shorter hospital stay. Nonetheless, the technique has not erased mortality, and one wonders about the ease of stitching the sinus wall from two small incisions.

Whatever the issues of surgical technique may be, the basic principle of smaller wounds is valid and must be respected by all pediatric neurosurgeons regardless of their adoption of an endoscopic or endoscope-assisted or open surgical concept.

The late correction as advocated by Simmons illustrates the advantages of performing surgery at this time, but this does involve a longer operative time, more blood loss, and prolonged hospital stay. The advantages are the immediate correction of the deformity and no need for the molding orthosis.

From the editors' point of view, the treatment or covering of the incision or bone edges with presumably active solutions or implants is not a favored strategy. Perhaps future innovation will provide more convincing agents for this purpose.

The postoperative care with helmet molding as an adjunct to surgical correction is advocated by both groups. Jimenez et al stress the importance of genetic pressure to resynostosis. The opening of the suture and skull to the growth pressure of the brain at a critical juncture of brain development during the first year of life may in fact give way to a healthy "counterpressure" that works in favor of a more normal skull shape. Helmets in addition to surgery may not be acceptable to all pediatric neurosurgeons taking care of scaphocephalic children. A study that may provide evidence for the beneficial effect of such adjunctive measures, for instance, comparing operated patients with and without molding helmet treatment, would be highly desirable to settle this question.

References

1. Renier D, Sainte-Rose C, Marchac D, Hirsch JF. Intracranial pressure in craniostenosis. J Neurosurg 1982;57(3):370–377
2. Shillito JJ Jr, Matson DD. Craniosynostosis: a review of 519 surgical patients. Pediatrics 1968;41(4):829–853
3. Hunter AG, Rudd NL. Craniosynostosis: 1. Sagittal synostosis: its genetics and associated clinical findings in 214 patients who lacked involvement of the coronal suture(s). Teratology 1976;14(2): 185–193
4. Jane JA, Edgerton MT, Futrell JW, Park TS. Immediate correction of sagittal synostosis. J Neurosurg 1978;49(5):705–710
5. Marsh JL, Jenny A, Galic M, Picker S, Vannier MW. Surgical management of sagittal synostosis: a quantitative evaluation of two techniques. Neurosurg Clin N Am 1991;2(3):629–640
6. Boop FA, Shewmake K, Chadduck WM. Synostectomy versus complex cranioplasty for the treatment of sagittal synostosis. Childs Nerv Syst 1996;12(7):371–375
7. Pensler JM, Ciletti SJ, Tomita T. Late correction of sagittal synostosis in children. Plast Reconstr Surg 1996;97(7):1362–1367, discussion 1368–1370
8. Maugans TA, McComb JG, Levy ML. Surgical management of sagittal synostosis: a comparative analysis of strip craniectomy and calvarial vault remodeling. Pediatr Neurosurg 1997;27(3): 137–148
9. Jane JA, Persing JA. Neurosurgical treatment of craniosynostosis. In: Cohen MM, ed. Craniosynostosis: Diagnosis, Evaluation, and Management. New York: Raven Press; 1986:249–320
10. Kimonis V, Gold JA, Hoffman TL, Panchal J, Boyadjiev SA. Genetics of craniosynostosis. Semin Pediatr Neurol 2007;14(3):150–161
11. Ririe DG, David LR, Glazier SS, Smith TE, Argenta LC. Surgical advancement influences perioperative care: a comparison of two surgical techniques for sagittal craniosynostosis repair. Anesth Analg 2003;97(3):699–703
12. Faberowski LW, Black S, Mickle JP. Blood loss and transfusion practice in the perioperative management of craniosynostosis repair. J Neurosurg Anesthesiol 1999;11(3):167–172
13. Burstein FD, Hudgins RJ, Cohen SR, Boydston WR. Surgical correction of severe scaphocephalic deformities. J Craniofac Surg 1994;5(4):228–235, discussion 236
14. Chadduck WM, Chadduck JB, Boop FA. The subarachnoid spaces in craniosynostosis. Neurosurgery 1992;30(6):867–871
15. Jane JA Jr, Lin KY, Jane JA Sr. Sagittal synostosis. Neurosurg Focus 2000;9(3):e3
16. Delahaye S, Bernard JP, Rénier D, Ville Y. Prenatal ultrasound diagnosis of fetal craniosynostosis. Ultrasound Obstet Gynecol 2003; 21(4):347–353
17. Gordon IR. Measurement of cranial capacity in children. Br J Radiol 1966;39:377–381
18. Shillito J Jr. A plea for early operation for craniosynostosis. Surg Neurol 1992;37(3):182–188
19. Alvarez-Garijo JA, Cavadas PC, Vila MM, Alvarez-Llanas A. Sagittal synostosis: results of surgical treatment in 210 patients. Childs Nerv Syst 2001;17(1–2):64–68
20. Pensler JM, Ciletti SJ, Tomita T. Late correction of sagittal synostosis in children. Plast Reconstr Surg 1996;97(7):1362–1367, discussion 1368–1370
21. Cooper GM, Curry C, Barbano TE, et al. Noggin inhibits postoperative resynostosis in craniosynostotic rabbits. J Bone Miner Res 2007; 22(7):1046–1054
22. Persing JA, Nichter LS, Jane JA, Edgerton MT Jr. External cranial vault molding after craniofacial surgery. Ann Plast Surg 1986;17(4): 274–283
23. Seymour-Dempsey K, Baumgartner JE, Teichgraeber JF, Xia JJ, Waller AL, Gateno J. Molding helmet therapy in the management of sagittal synostosis. J Craniofac Surg 2002;13(5):631–635
24. Kaufman BA, Muszynski CA, Matthews A, Etter N. The circle of sagittal synostosis surgery. Semin Pediatr Neurol 2004;11(4):243–248
25. Lauritzen CG, Davis C, Ivarsson A, Sanger C, Hewitt TD. The evolving role of springs in craniofacial surgery: the first 100 clinical cases. Plast Reconstr Surg 2008;19(30):588–592
26. Kapp-Simon KA. Mental development and learning disorders in children with single suture craniosynostosis. Cleft Palate Craniofac J 1998;35(3):197–203
27. Gewalli F, Guimarães-Ferreira JP, Sahlin P, et al. Mental development after modified pi procedure: dynamic cranioplasty for sagittal synostosis. Ann Plast Surg 2001;46(4):415–420
28. Murray DJ, Kelleher MO, McGillivary A, Allcutt D, Earley MJ. Sagittal synostosis: a review of 53 cases of sagittal suturectomy in one unit. J Plast Reconstr Aesthet Surg 2007;60(9):991–997
29. Panchal J, Marsh JL, Park TS, Kaufman B, Pilgram T. Photographic assessment of head shape following sagittal synostosis surgery. Plast Reconstr Surg 1999;103(6):1585–1591
30. Panchal J, Uttchin V. Management of craniosynostosis. Plast Reconstr Surg 2003;111(6):2032–2048, quiz 2049
31. Schmelzer RE, Perlyn CA, Kane AA, Pilgram TK, Govier D, Marsh JL. Identifying reproducible patterns of calvarial dysmorphology in nonsyndromic sagittal craniosynostosis may affect operative intervention and outcomes assessment. Plast Reconstr Surg 2007; 119(5):1546–1552
32. Williams JK, Ellenbogen RG, Gruss JS. State of the art in craniofacial surgery: nonsyndromic craniosynostosis. Cleft Palate Craniofac J 1999;36(6):471–485
33. Lajeunie E, Crimmins DW, Arnaud E, Renier D. Genetic considerations in nonsyndromic midline craniosynostosis: a study of twins and their families. J Neurosurg 2005;103(4):353–356
34. Agrawal D, Steinbok P, Cochrane DD, Renier D. Diagnosis of isolated sagittal synostosis: are radiographic studies necessary? Childs Nerv Syst 2006;22(4):375–378
35. Ruiz-Correa S, Sze RW, Starr JR, et al. New scaphocephaly severity indices of sagittal craniosynostosis: a comparative study with cranial index quantifications. Cleft Palate Craniofac J 2006;43(2):211–221
36. Weinzweig J, Baker SB, Whitaker LA, Sutton LN, Bartlett SP. Delayed cranial vault reconstruction for sagittal synostosis in older children:

an algorithm for tailoring the reconstructive approach to the craniofacial deformity. Plast Reconstr Surg 2002;110(2):397–408

37. Jimenez DF, Barone CM. Endoscopy-assisted wide-vertex craniectomy, "barrel-stave" osteotomies, and postoperative helmet molding therapy in the early management of sagittal suture craniosynostosis. Neurosurg Focus 2000;9(3):e2

38. Boulos PT, Lin KY, Jane JA Jr, Jane JA Sr. Correction of sagittal synostosis using a modified Pi method. Clin Plast Surg 2004; 31(3):489–498, vii

39. Persing JA, Edgerton MT, Park TS, Jane JA. Barrel stave osteotomy for correction of turribrachycephaly craniosynostosis deformity. Ann Plast Surg 1987;18(6):488–493

40. Fearon JA, McLaughlin EB, Kolar JC. Sagittal craniosynostosis: surgical outcomes and long-term growth. Plast Reconstr Surg 2006;117(2):532–541

41. Williams JK, Cohen SR, Burnstein FD, Hudgins R, Boydston W, Simms C. A longitudinal, statistical study of reoperation rates in craniosynostosis. Plast Reconstr Surg 1997;100(2):305–310

42. McCarthy JG, Bradley JP, Stelnicki EJ, Stokes T, Weiner HL, Simms C. Hung span method of scaphocephaly reconstruction in patients with elevated intracranial pressure. Plast Reconstr Surg 2002; 109(6):2009–2018

43. Arnaud E, Renier D, Marchac D. Prognosis for mental function in scaphocephaly. J Neurosurg 1995;83(3):476–479

44. Speltz ML, Kapp-Simon KA, Cunningham M, Marsh J, Dawson G. Single-suture craniosynostosis: a review of neurobehavioral research and theory. J Pediatr Psychol 2004;29(8):651–668

45. Anderson FM, Geiger L. Craniosynostosis: a survey of 204 cases. J Neurosurg 1965;22:229–240

46. Anderson FM, Johnson FL. Craniosynostosis: a modification in surgical treatment. Surgery 1956;40(5):961–970

47. Boop FA, Shewmake K, Chadduck WM. Synostectomy versus complex cranioplasty for the treatment of sagittal synostosis. Childs Nerv Syst 1996;12(7):371–375

48. Davis CH Jr, Alexander E Jr, Kelly DL Jr. Treatment of craniosynostosis. J Neurosurg 1969;30(5):630–636

49. Drake DB, Persing JA, Berman DE, Ogle RC. Calvarial deformity regeneration following subtotal craniectomy for craniosynostosis: a case report and theoretical implications. J Craniofac Surg 1993;4(2): 85–89, discussion 90

50. Epstein N, Epstein F, Newman G. Total vertex craniectomy for the treatment of scaphocephaly. Childs Brain 1982;9(5):309–316

51. Greene CS Jr, Winston KR. Treatment of scaphocephaly with sagittal craniectomy and biparietal morcellation. Neurosurgery 1988; 23(2):196–202

52. Klein MF. La craniostenose. Neurochirurgia (Stuttg) 1961;4:65–79

53. Kanev PM, Lo AK. Surgical correction of sagittal craniosynostosis: complications of the Pi procedure. J Craniofac Surg 1995;6(2): 98–102

54. McComb JG. Occipital reduction–biparietal widening technique for correction of sagittal synostosis. Pediatr Neurosurg 1994;20(1): 99–106

55. McLaurin RL, Matson DD. Importance of early surgical treatment of crainosynostosis: review of 36 cases treated during the first 6 months of life. Pediatrics 1952;10(6):637–652

56. Olds MV, Storrs B, Walker ML. Surgical treatment of sagittal synostosis. Neurosurgery 1986;18(3):345–347

57. Shillito J Jr. A plea for early operation for craniosynostosis. Surg Neurol 1992;37(3):182–188

58. Teng P. Premature synostosis of the sagittal suture, and its treatment: a modification of the linear craniectomy and the use of synthetic fabrics. J Neurosurg 1962;19:1094–1097

59. Jimenez DF, Barone CM. Endoscopic craniectomy for early surgical correction of sagittal craniosynostosis. J Neurosurg 1998;88(1): 77–81

10 Deformational Plagiocephaly

♦ Correction with Repositioning and with Cranial Remodeling Orthosis

Olivier Vernet, Sandrine de Ribaupierre, and Bénédict Rilliet

Etymologically, the term *plagiocephaly* has Greek roots, *plagios* meaning "oblique" and *kephale* meaning "head." Posterior plagiocephaly refers to a flattening of the occiput. It can be caused by lambdoid synostosis, which is an extremely rare condition. For the vast majority of affected infants, posterior plagiocephaly is the consequence of abnormal forces acting on an intrinsically normal, developing cranium. This situation has been referred to by many names, such as positional or deformational posterior plagiocephaly, benign positional molding, occipital plagiocephaly, and nonsynostotic occipital plagiocephaly.

In 1992 the American Academy of Pediatrics recommended that infants be placed on their backs to sleep, because prone and, to a lesser extent, side sleeping had been correlated with sudden infant death syndrome (SIDS).[1] Beginning in 1992, and following the "Back to Sleep" campaign,"[2] numerous craniofacial centers documented an exponential increase in the diagnosis of posterior positional plagiocephaly (PPP).[3-5] Following an initial period of diagnostic and surgical roaming,[6] it became obvious that this abnormal skull shape was not the result of a craniosynostosis, but rather the consequence of unrelieved pressure onto the occiput during infant sleep.

Incidence

Premature lambdoid fusion is extremely rare; whereas the overall incidence of craniosynostosis is 6 per 10,000 live births, posterior plagiocephaly secondary to isolated lambdoid premature fusion occurs in only 3 cases per 100,000 births.[7-9] In contrast, over the past decade there was an increasing incidence of PPP,[3-5] which was reported in up to 48% of live births.[7,10] Three quarters of those patients with PPP were boys, and a majority of infants had right-sided plagiocephaly.[2,4,7,11-19]

Pathophysiology

Regarding the pathophysiologic mechanism of PPP, it is admitted that external force applied consistently to a specific region of the infant's head deforms the skull. If PPP is present at birth, it is likely the result of in utero or intrapartum molding. Associated conditions include uterine constraint such as multiple-infant birth, oligohydramnios, uterine malformation, macrocephaly, cervical spine anomaly or brain injury with asymmetrical spasticity, and birth injury associated with forceps or vacuum-assisted delivery.[3,4,8,9,13,18-23] Most of these cranial deformities improve spontaneously during the first months of life, except if the infant continues to rest his or her head on the flattened side of the occiput. In this situation, the occipital plagiocephaly may be perpetuated or become more pronounced by gravitational forces.[24] Numerous babies, however, have at birth a round skull shape that may become flattened occipitally as a result of static supine positioning, because of the current advice to nurse them in a supine position to prevent SIDS and because neonates have limited cervical muscle strength.[1-4,19] Mulliken et al[19] discussed the unresolved controversy over whether torticollis is secondary to the abnormal head shape in PPP or is the cause of this cranial deformity. Because of the finding that an infant with PPP who lies supine on the flattened occiput can have either ipsilateral or contralateral shortening of the sternocleidomastoid muscle, these authors suggested that intrauterine (and cranial posture) was determinant.[19]

Diagnosis

It is important to distinguish lambdoid craniosynostosis from PPP, because the course and the management of these two conditions are clearly different. True synostosis is habitually present from birth and is progressive. It never improves spontaneously and confers the risk of intracranial hypertension, although this happens in < 10% of cases when only a single suture is involved.[25]

In contrast, PPP is often subtle and goes unnoticed or is absent at birth. It develops during the first months of age and confers no risk of raised intracranial pressure. Thus, the diagnosis of PPP is made primarily on the basis of history, with special attention to the antenatal period, looking for evidence of intrauterine constraint.

Simple physical examination usually confirms the diagnosis of PPP.[7] In the vertex view, patients presenting with PPP demonstrate a parallelogram-shaped head: there is a flattening of one side of the posterior cranium, along with contralateral parieto occipital and ipsilateral frontal bossing, and the ipsilateral ear is displaced anteriorly. A cheekbone prominence may be observed ipsilaterally to the flattened occiput. Lambdoid synostosis also produces a flat occiput. However, in this situation, the vertex view reveals a trapezium-shaped head: there is a unilateral occipitoparietal flattening associated with contralateral frontal bossing. In addition, the area of the fused lambdoid suture may present as a bony ridge, with a bony prominence in the mastoid region behind the ear, which is displaced posteriorly and inferiorly.[26] The severity of PPP may be assessed by anthropometric measurements using calipers: with the infant's head held in a neutral position, two transverse fronto-occipital diameters are measured obliquely from each supraorbital region, to the parietooccipital region at the midpoint of the flattened area (short axis) and the contralateral point of maximal parietooccipital convexity (long axis). Additionally, anterior displacement of the ear ipsilateral to the flattened occiput may be evaluated by measuring the distance between the external auditory meatus and the external canthus on both sides. The physical examination should be completed with an assessment of neck movements to confirm or rule out the presence of torticollis.

Normally, there is no need for complementary radiologic investigations. However, if available, skull radiographs reveal in PPP a sclerotic margin parallel to a patent lambdoid suture on the side of the occipital flattening. This aspect, sometimes called "lazy lambdoid," must not be confused with a true lambdoid synostosis, where the suture is no longer visible.[15] Perisutural sclerosis, sutural narrowing, and increased digitations are not signs of impending synostosis.[19,24]

Treatment

The natural history of PPP is difficult to establish in the absence of reliable and reproducible data, which would allow practitioners to grade its severity. PPP has likely existed for centuries, although at a lower rate than today. This condition was probably less recognized in the past than over this last decade. It is estimated that > 70% of cases improve spontaneously.[11] This improvement may be encouraged by regular change in sleeping position and physiotherapy.[11,24,27] Severe positional skull deformations, however, may not always correct satisfactorily.[3,28,29] Even though there is little information about the true risks of leaving this condition untreated,[7] PPP is probably essentially a cosmetic problem without significant neurologic consequence.[3,11,29]

In the 1990s, when this condition became more recognized, surgical management was the chief response[6,11] until cranial remodeling helmets were developed.[12,30] The role of different therapeutic modalities has to be determined, and the management of infants with PPP remains controversial.

Repositioning

In the initial management of PPP, preventive counseling is of paramount importance. Because most of these occipital deformities develop during the first 2 months of age when the skull is maximally deformable, parents should be counseled shortly after birth. According to recommendations from the American Academy of Pediatrics, they should be encouraged to alternate the supine head position of the infant nightly. When awake and being observed, the infant should spend time in the prone position, with minimal time in a car seat (when not a passenger in a vehicle).[23] It is not uncommon that occipital flattening is either absent or subtle in the neonatal period. If the parents were not taught these preventive strategies, PPP may develop progressively and be noticed later on, usually by 2 to 3 months, at the first visit to the pediatrician. Once deformational posterior plagiocephaly is diagnosed, parents should be made aware of this condition and be given the same preventive counseling, to minimize progression of PPP. In addition, the infant's room should be arranged so that the crib is placed to require the child to turn away from the flat side to see objects of interest in the room (e.g., parents, window, door, and toys). The prone position should continue to be encouraged when the infant is awake and being observed. If torticollis is present, physiotherapy may be considered and/or parents should be trained to perform neck-stretching exercises. According to the American Academy of Pediatrics, these exercises should be done with each diaper change: one hand is placed on the child's chest, and the other gently rotates the infant's head so that the child's chin touches the shoulder. This is held for 10 seconds. The head is then rotated toward the opposite side for 10 seconds. Next, the child's head is tilted so that the ear touches the shoulder for ~10 seconds; this exercise is repeated for the opposite side. This will stretch the sternocleidomastoid and trapezius muscles.[23]

Only a few studies have demonstrated the effectiveness of these repositioning adjustments and exercises.[22,24,27] In 1997 Moss, in a series of 66 infants with mild to moderate PPP (difference between fronto-occipital diameters of ≤ 12 mm), reported that repositioning infants may produce improvement similar to that reported with cranial orthosis.[24]

Dynamic Cranial Orthosis

If there is progression or lack of improvement of PPP after a trial of physiotherapy, osteopathy, crib positioning, and neck-stretching exercises conducted for a 2-month period, then helmet therapy should be considered, particularly if the difference between fronto-occipital diameters > 1 cm. The treatment by dynamic cranial orthosis was inspired by ancestral ethnic practices aimed at intentionally deforming human skulls.[31]

As others have done over this last decade,[12,17–20,28,30] the authors of this chapter have used helmet therapy to correct PPP and reported their experience with this technique in 260 infants.[32] We used a thermoplastic construct consisting of a semirigid styrene outer shell thermobonded to a polyurethane foam inner lining (**Fig. 10.1**). The first step to building this helmet is to take a plaster of paris impression of the infant's head, which should be covered with a jersey sock. This impression is filled with plaster to create a positive mold that is corrected by applying a crescent-shaped silicone module over the occipital flattening. A cranial remodeling orthosis is then created over this corrected mold. Pressure is directed to constrain growth at the ipsilateral frontal and contralateral parietooccipital bulging, whereas a cavity is created over the adjacent flattened area, to promote remodeling. The helmet is worn up to 21 hours a day. Average duration of treatment in this study group was 13 weeks. There was a tendency toward shorter treatment over the years. As reported elsewhere, excellent results were obtained with this treatment, as judged by the parents and

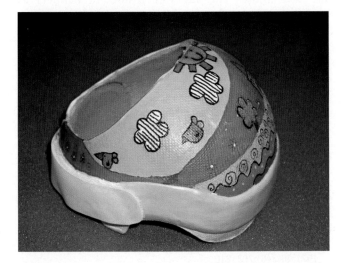

Fig. 10.1 Cranial remodeling orthosis consisting of a semirigid styrene outer shell thermobonded to a polyurethane foam inner lining.

the physicians.[12,17–20,28,30] Objectively, this favorable impression was confirmed by serial photographs (**Fig. 10.2**) and anthropometric measurements showing a symmetrization of the external auditory meatus to external canthus distances, as well as fronto-occipital diagonals. In our experience, such an orthosis was available for a 3-month period. Cranial orthosis did not restrict cranial growth; serial measurements of head circumference thus showed that every patient remained on his or her usual percentile curve.

Cranial remodeling orthosis is a valuable treatment option for infants who do not satisfactorily correct their PPP with repositioning adjustments and exercises. It was observed that the earlier the helmet is applied, the quicker and more complete will be the correction.[12,17] In practice, the ideal period of time to initiate this treatment is from 4 to 6 months of age. Before 4 months of age, experience has shown that the infants have usually not enough cervical muscle strength to tolerate the helmet. After 1 year of age, because the cranial growth lessens, and the skull has thickened, the correction with an orthosis is longer and less impressive.[19] In addition, older children do not tolerate helmets as well. In practice, we do not propose treatment after 1 year of age, except as an ultimate attempt to avoid a surgical correction. In such rare cases, however, favorable results were reported in a small series.[33] The treatment with cranial remodeling orthosis is efficient, well tolerated, and has no morbidity.

Only one study, although not randomized, has shown that infants treated with helmet therapy seemed to improve more rapidly and completely than those treated with crib positioning alone.[19]

Conclusion

The recommendation that neonates be placed exclusively on the back to prevent SIDS has led to an increase in the incidence of PPP. An infant born with deformational posterior flattening or who develops it in the postnatal period should first be seen by the pediatrician. Preventive counseling, repositioning adjustments, and exercises should be taught to the parents. If occipital flattening persists after a trial of exercises and crib repositioning for 2 months, helmet therapy is recommended, particularly if the difference between the fronto-occipital diagonals still exceeds 1 cm. This treatment is rapid and effective if started between 4 to 6 months of age. However, it can be conducted until 1 year of age. Helmet therapy is diminishingly effective if instituted after 1 year of age. This therapeutic option should always be used before surgical intervention is considered for patients recognized with PPP in the first year of life, knowing that this type of surgery would be a cosmetic procedure, frequently requiring blood transfusion, and not without risk in view of the proximity of posterior dural sinuses.

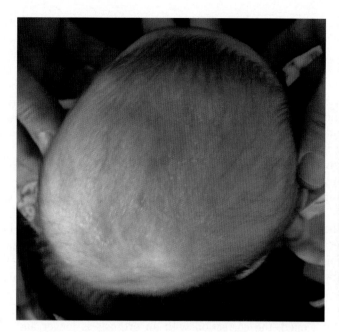 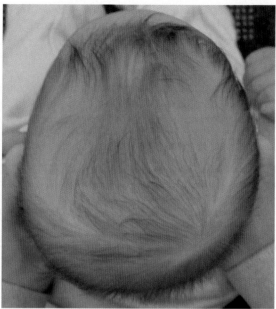

A   B

Fig. 10.2 (A) Vertex view of the skull of a 4-month-old infant with right posterior positional plagiocephaly. **(B)** Vertex view of the skull of the same infant, age 7 months, treated at 3 months with a cranial remodeling orthosis.

♦ Lessons Learned

This chapter illustrates the controversy surrounding the management of plagiocephaly. This condition was rare prior to the "Back to Sleep" campaign. The authors emphasize the importance of distinguishing positional plagiocephaly from the rare lambdoid craniosynostosis. The diagnosis is typical based on the patient's history and physical examination. There is little need for advanced imaging studies, such as radiographs and computed tomography scans. The treatment is simple, with either repositioning or molding orthosis. The authors discuss their treatment algorithm with repositioning followed by molding orthosis in children younger than 1 year of age. The issue arises in those children who present later in life at 13 months of age or older. The optimal question is unanswered as to the best treatment in these children. We should also understand that there have been few studies that have shown the superior results of helmets as compared with simple repositioning.

References

1. American Academy of Pediatrics. American Academy of Pediatrics AAP Task Force on Infant Positioning and SIDS: positioning and SIDS. Pediatrics 1992;89(6 Pt 1):1120–1126
2. Havens DH, Zink RL. The "Back to Sleep" campaign. J Pediatr Health Care 1994;8(5):240–242
3. Kane AA, Mitchell LE, Craven KP, Marsh JL. Observations on a recent increase in plagiocephaly without synostosis. Pediatrics 1996;97(6 Pt 1):877–885
4. Argenta LC, David LR, Wilson JA, Bell WO. An increase in infant cranial deformity with supine sleeping position. J Craniofac Surg 1996;7(1):5–11
5. Turk AE, McCarthy JG, Thorne CH, Wisoff JH. The "Back to Sleep campaign" and deformational plagiocephaly: is there cause for concern? J Craniofac Surg 1996;7(1):12–18
6. Ortega B. Unkind cut: some physicians do unnecessary surgery on heads of infants. Wall Street Journal. February 23, 1996
7. Rekate HL. Occipital plagiocephaly: a critical review of the literature. J Neurosurg 1998;89(1):24–30
8. Shuper A, Merlob P, Grunebaum M, Reisner SH. The incidence of isolated craniosynostosis in the newborn infant. Am J Dis Child 1985; 139(1):85–86
9. French LR, Jackson IT, Melton LJ III. A population-based study of craniosynostosis. J Clin Epidemiol 1990;43(1):69–73
10. Watson GH. Relation between side of plagiocephaly, dislocation of hip, scoliosis, bat ears, and sternomastoid tumours. Arch Dis Child 1971;46(246):203–210
11. Jones BM, Hayward R, Evans R, Britto J. Occipital plagiocephaly: an epidemic of craniosynostosis? BMJ 1997;315(7110):693–694

12. Littlefield TR, Beals SP, Manwaring KH, et al. Treatment of craniofacial asymmetry with dynamic orthotic cranioplasty. J Craniofac Surg 1998;9(1):11–17, discussion 18–19

13. Golden KA, Beals SP, Littlefield TR, Pomatto JK. Sternocleidomastoid imbalance versus congenital muscular torticollis: their relationship to positional plagiocephaly. Cleft Palate Craniofac J 1999;36(3): 256–261

14. Slate RK, Posnick JC, Armstrong DC, Buncic JR. Cervical spine subluxation associated with congenital muscular torticollis and craniofacial asymmetry. Plast Reconstr Surg 1993;91(7):1187–1195, discussion 1196–1197

15. Pople IK, Sanford RA, Muhlbauer MS. Clinical presentation and management of 100 infants with occipital plagiocephaly. Pediatr Neurosurg 1996;25(1):1–6

16. Dias MS, Klein DM, Backstrom JW. Occipital plagiocephaly: deformation or lambdoid synostosis? 1. Morphometric analysis and results of unilateral lambdoid craniectomy. Pediatr Neurosurg 1996;24(2):61–68

17. Kelly KM, Littlefield TR, Pomatto JK, Ripley CE, Beals SP, Joganic EF. Importance of early recognition and treatment of deformational plagiocephaly with orthotic cranioplasty. Cleft Palate Craniofac J 1999;36(2):127–130

18. Kelly KM, Littlefield TR, Pomatto JK, Manwaring KH, Beals SP. Cranial growth unrestricted during treatment of deformational plagiocephaly. Pediatr Neurosurg 1999;30(4):193–199

19. Mulliken JB, Vander Woude DL, Hansen M, LaBrie RA, Scott RM. Analysis of posterior plagiocephaly: deformational versus synostotic. Plast Reconstr Surg 1999;103(2):371–380

20. Clarren SK. Plagiocephaly and torticollis: etiology, natural history, and helmet treatment. J Pediatr 1981;98(1):92–95

21. Littlefield TR, Kelly KM, Pomatto JK, Beals SP. Multiple-birth infants at higher risk for development of deformational plagiocephaly. Pediatrics 1999;103(3):565–569

22. Tinuper P, Plazzi G, Provini F, et al. Facial asymmetry in partial epilepsies. Epilepsia 1992;33(6):1097–1100

23. Persing J, James H, Swanson J, Kattwinkel J; American Academy of Pediatrics Committee on Practice and Ambulatory Medicine, Section on Plastic Surgery and Section on Neurological Surgery. Prevention and management of positional skull deformities in infants. Pediatrics 2003;112(1 Pt 1):199–202

24. Moss SD. Nonsurgical, nonorthotic treatment of occipital plagiocephaly: what is the natural history of the misshapen neonatal head? J Neurosurg 1997;87(5):667–670

25. Gault DT, Renier D, Marchac D, Jones BM. Intracranial pressure and intracranial volume in children with craniosynostosis. Plast Reconstr Surg 1992;90(3):377–381

26. Huang MH, Mouradian WE, Cohen SR, Gruss JS. The differential diagnosis of abnormal head shapes: separating craniosynostosis from positional deformities and normal variants. Cleft Palate Craniofac J 1998;35(3):204–211

27. Hellbusch JL, Hellbusch LC, Bruneteau RJ. Active counter-positioning treatment of deformational occipital plagiocephaly. Nebr Med J 1995;80(12):344–349

28. Clarren SK, Smith DW, Hanson JW. Helmet treatment for plagiocephaly and congenital muscular torticollis. J Pediatr 1979;94(1): 43–46

29. Danby PM. Plagiocephaly in some 10-year-old children. Arch Dis Child 1962;37:500–504

30. Ripley CE, Pomatto J, Beals SP, Joganic EF, Manwaring KH, Moss SD. Treatment of positional plagiocephaly with dynamic orthotic cranioplasty. J Craniofac Surg 1994;5(3):150–159, discussion 160

31. Gerszten PC, Gerszten E. Intentional cranial deformation: a disappearing form of self-mutilation. Neurosurgery 1995;37(3):374–381, discussion 381–382

32. de Ribaupierre S, Vernet O, Rilliet B, Cavin B, Kalina D, Leyvraz PF. Posterior positional plagiocephaly treated with cranial remodeling orthosis. Swiss Med Wkly 2007;137(25–26):368–372

33. Littlefield TR, Pomatto JK, Kelly KM. Dynamic orthotic cranioplasty: treatment of the older infant: report of four cases. Neurosurg Focus 2000;9(3):e5

11 Intracranial Suppuration

◆ Conservative Management

D. Douglas Cochrane, S. Dobson, and Paul Steinbok

Cases

Case 1

A previously healthy 4-year-old girl developed a mild upper respiratory tract infection 5 days prior to presentation with frontal morning headache, vomiting, earache, and fever varying from 38.0 to 39.5°C (100.4–103.1°F). Clinical examination revealed a febrile, alert, and neurologically intact child with chronic otitis media, left-sided conductive hearing loss, and retroauricular tenderness. Myringotomies and left mastoid drainage were performed. Mixed anaerobic organisms and *Pseudomonas* species were cultured (**Fig. 11.1**).

Case 2

An alert 14-year-old male patient presented with frontal headache, nasal congestion, and a first-ever generalized seizure. Following the postictal period, clinical examination

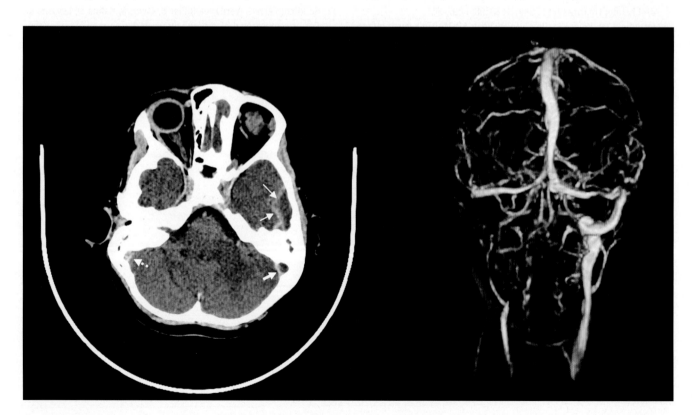

Fig. 11.1 Axial computed tomography (CT) scan with contrast (*left*) with *thin arrows* outlining the extradural temporal and subtemporal abscess collection. *Solid thick arrow* shows the filling defect in the left transverse-sigmoid sinus complex compared with the patent sinus (*right, dotted thick arrow*).

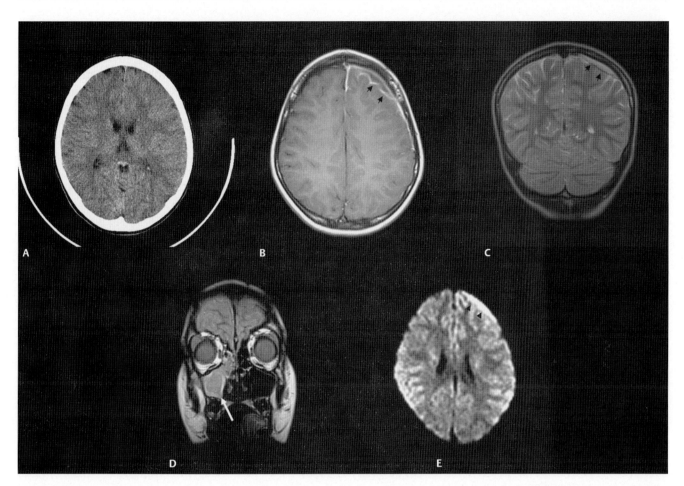

Fig. 11.2 (A) CT scan without contrast shows obliteration of the cortical subarachnoid space over the left frontal lobe, suggesting a subtle mass effect on the left hemisphere. **(B)** Axial and **(C)** coronal magnetic resonance imaging (MRI) confirmed that the mass was due to a thin extra-axial collection (*arrowheads*). **(D)** Lower left coronal MRI showing mucosal thickening in a fluid-filled maxillary sinus (*arrow*). **(E)** Diffusion axial image with high-intensity signal in the collection (*arrowheads*).

revealed him to be neurologically intact with mild fever (38.5°C [101.3°F]) and to have purulent nasal discharge.

Endoscopic sinus drainage of the right maxillary sinus grew mixed organisms, predominantly aerobic and anaerobic *Streptococcus* (**Fig. 11.2**).

Surgery of intracranial infections laid the foundation for clinical neurosurgery as it is known today. The first successful craniectomies and craniotomies for nontraumatic mass lesions were performed for these disorders. Although chronic infections in bone and intra- and extradural spaces were controllable with surgery, acute infections, particularly in the subdural space, had to await the availability of effective antimicrobial agents to be effectively treated.[1] With sulfonamides and penicillin, in addition to surgical drainage, subdural empyema became potentially curable. Guided by neuroradiologic investigations, initially angiography, and now computed tomography (CT) and magnetic resonance imaging (MRI), the focus of treatment has shifted to early recognition, accurate and specific bacteriologic diagnosis, and directed surgical intervention.

The neurosurgical management of intracranial suppuration is designed to (1) obtain adequate specimens of purulent material for accurate bacteriologic diagnosis and to direct antimicrobial therapy where accurate cultures cannot be obtained by other means; (2) evacuate sizable collections of liquefied pus from any and all extra- and intradural spaces affected and to lower intracranial pressure and minimize cerebral distortion; (3) débride sequestered bone; (4) decompress and, if needed, irrigate the ventricular system in the event of rupture of the abscess into the ventricular system; and (5) control hydrocephalus, if present. In the absence of these indications, neurosurgical intervention may not be necessary.

Principles of Management

The rationale and nature of neurosurgical intervention necessary to manage patients with intracranial suppuration are dependent upon the principles outlined in the following sections that describe the impact of current neuroimaging for early diagnosis and assessment of the response to therapy, the need for accurate bacteriologic diagnosis and administration of effective antibiotics, and the requirement to evacuate sizable collections of pus.

Impact of Neuroimaging: Early Diagnosis and Assessment of Response to Therapy

The pathologic and imaging evolution of brain abscess is outlined in **Table 11.1.** Experimental studies in primates suggest that brain abscess formation occurs in an area of preexisting necrosis or injury caused by direct traumatic injury, hemorrhage, infarction secondary to thrombophlebitis, or relative hypoxia in watershed areas.[2,3] Seeding with organisms sets the stage for the development of septic cerebritis occurring within the white matter. Cerebritis is characterized by an acute inflammatory response, vascular dilatation, diapedesis, microthrombosis, and small vessel rupture. Edema and polymorphonuclear infiltration with a surrounding microglial response occur. The center of the lesion then undergoes liquefaction.

By 10 to 13 days, early encapsulation is seen in experimental brain abscesses.[4,5] A peripheral zone of inflammatory cells, neovascularization, and fibroblasts surround a central necrosis. The latter cells produce a dense collagenous capsule. The capsule is surrounded by edema and reactive gliosis. Capsule formation is thinnest adjacent to the ventricle and thicker on the side of the more luxuriantly vascularized cortex. Grant, in a clinical study of patients with brain abscess during the preantibiotic era, demonstrated the presence of a capsule in every patient after a period of 6 weeks.[6]

In immune-suppressed animals, there is a decrease and delay in collagen formation, a reduction in polymorphonuclear leukocytes and macrophages, a longer persistence of organisms, and an increase in gliosis.[9]

Early cerebritis is characterized on CT scan by an ill-defined, low-density change within the parenchyma. Enhancement occurs after contrast medium administration. Subsequently, imaging will show the classic ring-enhancing lesion with surrounding edema. Ring enhancement may or may not correlate with capsule formation. Differentiation of capsule formation from enhancing cerebritis may be made using delayed (30–60 minutes) scanning after contrast medium administration. On CT, ring contrast enhancement reflects the degree of neovascularization and capsule maturation. Calcification is common in abscesses in neonates.[7,8]

The administration of corticosteroids to a patient whose lesion is in the cerebritis stage may result in definite reduction in contrast medium enhancement. Contrast medium enhancement in well-encapsulated lesions is not reduced.[4]

Table 11.1 Stages of Cerebral Abscess Formation and Imaging Findings Based on Experimental and Clinical Observations

Stage	Duration (Days)	Pathology	CT	MRI	DWI
Early cerebritis	1–3	Bacterial invasion in an area of injury followed by an acute inflammatory response, vascular dilatation, diapedesis, microthrombosis, and small vessel rupture	Local edema without CE	Low signal on T1 with mass effect and edema	Increased signal intensity on DWI and low ADC values
Late cerebritis	4–9	Edema and polymorphonuclear infiltration with a surrounding microglial response followed by liquefactive necrosis of the center of the lesion	Ill-defined capsule rim with CE of contents		
Early capsule	10–14	Central necrosis is bounded by a peripheral zone of inflammatory cells, neovascularization, and fibroblasts, which create the capsule	Distinctly enhancing capsule Low-density center Peripheral edema	T1: low to intermediate intensity FLAIR Isodense relative to gray matter CE T1: ring enhancement Perifocal edema	Low ADC in the cavity
Late capsule	14 or later	Capsule thickening Increasing gliosis. Calcification in neonates			

Abbreviations: ADC, apparent diffusion coefficient; CE, contrast enhancement; CT, computed tomography; DWI, diffusion weighted imaging; FLAIR, fluid attenuation inversion recovery; MRI, magnetic resonance imaging.

Source: Compiled from references [5, 9, 21–25]

Increased uptake of contrast material by the ependyma may indicate the presence of primary ventriculitis or that due to intraventricular rupture.

CT and MRI are required for accurate preoperative localization of the epidural, subdural, and/or parenchymal collections and for monitoring resolution of the infection. Contrast medium enhancement of the dura, empyema wall, and abscess capsule is usually seen, and complicating cerebral edema, venous infarction, and parenchymal abscess formation may be revealed.[10–12]

CT may not be diagnostic, revealing only hemispheral swelling in subdural empyema;[13] however, contrast medium–enhanced MRI will usually reveal the extra-axial collections, as well as areas of underlying tissue and vascular injury.[10] Whether imaging is done using CT or MRI, coronal and sagittal views are helpful in revealing collections at the skull base and at the vertex and in defining the relationship of the intracranial collection(s) to the involved sinuses.

MR images have typical characteristics on T1 weighting (central hypointensity surrounded by a ring of enhancement after gadolinium administration) and T2 weighting (hyperintense area of pus, surrounded by hypointense capsule, enveloped within surrounding edema).[14,15] MR spectroscopy has an evolving role in the differentiation of abscess from tumor,[16,17] in the differential diagnosis of brain lesions in patients with acquired immunodeficiency syndrome (AIDS),[18] and in staging abscess development.[19]

The use of diffusion weighted imaging (DWI) and the corresponding apparent diffusion coefficient (ADC) maps has greatly improved the ability to differentiate cerebral infections from other cystic cerebral lesions presenting as nonspecific ring enhancement[20] and to demonstrate treatment success and failure.[21–25]

DWI is based on detecting the microscopic motion of water molecules and depends mostly on the water located in the extracellular space. ADC maps are used to quantify the degree of water motion. The degree of viscosity, the causative organism, and the level of protein in the abscess cavity may affect DWI findings and ADC values. Cerebral abscesses contain inflammatory cells, a matrix of proteins, cellular debris, and bacteria in high-viscosity pus; all of these factors restrict water motion.[21] Restricted water motion in cerebral abscesses has increased signal intensity on trace DWI and low ADC values. Because water movement is less restricted in necrotic tumors, most show mildly increased diffusion with low to intermediate signal intensity on trace DWI and high ADC values.[21] In one series, the sensitivity of DWI for the differentiation of brain abscesses from nonabscesses was 96%; specificity, 96%; positive predictive value, 98%; negative predictive value, 92%; and accuracy of the test, 96%.[24]

Changes in the signal intensity have been correlated to successful treatment.[21,22] Persisting or reappearing high signal intensity in the abscess cavity on trace DW images and low ADC values indicating restricted diffusion were seen in cases of treatment failure and were correlated with pus accumulation. Changes in the capsule interface may also be important.[23,26] Sensitivity and specificity have been reported by Reddy and colleagues.[24]

Nonpyogenic parasitic and fungal abscesses may show increased ADC in the cavity compared with bacterial abscesses.[22,27] Although overlap in values occurs with bacterial abscesses, other features are important in distinguishing fungal abscesses, including multiplicity, size, deep nuclear location, and signal heterogeneity on T2 and DWI.

On DWI, subdural empyema exhibits areas of high signal similar to that produced by most brain abscesses, with the high signal resulting from the high viscosity of the infected fluid.[21] DWI may be used as a simple method of making a reliable diagnosis if an area of abnormal high signal is found. Sterile effusions sometimes give signal similar to that of empyema, and benign effusions often appear as areas of low signal similar to that of cerebrospinal fluid (CSF).

The degree of enhancement of dura, empyema, or abscess wall on CT or MRI varies over the course of treatment and is a reflection of the inflammatory response and not whether the collection has been sterilized. In limited case observations, the DWI signal intensity from epidural abscesses was variable.[28]

In infants with meningitis-associated subdural empyema, cranial ultrasonography (or CT or MRI) usually reveals unilateral or bilateral frontoparietal extra-axial collections with echogenic boundaries.[29,30]

Plain film studies supplement the information obtained by CT (and MRI) in patients with otorhinologic-associated intracranial suppuration, by demonstrating opacification of one or more sinuses[13] and/or revealing a foreign body, skull fracturing, pneumocephalus, or gas within the abscess cavity.

Accurate Bacteriologic Diagnosis and Appropriate Antimicrobials

Pathogen Identification

Bacteriologic identification can be obtained from various sources in the acutely unwell patient (**Table 11.2**). Blood cultures may reveal the causative organism in epidural abscess or subdural empyema but are rarely positive in brain abscess.[31] In patients with sinogenic suppuration, pus collected at the time of sinus or ear drainage will usually reveal the causative organisms unless antibiotic treatment has been started.

The culture of purulent material obtained at the time of surgical drainage provides the best opportunity for microbiologic diagnosis. Proper handling of the specimen and appropriate aerobic and anaerobic culture techniques result in positive cultures in the majority of cases. Gram staining of the pus can guide therapy in the presence of a negative culture.

Table 11.2 Bacterial Etiology and Suggested Initial Antibiotic Choices

Underlying Condition	Usual Organisms	Initial Antibiotic Choice*
Otorhinological disease	Aerobic and anaerobic *Streptococcus* S. aureus Other anaerobes *Pseudomonas aeruginosa*	Penicillinase-resistant synthetic penicillin + third-generation cephalosporin + metronidazole† or meropenem‡
Head injury or operation	*Staphylococcus aureus* Gram negatives	Penicillinase-resistant synthetic penicillin + third-generation cephalosporin or meropenem‡
Meningitis in infancy	Usually sterile unless secondarily infected	Third-generation cephalosporin ± vancomycin
Unknown	Unknown	Penicillinase-resistant synthetic penicillin + third-generation cephalosporin + metronidazole

Drug Doses		
Cloxacillin	200 mg/kg/day divided q6hr	
Vancomycin	60 mg/kg/day divided q6hr	
Cefotaxime	300 mg/kg/day divided q8hr	
Ceftriaxone	100 mg/kg/day divided q12hr	
Ceftazidime	225 mg/kg/day divided q8hr	
Metronidazole	30 mg/kg/day divided q8hr	
Meropenem	120 mg/kg/day divided q6hr	

*If a gram-positive organism has the potential for resistance to β-lactam antibiotics, or if allergy to β-lactam antibiotics is suspected, substitute vancomycin for penicillinase-resistant synthetic penicillin.

†Third-generation cephalosporin (e.g., cefotaxime and ceftriaxone); ceftazidime if *P. aeruginosa* is suspected in the setting of chronic otitis media.

‡Meropenem if

• Previous third-generation cephalosporin therapy has been given

• Prolonged hospitalization

• Prolonged ventilatory support

• Burns

The spectrum of organisms cultured from sites of intracranial suppuration has changed (**Table 11.2**). This is a reflection of improved bacteriologic isolation techniques, aggressive treatment of primary infections, and a decreased incidence of nonmissile compound brain wounds. In most series, the incidence of *Staphylococcus aureus* has decreased and that of anaerobes has increased.[32]

Cultures from suppuration associated with sinusitis commonly show the growth of organisms responsible for chronic sinusitis, including aerobic and/or anaerobic *Streptococcus* (made up of the Viridans group streptococci and the *Streptococcus anginosus* group) or other anaerobes. *S. aureus,* aerobic and anaerobic *Streptococcus, Pseudomonas aeruginosa,* facultative gram-negative organisms, and other anaerobes are causative in those infections of mastoid or middle ear origin, whereas those secondary to trauma, surgery, or primary calvarial osteomyelitis are due to *Staphylococcus, Streptococcus,* or gram-negative organisms. Skin flora of low pathogenicity, including coagulase-negative *Staphylococcus, Corynebacterium,* and *Propionibacterium* acnes, have been reported in postoperative/traumatic epidural abscesses.[33]

Reflecting their role in the pathogenesis of sinusitis, anaerobes play a definite part in the pathogenesis of subdural

suppuration.[34] Anaerobic or microaerophilic *Streptococcus, Bacteroides* species, *Fusobacterium, Peptostreptococcus,* and *Clostridium perfringens*[35] have been reported. *Salmonella* has been reported in the immunologically compromised host. Subdural fluid collections complicating meningitis in infants, although usually sterile, may culture the organism responsible for the meningitis. Specimens from subdural empyema are sterile in up to 25% of patients.[34,36]

Anaerobic organisms isolated from brain abscess pus include *Bacteroides, Peptostreptococcus, Fusobacterium, Veillonella, Propionibacterium,* and *Actinomyces.* Aerobic organisms include *Staphylococcus, Streptococcus, Enterobacteriaceae,* and *Haemophilus.* In at least one third of brain abscesses, the pus will culture multiple organisms. This is particularly common in otitic abscesses. In patients with cyanotic congenital heart disease, Viridans *Streptococcus,* anaerobic *Streptococcus,* and occasionally *Haemophilus* species are seen. No growth is reported from up to 25 to 30% of properly handled specimens.[37–39]

The bacteriologic diagnosis often points to the originating infection. *S. aureus* abscess formation occurs most commonly after compound skull fracturing, after operative intervention, or as a result of a retained foreign body.[40] Gram-negative organisms, including *Bacteroides* and *Haemophilus,* are commonly isolated from otogenic abscesses. Most brain abscesses that complicate paranasal sinus infection will culture aerobic and/or anaerobic streptococci.

The nature of the offending organism may influence the development of the abscess capsule. *Bacteroides* excretes a collagenase that inhibits capsule formation, resulting in the development of small daughter abscesses. Propagation of edema is aided by bacterial production of hyaluronidase and heparinase.

Brain abscess formation in the neonate is usually caused by *Proteus mirabilis* or *Citrobacter diversus.*[41] Individual case reports and series have also reported *Salmonella, Serratia, Enterobacter,* and *Staphylococcus* as causative organisms. Meningitis caused by *Citrobacter, Proteus, Serratia,* or *Enterobacter* is complicated by abscess formation in a high percentage of patients.[42,43]

Fungal brain abscesses most commonly develop in patients with impaired host defenses, particularly those with AIDS, or who are immunologically suppressed after organ transplantation or chemotherapy for malignancy. *Candida, Aspergillus, Nocardia,* and *Cryptococcus* are the most common responsible fungal organisms. Pathogenic fungi, acquired through either inhalation or implantation, can result in brain abscess formation. This is most commonly seen with *Histoplasma, Coccidioides,* and *Blastomyces* and the zygomycetes (*Mucor* and *Rhizopus*).

Toxoplasma gondii is the leading cause of brain abscess in patients with AIDS. *Entamoeba histolytica* brain abscess usually occurs in the presence of involvement in extracranial sites. Helminthic brain abscess is rare.[39,41]

Antibiotic Treatment

Systemic antibiotic treatment (see **Table 11.2**) should be started as soon as the diagnosis of epidural abscess, subdural empyema, or brain abscess is considered. Antibiotics administered before surgery, although achieving some penetration of bone, are unlikely to interfere with culture information from the pus.

The microbial spectrum of brain abscess varies with the primary site of infection. If this is known, the initial choice of antibiotics can be directed to the most likely organisms. For abscesses arising as a result of sinusitis where streptococcal species are the most likely organisms, penicillin or a third-generation cephalosporin (e.g., cefotaxime) and metronidazole provide basic coverage. The majority of infratentorial subdural empyemas are otogenic in origin,[36] and because chronic otitis media or mastoiditis is often associated with *P. aeruginosa* and *Enterobacteriaceae,* coverage should include a third-generation cephalosporin, such as ceftazadime. Metastatic abscesses require a regimen based on the likely site of primary infection. In particular circumstances where multiresistant, gram-negative organisms might be suspected (see **Table 11.2**), a carbapenem antibiotic, such as meropenem, can be used as monotherapy, as it also covers *S. aureus* and anaerobes.

S. aureus is commonly identified in an abscess after trauma. Compound wounds, in particular those contaminated with soil, may contain facultative gram-negative organisms or *Clostridium* species. In these situations, a penicillinase-resistant penicillin and a third-generation cephalosporin provide initial coverage. Postoperative brain abscess is rare and usually due to *S. aureus* or *S. epidermidis.* Vancomycin should be considered, given the resistance of nosocomial organisms to penicillinase-resistant penicillins. Abscesses secondary to animal bites contain a mixed flora, including *Pasteurella multocida* and a variety of *Haemophilus* species.[44]

In the absence of a likely primary source of infection, the initial choice of antibiotics should include agents to cover *Streptococcus* (aerobic and anaerobic), other anaerobes, and the less common *Staphylococcus.* A penicillinase-resistant synthetic penicillin, a third-generation cephalosporin, and metronidazole should be instituted empirically pending results of Gram staining and culture.

The optimal duration of parenteral antibiotic therapy is not known, although 6 to 8 weeks of intravenous therapy has been empirically recommended. Certainly, treatment should be continued until systemic evidence of infection has resolved and the abscess collections have been shown to be decreasing in size.[45–49] In some situations a shorter course may be sufficient. Depending on the organisms cultured, their sensitivity to the prescribed antibiotic regimen, and the response to therapy, some authors recommend an additional 2 to 3 months of oral antimicrobial therapy to prevent recurrence.[43]

Evacuation of Sizable Collections of Liquefied Pus

The need to evacuate collections of pus is dependent upon the patient's clinical condition, degree of cerebral distortion, and the need for bacteriologic diagnosis. Neurosurgical drainage is not always required. Drainage of the epidural abscess may occur spontaneously or as a result of sinus drainage procedures.[50–52] When necessary, and with the aid of modern imaging and stereotaxic localization, a more conservative approach can be taken to bone removal to achieve diagnostic and therapeutic drainage by targeting collections with precision. The extent of bone removal is determined by the degree of osteomyelitis and bone sequestration, as in some epidural abscesses; the need to reach the subdural space widely, as in hemispheral, parafalcine, and infratentorial subdural empyema; or the need to address multiple separated lesions within the brain and subdural space concurrently.

Neurosurgical Intervention

When Is Neurosurgical Intervention Not Required?

In many patients with sinogenic or hematogenic intracranial suppuration, accurate bacteriologic identification can be obtained from the purulent material obtained from the sinuses or from blood cultures. Wound cultures in the case of penetrating or postoperative wound infections may also suffice. Empirical antibiotic treatment, based on the known or presumed source, may be started in patients with multiple or deeply seated brain abscesses.[21,23,53,54]

In the early stages of intracranial suppuration, prior to the liquefaction of purulent material, surgical drainage may not retrieve diagnostic tissue and is likely to result in further parenchymal injury. Cerebritis is by definition a nonliquefied state, and treatment of infection early in the course needs only presumptive diagnosis and empirical antibiotics.[19]

Selected minimally symptomatic patients presenting with small collections may be treated with antibiotics alone, if appropriate bacteriologic identification and sensitivity testing are completed[52,53] and if adequate sinus drainage can be achieved by either medical or surgical means. Transient symptomatic worsening over the first 48 hours of treatment may occur and is not necessarily reason to abort conservative therapy, but clinical improvement is to be expected within 2 weeks of the initiation of therapy.[53] Neuroimaging performed after 2 weeks of treatment should show the collections to be the same size or smaller and at 6 weeks should demonstrate complete resolution of the epidural infection. Diffusion weighted MRI may also play a role in defining the response to treatment.[21–23,26]

Mauser et al and Leys et al have reported the successful treatment of subdural empyema without operative intervention.[55,56] Empirical antimicrobial therapy or an antibiotic regime based on positive blood or CSF cultures was administered intravenously for 6 weeks, followed by oral therapy until the CT scan was normal. In a subsequent study, Leys et al compared medical (antibiotic and intracranial pressure control) treatment with medical plus either aspiration or excision in patients with single hemispheric abscesses or subdural abscesses measuring from 1 to 5 cm in size.[57] The prognosis for survival was no different in the three groups; however, those treated medically without either aspiration or excision showed a lower incidence of posttreatment seizures and residual neurologic deficit. These authors suggest that surgery is always indicated for lesions > 5 cm in diameter, those in the posterior fossa, and those that increase in size while undergoing medical treatment. Empirical medical management can be considered for lesions < 5 cm that show response to antibiotic treatment.

In our experience, débridement of sequestered bone is required only when infection follows craniotomy as a primary operation, when it was part of any approach to address infection, or in the setting of postoperative infection of penetrating wounds.

Intracranial pressure monitoring or CSF drainage is not commonly needed as part of the management of pediatric patients with intracranial suppuration except in the setting of infratentorial subdural empyema or cerebellar abscess.

Dural venous sinus thrombosis, a common accompaniment of mastoiditis and extradural abscess, does not require surgical intervention (either thrombectomy or needle aspiration) in the face of adequate antibiotic treatment.[58,59]

When Is Neurosurgical Intervention Needed, and in What Form?

Targeted Access and Drainage

Neurosurgical treatment is required for patients who (1) are stuporous or comatose; (2) are deteriorating in neurologic status despite nonoperative management; (3) exhibit marked mass effect on CT or MRI; (4) show no improvement with 1 to 2 weeks of antibiotic therapy, whether drained initially or not; and/or (5) indicate that intervention is necessary to obtain purulent material for culture, the results of which will direct antibiotic treatment. It should be noted that the mass effect and cerebral irritation seen with subdural empyema usually exceed that visualized on preoperative imaging studies, so that the threshold for surgical drainage is less than in the case of extradural abscess or many brain abscesses.

Surgical management of extradural abscess is less complex than that necessary for intradural collections. Limited bone removal either by craniotomy (osteoplastic or free flap), craniectomy, bur hole, removal of a previously created bone flap, or depressed fracture fragments should be planned to allow access to the collection. If bone is sequestered and devascularized as a result of the operation or skull fracturing, removal is required. The finding of pus in the diploic space of vascularized bone at the time of operation does not necessarily mandate bone removal if the skull appears otherwise normal. The epidural abscess should be drained and the space thoroughly irrigated, and a suction drain may be placed.

In the case of intradural suppuration, the absence of definitive cultures and mass effect associated with clinical symptoms[57] prompts a surgical procedure for bacteriologic diagnosis and evacuation of liquefied pus.[36,60] The operative approach, positioning, draping, and bur hole localization are chosen to allow direct extracerebral access to the imaged collections while permitting a craniotomy to be performed if required. After the placement of the bur hole(s) or small craniectomy(ies), the dura is opened, the collection is opened, and aerobic and anaerobic cultures are obtained. The subdural space is then drained of liquefied pus and irrigated through the bur hole(s) with antibiotic (bacitracin)–containing saline solution, until the returns are clear. No attempt is made to remove formed adherent pus from the arachnoid. If drainage is not believed to be adequate, as may be the case with an interhemispheric collection, a craniotomy flap is turned and the subdural space inspected and pus evacuated.[61–63] In the absence of osteomyelitis and extradural abscess formation, the bone flap is replaced at the end of the procedure. Drains are not used to irrigate the subdural space after wound closure.

Regardless of the technique of empyema drainage, reoperation is not infrequently needed prior to bringing the infection under control. Nathoo et al reported on average 1.9 operations per patient,[64] and 30% of Venkatesh et al series of children with infratentorial collections required multiple operations.[36]

In infants whose subdural empyema is associated with chronic subdural hematoma, intermittent transfontanelle needle drainage is likely to be all that is required in most patients.[49,65] Occasionally, craniotomy has been reported as necessary.[66]

The majority of infants who develop subdural collections as a complication of *Haemophilus influenzae* meningitis (type B) will not require surgical intervention. If the mass effect of the subdural collection is sizable and the clinical condition of the infant fails to improve as expected, transfontanelle needle or bur hole drainage is usually successful. Cultures of the subdural material are usually sterile.

For parenchymal abscesses, aspiration with or without catheter drainage is the oldest successful method and has been used with good results.[6,67–72] Abscess aspiration can be performed using a variety of techniques. Free-hand CT or ultrasound-guided aspiration assists with the accurate placement of a drainage needle or catheter in most superficial cerebral abscesses. Deeply seated abscesses can be reached safely using frame-based or frameless stereotactic techniques with or without intraoperative MRI or ultrasound guidance.[73–75]

After localization, the procedure consists of making a bur hole over the most insensitive portion of the cortex where the abscess is superficial, opening the dura, and making a small cortical incision. The abscess is palpated with a brain cannula and punctured with a small soft catheter over a stylet. The catheter is anchored loosely with a suture through the scalp. Pus usually flows spontaneously from the tube. Gentle aspiration with a syringe can be performed at the operating table, and saline irrigation is used to help empty the cavity. The catheter is left in place until drainage ceases and is then removed. Repeated aspirations may be needed as the infection is brought under control. The only contraindication to aspiration is a bleeding diathesis. Repeat aspiration is needed in ~20% of patients treated with aspiration only.[33,76]

Recent advances in endoscopic technology allow the direct visualization of the abscess cavity and more complete irrigation.[60,77]

Intraventricular rupture of parenchymal abscesses, particularly those that are deep-seated or located adjacent to the occipital horn, is not always fatal but does worsen the prognosis. To prevent this event, aggressive antimicrobial therapy and early drainage are recommended[4,78] because a delay in surgical intervention is believed to contribute to the likelihood of intraventricular rupture.

Abscess Excision

Formal craniotomy and excision of abscess are less frequently required now than in the past, given the effectiveness of antibiotics and the ability to confirm the response to therapy with CT and MRI. Excision is indicated for patients who have multiloculated abscesses where aspiration has failed, abscesses containing gas within the cavity (reflecting either gas-forming organisms or a dural fistula), recurrent bacterial abscesses that do not respond to antibiotic treatment and drainage, and when the diagnosis or the bacteriology remains in doubt (*Nocardia* or fungal abscesses).[32,79–82] Abscess formation in intracranial dermoid tumors[83–85] and complicating hemorrhage from cavernous hemangioma[86] should be excised with the primary pathology. Current series report < 20% of patients undergoing excision.[76]

Ventricular Drainage and Shunting

The need for permanent CSF diversion in patients recovering from intracranial abscess is infrequent. It is most commonly seen following infratentorial subdural empyema. Permanent shunting has been needed in ~20 to 25% of patients.[36,87]

Conclusion

Epidural abscess, subdural empyema, and brain abscesses are classic neurosurgical complications of otorhinologic, middle ear, and posttraumatic infections and immunosuppression. Each may present as a neurologic emergency and require a high index of diagnostic suspicion and early recognition to minimize mortality and morbidity. To facilitate recovery from neurologic deficit, aggressive treatment must include antibiotic administration with coverage for aerobic and anaerobic organisms and, in most patients, selective drainage for bacteriologic diagnosis and removal of suppurative collections guided by appropriate neuroimaging. Empirical antibiotic therapy without surgical drainage may be appropriate in patients with small collections. The availability of CT and MRI scanning has resulted in earlier and more precise diagnosis of intracranial suppuration, allowing nonneurosurgical or minimally invasive neurosurgical treatment in a larger percentage of patients.

♦ Open Craniotomy and Drainage

Saadi Ghatan

Timely recognition and appropriate, aggressive therapy are crucial in the treatment of infections of the central nervous system (CNS) in pediatric patients. In children, purulent infections within the cranial vault can have catastrophic consequences if they are not recognized and treated expeditiously. Advances in diagnosis and treatment have lowered the morbidity and mortality rates associated with epidural abscess, subdural empyema, and brain abscess, the three suppurative entities explored here. A description of their predisposing factors, etiologies, and natural history, as well as the therapeutic options available to treat each condition, is provided for these acute neurosurgical diseases, where both diagnostic and therapeutic maneuvers are necessary. Some form of surgical intervention (otolaryngology or neurosurgery) is usually indicated in each of these conditions, and neurosurgical intervention is nearly inevitable in cases of subdural empyema and brain abscess, where the risk of morbidity and mortality is greatly increased.

Suppurative Infections: General Considerations

Fortunately, epidural abscess, subdural empyema, and brain abscess are rare entities in pediatric neurosurgery and historically have been thought to make up only a small percentage of cases treated in a busy pediatric neurosurgery practice.[88,89] Nevertheless, children are particularly susceptible to suppurative infections due to their association with conditions such as sinusitis and mastoiditis and uniquely pediatric problems such as congenital heart disease. Undoubtedly, they are recognized more frequently with modern imaging techniques, and their incidence and therefore prevalence will be higher in more frequently encountered immunocompromised children in the setting of organ transplantation, children undergoing chemotherapy for neoplastic processes, and those with AIDS.[90]

Because hematologic analysis is of little use in CNS infection, and because CSF analysis is mostly contraindicated in suppurative intracranial infection due to mass effect and raised intracranial pressure, diagnostic imaging, along with its accurate interpretation, is the mainstay of work-up for subdural empyema and epidural and intracerebral abscess. Contrast-enhanced CT is readily available and simple to obtain in children without the need for sedation. MRI is more sensitive, particularly in the detection of multiple abscesses, CSF involvement, or subdural empyema,[91] but inherent difficulties with availability and logistics, given the need for sedation in younger children and occasionally critically ill patients, are well recognized.

Subdural Empyema

Representing only a minority of intracranial suppurative infections,[92] subdural empyema can be lethal or rapidly lead to severe morbidity if diagnosis and treatment are delayed and uniformly fatal if left untreated.[93] In comparison with cranial epidural or brain abscess, the rationale for rapid neurosurgical evacuation of a subdural empyema is most clearly and commonly made for both diagnostic and therapeutic reasons.

Defined as a purulent infection between the dura and subarachnoid space, subdural empyema can be found anywhere in the cranial vault, but it most commonly occurs over the cerebral convexities. The source of infection in the pediatric population varies according to age. In most children, cases of subdural empyema occur as a complication of otogenic or sinus disease;[94–97] infants with meningitis develop empyema in ~2% of cases, and purulent transformation of the sterile subdural effusions is not uncommon.[89] Otogenic and sinus infections are thought to seed the subdural space through hematogenous spread along bridging veins or via invasion and erosion of adjacent bone and dura. Most often, cultures from subdural empyema reveal a polymicrobial infection that includes anaerobes.[98]

Because early and prompt recognition of subdural empyema is crucial, an understanding of the clinical symptoms and signs in conjunction with the pathophysiology of this condition is essential. Early signs are similar to those of meningitis due to spread through the subdural space: fever, headache, and nuchal rigidity rapidly lead to an altered level of consciousness secondary to inflammation of the brain parenchyma, cerebral edema, and mass effect of the collection with resultant elevated intracranial pressure. Seizures and focal neurologic deficits occur due to mass effect, venous thrombosis, and infarction.[99] Hematologic work-up may reveal a peripheral leukocytosis, an elevated erythrocyte sedimentation rate (ESR), and an elevation in C-reactive protein (CRP), all of which are nonspecific. Neuroimaging, therefore, is essential.

CT and MRI scans can provide definitive diagnoses. Small subdural empyemas on noncontrast CT may be subtle and difficult to recognize, but they distinguish themselves from other suppurative intracranial infections by not crossing the midline, and instead can occupy the interhemispheric fissure (**Fig. 11.3**). They appear as isointense

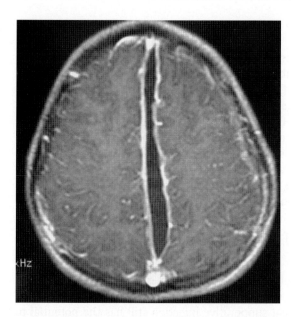

Fig. 11.3 Subdural empyema. A 5-year-old presented with headaches, nausea, vomiting, and lethargy. T1-weighted MRI showed multifocal collections of subdural fluid consistent with empyema with surrounding enhancement and mass effect.

or hypointense extra-axial collections with rim enhancement,[100] with sulcal effacement and edema. MRI is the study of choice for the detection of empyema among small subdural fluid collections, revealing isointense signal on T1-weighted images and high signal on T2-weighted images,[101] and DWI can distinguish between empyema and effusion.[102]

Once recognized, subdural empyema is a surgical emergency until proven otherwise. Although the literature may reveal an alternative medical approach in the management of a clinically stable, neurologically normal patient with a small empyema,[103–105] there is overwhelming clinical evidence that surgical management is beneficial from a diagnostic and therapeutic perspective.[89,93,106] Disadvantages of nonsurgical medical management include the need for a longer period of therapy, closer and more rigid neuroradiologic monitoring, and a lack of knowledge about the organism and its medical sensitivity.[89]

The need for aggressive surgical therapy is particularly important in reference to the location of the empyema.[106] In the posterior fossa, subdural empyema is mostly of otogenic origin and leads to rapid deterioration due to hydrocephalus and brainstem compression. In the pediatric population in particular, early diagnosis and aggressive surgical management are strongly advocated.[106] Although it is important to address the source of the infection,[103] craniotomy has been found to be superior to sinus or otologic surgery, bur holes, or small craniectomies.[92,93,103,107–110] A

large study of nearly 700 patients in the era of CT revealed superior outcomes with extensive craniotomy to allow complete evacuation of purulent material and decompress the swollen hemisphere.[93]

Brain Abscess

As with subdural empyema, children with brain abscess require neurosurgical and infectious disease specialists to manage their care: depending on risk factors, location, and size of the abscess, delays in recognition and effective treatment can lead to major morbidity and death. Improvements in diagnostic imaging and antibiotic effectiveness have made the treatment of brain abscess more effective and less invasive, but it still remains a dangerous neurosurgical condition with major short- and long-term morbidity, including seizures[111] and cognitive[112,113] and fixed focal neurologic deficits. Furthermore, definitive statements about a decrease in the incidence or prevalence of brain abscess in the pediatric population that have accompanied these advances in diagnosis and therapy cannot be made;[90] if anything, better diagnostic imaging has led to the detection of more abscesses, and more children are immunosuppressed due to cancer chemotherapy, organ transplantation, and AIDS.

Given that clinical presentation of brain abscess can be varied and dependent upon the size, location, and stage of disease, an understanding of the risk factors for abscess in children is imperative. A high index of suspicion for brain abscess should be maintained in children with congenital heart disease, chronic sinusitis/otitis, penetrating head injury, and cranial dermal sinus tract who have otherwise unexplained fever and/or neurologic symptoms and signs. Presentation may vary with age: infants may present with an enlarged head circumference and bulging fontanelle without localizing signs, whereas older children may present with focal deficits particular to the location of the abscess. Seizures are common both at presentation and in the long term, with up to 70% of patients being affected, particularly when the abscess localized to the frontal lobes.[111]

Diagnosis of brain abscess is made with CT or MRI, and imaging features depend on the stage of abscess evolution. Data from animal models and humans, correlated with CT[114,115] and MR[116] images, have defined abscess development, which can be divided into four stages: (1) early cerebritis (days 1–3), (2) late cerebritis (days 4–10), (3) early capsule formation (days 11–14), and (4) late capsule formation (> 2 weeks).[116] Edema is common in stages 1 to 3, and ring enhancement is present in later stages.[101]

Improvements in diagnostic imaging have further facilitated advances in the surgical management of brain abscess, allowing a minimally invasive approach through image-guided stereotactic aspiration methods. Although abscess during early cerebritis may be better managed medically due to risks of hemorrhage,[117] both diagnostic and therapeutic efficacy is significantly enhanced through a surgical approach. Surgical management can be divided into two categories: stereotactic aspiration and craniotomy. Both techniques have been refined with the introduction of frameless stereotaxis over the past decade. Multiple small abscesses are sampled and drained with the stereotactic approach through a small bur hole, whereas larger abscesses that come to the surface may be excised completely and directly targeted through a smaller incision and craniotomy.

In infants, abscesses can be managed with needle aspiration through the fontanelle, guided by ultrasound,[118] frameless stereotactic skull base arrays (BrainLab, BrainLab AG, Feldkirchen, Germany) (author's unpublished experience), or electromagnetic frameless stereotaxis (AxiEM Stealth, Medtronic, Louisville, Colorado)[119] without the need for cranial fixation of the underdeveloped skull in this age group. Given the accuracy of frameless stereotaxis, younger children and adolescents no longer require placement in stereotactic head frames. Furthermore, the use of the endoscope can be directed with neuronavigation into large and potentially multiloculated collections for lysis and irrigation.[120]

Timing and the modality of surgical intervention must be made on a case-by-case basis, based on lesion location, stage, and the patient's clinical condition. Abscesses that are near the ventricle (**Fig. 11.4**) require more urgent management,

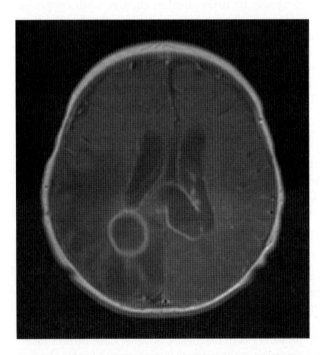

Fig. 11.4 Brain abscess. A 3-month-old presented with fever and malaise. Periventricular abscess with edema is seen after surgery in infancy for jejunal atresia and presumed hematogenous seeding to the brain.

given the risk of rupture with ensuing life-threatening ventriculitis.[121] Large abscesses with edema and mass effect threatening herniation are a surgical emergency, whereas smaller abscesses found incidentally on imaging (e.g., in the setting of congenital heart disease or immunosuppression due to cancer chemotherapy) can be managed with less urgency. Even in such cases, where neurologic symptoms or signs are absent, the most important microbiological investigation is culture of the abscess fluid or pus.[122] As with subdural empyema, posterior fossa abscesses are better managed with craniotomy than by stereotactic or bur hole aspiration.[123]

Cranial Epidural Abscess

Although cranial epidural abscess may not present as acutely or severely in comparison with subdural empyema, brain abscess, or even its spinal epidural counterpart, this intracranial suppurative infection still has the potential to lead to catastrophic complications and must be considered a primarily neurosurgical disease. Most cases of epidural abscess are associated with frontal sinusitis or cranial osteomyelitis (Pott's puffy tumor) or arise from an otogenic source, as in subdural empyema.[89,94,124,125] Other reported causes are skull fracture, hematogenous spread, poor dentition, and iatrogenic etiologies after craniotomy.[89]

In the most common presentations, where there is sinusitis, otitis, or another bony infection as the source of infection, bacteria appear to spread along the valveless diploic veins or by direct extension through areas of frank osteomyelitis. Boys and younger adolescent male patients appear to be particularly susceptible due to a peak in vascularity of the diploic system between 7 and 20 years.[126] Infections are usually polymicrobial, and bacterial species commonly found in epidural abscess mimic those in empyema, with streptococci, *H. influenzae,* and anaerobic species being the most common, with staphylococcal and enterococcal species seen in a minority of cases.[97,99] The hypoxic environment of the frontal sinuses, in particular, favors anaerobic species.

Because the infection occurs in the potential space between the dura and the skull, symptom onset is typically insidious, in contrast to subdural infection. Presenting symptoms are usually headache, fever, and localized pain accompanied by swelling and tenderness on exam. However, focal neurologic deficits can still result, but usually later in the course of the disease when the epidural collection has generated sufficient mass effect, direct compression of neural structures, or venous compression leading to infarction, as with subdural empyema above.

In contrast to subdural empyema, definitive diagnosis can be made with CT scans, with well-localized, crescent-shaped (lentiform) collections analogous to epidural hematomas seen in the setting of trauma (**Fig. 11.5**). Furthermore, epidural abscesses can cross the midline, whereas subdural empyema does not, and surrounding brain appears normal in the former and not in the latter in the early stages of disease.[101] On MRI there is often dural thickening.[127]

Following the same rationale for treatment of subdural empyema and brain abscess above, it is safer, more expeditious, and cost-effective to involve some form of surgical therapy in the diagnosis and management of epidural abscess. Heran et al proposed "conservative" neurosurgical management of epidural hematoma in a series of children with isolated epidural abscess over a 20-year period.[128] Of eight patients treated with this condition, four had endonasal or otologic procedures as the surgical intervention in their disease, despite symptomatic worsening after the procedure had been completed, a culture obtained, and antibiotic therapy initiated. With improvements in endoscopic techniques and antibiotic efficacy, this was achieved in the latter four patients in their series of eight. This series is small and underscores the need for prudent and expeditious neurosurgical treatment if there is clinical deterioration or a "more exuberant collection of pus in the epidural space."[129] Neurosurgical management provides immediate diagnostic and therapeutic benefit and allows débridement of infected bony margins and/or cranialization of an infected sinus when indicated.

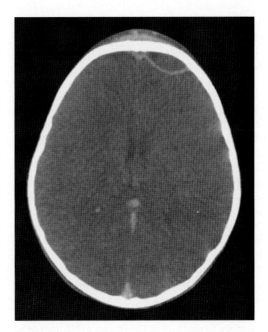

Fig. 11.5 Cranial epidural abscess and Pott's puffy tumor. A 6-year-old girl presented with fever and a tender, swollen forehead. Significant soft tissue swelling of the region of the forehead overlying a lentiform collection representing an epidural abscess is seen. On bone window and at surgery, osteomyelitis of the frontal bone was visualized as a complication of frontonasal sinusitis.

♦ Lessons Learned

Ghatan informs us about the urgency for the prompt diagnosis and management for intracranial infections. Children are particularly susceptible to suppurative infections from the common infectious processes such as sinusitis and mastoiditis. The proponent for aggressive and prompt surgery is to prevent progression of these infections and potential morbidity that had previously been reported. Cochrane and colleagues remind us that neurologic surgery began, among other things, with the treatment of intracranial infection, and that in the early days this was often fatal due to the lack of antimicrobial agents. The pathogenetic evolution of the infection from cerebritis to abscess and its imaging equivalents are presented in an appropriate overview. Furthermore, we learn that the microbial spectrum has evolved over the years in that *S. aureus* has become less frequently found, whereas anaerobes are increasingly responsible for intracranial infection. The authors state something that many infectious disease specialists may dispute, that is, the contention that preoperatively started antibiotics will not significantly affect the yield of microbial culturing.

We are also reminded that there is little evidence on the duration of antimicrobial therapy. This is all experience based, with intravenous antibiotic treatment generally recommended for 6 to 8 weeks, followed by oral treatment for 2 to 3 months.

References

1. Schiller F, Cairns H, Russell DS. The treatment of purulent pachymeningitis and subdural suppuration with special reference to penicillin. J Neurol Neurosurg Psychiatry 1948;11(3):143–182
2. Wood JH, Doppman JL, Lightfoote WE II, Girton M, Ommaya AK. Role of vascular proliferation on angiographic appearance and encapsulation of experimental traumatic and metastatic brain abscesses. J Neurosurg 1978;48(2):264–273
3. Wood JH, Lightfoote WE II, Ommaya AK. Cerebral abscesses produced by bacterial implantation and septic embolisation in primates. J Neurol Neurosurg Psychiatry 1979;42(1):63–69
4. Britt RH, Enzmann DR. Clinical stages of human brain abscesses on serial CT scans after contrast infusion: computerized tomographic, neuropathological, and clinical correlations. J Neurosurg 1983; 59(6):972–989

5. Britt RH, Enzmann DR, Yeager AS. Neuropathological and computerized tomographic findings in experimental brain abscess. J Neurosurg 1981;55(4):590–603

6. Grant F. The mortality from abscess of the brain. JAMA 1932;99: 550–556

7. Stephanov S. Experience with multiloculated brain abscesses. J Neurosurg 1978;49(2):199–203

8. Zimmerman RA, Patel S, Bilaniuk LT. Demonstration of purulent bacterial intracranial infections by computed tomography. AJR Am J Roentgenol 1976;127(1):155–165

9. Obana WG, Britt RH, Placone RC, Stuart JS, Enzmann DR. Experimental brain abscess development in the chronically immunosuppressed host: computerized tomographic and neuropathological correlations. J Neurosurg 1986;65(3):382–391

10. Baum PA, Dillon WP. Utility of magnetic resonance imaging in the detection of subdural empyema. Ann Otol Rhinol Laryngol 1992; 101(10):876–878

11. Borovich B, Braun J, Honigman S, Joachims HZ, Peyser E. Supratentorial and parafalcial subdural empyema diagnosed by computerized tomography: case report. J Neurosurg 1981;54(1): 105–107

12. Komori H, Takagishi T, Otaki E, et al. The efficacy of MR imaging in subdural empyema. Brain Dev 1992;14(2):123–125

13. Hodges J, Anslow P, Gillett G. Subdural empyema—continuing diagnostic problems in the CT scan era. Q J Med 1986;59(228): 387–393

14. Pyhtinen J, Pääkkö E, Jartti P. Cerebral abscess with multiple rims of MRI. Neuroradiology 1997;39(12):857–859

15. Weingarden SI, Swarczinski C. Non-granulomatous spinal epidural abscess: a rehabilitation perspective. Paraplegia 1991;29(9): 628–631

16. Martínez-Pérez I, Moreno A, Alonso J, et al. Diagnosis of brain abscess by magnetic resonance spectroscopy: report of two cases. J Neurosurg 1997;86(4):708–713

17. Silberstein M. H-1 MR spectroscopy in differentiation of brain abscess and brain tumor. Radiology 1998;206(3):847

18. Chang L, Miller BL, McBride D, et al. Brain lesions in patients with AIDS: H-1 MR spectroscopy. Radiology 1995;197(2):525–531

19. Jaggi RS, Husain M, Chawla S, Gupta A, Gupta RK. Diagnosis of bacterial cerebellitis: diffusion imaging and proton magnetic resonance spectroscopy. Pediatr Neurol 2005;32(1):72–74

20. Guzman R, Barth A, Lövblad KO, et al. Use of diffusion-weighted magnetic resonance imaging in differentiating purulent brain processes from cystic brain tumors. J Neurosurg 2002;97(5):1101–1107

21. Cartes-Zumelzu FW, Stavrou I, Castillo M, Eisenhuber E, Knosp E, Thurnher MM. Diffusion-weighted imaging in the assessment of brain abscesses therapy. AJNR Am J Neuroradiol 2004;25(8): 1310–1317

22. Chen SC, Chung HW. Diffusion-weighted imaging parameters to track success of pyogenic brain abscess therapy. AJNR Am J Neuroradiol 2004;25(8):1303–1304

23. Duprez TP, Cosnard G, Hernalsteen D. Diffusion-weighted monitoring of conservatively treated pyogenic brain abscesses: a marker for antibacterial treatment efficacy. AJNR Am J Neuroradiol 2005; 26(5):1296–1298, author reply 1300–1301

24. Reddy JS, Mishra AM, Behari S, et al. The role of diffusion-weighted imaging in the differential diagnosis of intracranial cystic mass lesions: a report of 147 lesions. Surg Neurol 2006;66(3):246–250, discussion 250–251

25. Fanning NF, Laffan EE, Shroff MM. Serial diffusion-weighted MRI correlates with clinical course and treatment response in children with intracranial pus collections. Pediatr Radiol 2006;36(1): 26–37

26. Fertikh D, Krejza J, Cunqueiro A, Danish S, Alokaili R, Melhem ER. Discrimination of capsular stage brain abscesses from necrotic or cystic neoplasms using diffusion-weighted magnetic resonance imaging. J Neurosurg 2007;106(1):76–81

27. Mueller-Mang C, Castillo M, Mang TG, Cartes-Zumelzu F, Weber M, Thurnher MM. Fungal versus bacterial brain abscesses: is diffusion-weighted MR imaging a useful tool in the differential diagnosis? Neuroradiology 2007;49(8):651–657

28. Tsuchiya K, Osawa A, Katase S, Fujikawa A, Hachiya J, Aoki S. Diffusion-weighted MRI of subdural and epidural empyemas. Neuroradiology 2003;45(4):220–223

29. Gray PH, O'Reilly C. Neonatal proteus mirabilis meningitis and cerebral abscess: diagnosis by real-time ultrasound. J Clin Ultrasound 1984;12(7):441–443

30. Nielsen HC, Shannon K. Use of ultrasonography for diagnosis and management of neonatal brain abscess. Pediatr Infect Dis 1983; 2(6):460–461

31. Idriss ZH, Gutman LT, Kronfol NM. Brain abscesses in infants and children: current status of clinical findings, management and prognosis. Clin Pediatr (Phila) 1978;17(10):738–740, 745–746

32. Garfield J. Management of supratentorial intracranial abscess: a review of 200 cases. BMJ 1969;2(5648):7–11

33. Tseng JH, Tseng MY. Brain abscess in 142 patients: factors influencing outcome and mortality. Surg Neurol 2006;65(6):557–562, discussion 562

34. Yoshikawa TT, Chow AW, Guze LB. Role of anaerobic bacteria in subdural empyema: report of four cases and review of 327 cases from the English literature. Am J Med 1975;58(1):99–104

35. Meschia JF, Bhat RK, Dwinnell B, MacKenzie T, Slogosky S, Schneck S. *Clostridium perfringens* subdural empyema and meningitis. Neurology 1994;44(7):1357–1358

36. Venkatesh MS, Pandey P, Devi BI, et al. Pediatric infratentorial subdural empyema: analysis of 14 cases. J Neurosurg 2006;105(5, Suppl): 370–377

37. Alderson D, Strong AJ, Ingham HR, Selkon JB. Fifteen-year review of the mortality of brain abscess. Neurosurgery 1981;8(1):1–6

38. Heineman HS, Braude AI, Osterholm JL. Intracranial suppurative disease: early presumptive diagnosis and successful treatment without surgery. JAMA 1971;218(10):1542–1547

39. Mathisen GE, Johnson JP. Brain abscess. Clin Infect Dis 1997;25(4): 763–779, quiz 780–781

40. Chibbaro S, Tacconi L. Orbito-cranial injuries caused by penetrating non-missile foreign bodies: experience with eighteen patients. Acta Neurochir (Wien) 2006;148(9):937–941, discussion 941–942

41. Woods CR Jr. Brain abscess and other intracranial suppurative complications. Adv Pediatr Infect Dis 1995;10:41–79

42. Bell WE, McGuinness GA. Suppurative central nervous system infections in the neonate. Semin Perinatol 1982;6(1):1–24

43. Renier D, Flandin C, Hirsch E, Hirsch JF. Brain abscesses in neonates: a study of 30 cases. J Neurosurg 1988;69(6):877–882

44. Steinbok P, Flodmark O, Scheifele DW. Animal bites causing central nervous system injury in children: a report of three cases. Pediatr Neurosci 1985–1986;12(2):96–100

45. Bok AP, Peter JC. Subdural empyema: burr holes or craniotomy? A retrospective computerized tomography-era analysis of treatment in 90 cases. J Neurosurg 1993;78(4):574–578

46. Dill SR, Cobbs CG, McDonald CK. Subdural empyema: analysis of 32 cases and review. Clin Infect Dis 1995;20(2):372–386

47. Khan M, Griebel R. Subdural empyema: a retrospective study of 15 patients. Can J Surg 1984;27(3):283–285, 288

48. Pathak A, Sharma BS, Mathuriya SN, Khosla VK, Khandelwal N, Kak VK. Controversies in the management of subdural empyema. A study of 41 cases with review of literature. Acta Neurochir (Wien) 1990;102(1-2):25–32

49. Smith HP, Hendrick EB. Subdural empyema and epidural abscess in children. J Neurosurg 1983;58(3):392–397

50. Gök A, Kanlikama M, Ozsaraç C. Congenital cholesteatoma with spontaneous epidural abscess, sinus thrombosis and cutaneous fistula. Neurosurg Rev 1996;19(3):189–191

51. Nathoo N, Nadvi S, van der Merwe R. Spontaneous drainage of an infratentorial extradural empyema: case report. Br J Neurosurg 1997;11(1):75–77

52. Nathoo N, Nadvi SS, van Dellen JR. Cranial extradural empyema in the era of computed tomography: a review of 82 cases. Neurosurgery 1999;44(4):748–753, discussion 753–754

53. Heran NS, Steinbok P, Cochrane DD. Conservative neurosurgical management of intracranial epidural abscesses in children. Neurosurgery 2003;53(4):893–897, discussion 897–898

54. Mauser HW, van Nieuwenhuizen O, Tummers FC, Willemse J. Conservative and surgical management of focal cerebral infection. Clin Neurol Neurosurg 1985;87(3):199–204

55. Mauser HW, Ravijst RA, Elderson A, van Gijn J, Tulleken CA. Nonsurgical treatment of subdural empyema: case report. J Neurosurg 1985;63(1):128–130

56. Leys D, Destee A, Petit H, Warot P. Management of subdural intracranial empyemas should not always require surgery. J Neurol Neurosurg Psychiatry 1986;49(6):635–639

57. Leys D, Christiaens JL, Derambure P, et al. Management of focal intracranial infections: is medical treatment better than surgery? J Neurol Neurosurg Psychiatry 1990;53(6):472–475

58. Agarwal A, Lowry P, Isaacson G. Natural history of sigmoid sinus thrombosis. Ann Otol Rhinol Laryngol 2003;112(2):191–194

59. Cochrane DD, Almqvist P, Dobson S. Intracranial epidural and subdural infections. In: Albright L, Pollack IF, Adelson P, eds. Principles and Practice of Pediatric Neurosurgery. 2nd ed. New York: Thieme; 2008:1148–1161

60. Longatti P, Perin A, Ettorre F, Fiorindi A, Baratto V. Endoscopic treatment of brain abscesses. Childs Nerv Syst 2006;22(11):1447–1450

61. Borzone M, Capuzzo T, Rivano C, Tortori-Donati P. Subdural empyema: fourteen cases surgically treated. Surg Neurol 1980;13(6):449–452

62. Miller ES, Dias PS, Uttley D. Management of subdural empyema: a series of 24 cases. J Neurol Neurosurg Psychiatry 1987;50(11):1415–1418

63. Shaw MDM. Brain abcess and other inflammatory conditions. In: Miller JD, ed. Northfield's Surgery of the Central Nervous System. Edinburgh: Blackwell Scientific Publications; 1987:526–530

64. Nathoo N, Nadvi SS, van Dellen JR, Gouws E. Intracranial subdural empyemas in the era of computed tomography: a review of 699 cases. Neurosurgery 1999;44(3):529–535, discussion 535–536

65. Pattisapu JV, Parent AD. Subdural empyemas in children. Pediatr Neurosci 1987;13(5):251–254

66. Feuerman T, Wackym PA, Gade GF, Dubrow T. Craniotomy improves outcome in subdural empyema. Surg Neurol 1989;32(2):105–110

67. Macewen W. Pyogenic Infective Diseases of the Brain and Spinal Cord. Glasgow: James Maclehose & Sons; 1893

68. Mount LA. Conservative surgical therapy of brain abscesses. J Neurosurg 1950;7(5):385–389

69. Selker RG. Intracranial abscess: treatment by continuous catheter drainage. Childs Brain 1975;1(6):368–375

70. Ballantine HT Jr, White JC. Brain abscess: influence of the antibiotics on therapy and mortality. N Engl J Med 1953;248(1):14–19

71. Dandy W. Treatment of chronic abscess of the brain by tapping. JAMA 1926;87:1477–1478

72. Jooma OV, Pennybacker JB, Tutton GK. Brain abscess: aspiration, drainage, or excision? J Neurol Neurosurg Psychiatry 1951;14(4):308–313

73. Broggi G, Franzini A, Peluchetti D, Servello D. Treatment of deep brain abscesses by stereotactic implantation of an intracavitary device for evacuation and local application of antibiotics. Acta Neurochir (Wien) 1985;76(3-4):94–98

74. Walsh PR, Larson SJ, Rytel MW, Maiman DJ. Stereotactic aspiration of deep cerebral abscesses after CT-directed labeling. Appl Neurophysiol 1980;43(3-5):205–209

75. Wild AM, Xuereb JH, Marks PV, Gleave JR. Computerized tomographic stereotaxy in the management of 200 consecutive intracranial mass lesions: analysis of indications, benefits and outcome. Br J Neurosurg 1990;4(5):407–415

76. Hakan T, Ceran N, Erdem I, Berkman MZ, Göktaş P. Bacterial brain abscesses: an evaluation of 96 cases. J Infect 2006;52(5):359–366

77. Fritsch M, Manwaring KH. Endoscopic treatment of brain abscess in children. Minim Invasive Neurosurg 1997;40(3):103–106

78. Takeshita M, Kagawa M, Yato S, et al. Current treatment of brain abscess in patients with congenital cyanotic heart disease. Neurosurgery 1997;41(6):1270–1278, discussion 1278–1279

79. Liske E, Weikers NJ. Changing aspects of brain abscesses: review of cases in Wisconsin 1940 through 1962. Neurology 1964;14:294–300

80. Morgan H, Wood MW, Murphey F. Experience with 88 consecutive cases of brain abscess. J Neurosurg 1973;38(6):698–704

81. Van Alphen HA, Dreissen JJ. Brain abscess and subdural empyema: factors influencing mortality and results of various surgical techniques. J Neurol Neurosurg Psychiatry 1976;39(5):481–490

82. Young RF, Frazee J. Gas within intracranial abscess cavities: an indication for surgical excision. Ann Neurol 1984;16(1):35–39

83. Akhaddar A, Jiddane M, Chakir N, El Hassani R, Moustarchid B, Bellakhdar F. Cerebellar abscesses secondary to occipital dermoid cyst with dermal sinus: case report. Surg Neurol 2002;58(3-4):266–270

84. Erdem G, Topaloğlu H. Abscess formation in posterior fossa dermoid cysts. Childs Nerv Syst 1997;13(6):297

85. Schijman E, Monges J, Cragnaz R. Congenital dermal sinuses, dermoid and epidermoid cysts of the posterior fossa. Childs Nerv Syst 1986;2(2):83–89

86. Borsaru AD, Naidoo P. Pyogenic abscess complicating a resolving cerebral haematoma secondary to a cavernous haemangioma: computed tomography and magnetic resonance imaging findings. Australas Radiol 2005;49(2):144–150

87. Nathoo N, Nadvi SS, van Dellen JR. Infratentorial empyema: analysis of 22 cases. Neurosurgery 1997;41(6):1263–1268, discussion 1268–1269

88. Cheek WR. Suppurative central nervous system infections. In: Cheek WR, ed. Pediatric Neurosurgery: Surgery of the Developing Nervous System. 3rd ed. Philadelphia: WB Saunders; 1994:497–511

89. Mutluer S. Bacterial infections of the central nervous system. In Choux M, Di Rocco C, Hockley A, et al, eds. Pediatric Neurosurgery. London: Churchill Livingstone; 1999:617–636

90. Frazier JL, Ahn ES, Jallo GI. Management of brain abscesses in children. Neurosurg Focus 2008;24(6):E8

91. Smith RR. Neuroradiology of intracranial infection. Pediatr Neurosurg 1992;18(2):92–104

92. Smith HP, Hendrick EB. Subdural empyema and epidural abscess in children. J Neurosurg 1983;58(3):392–397

93. Nathoo N, Nadvi SS, Gouws E, van Dellen JR. Craniotomy improves outcomes for cranial subdural empyemas: computed tomography-era experience with 699 patients. Neurosurgery 2001;49(4):872–877, discussion 877–878

94. Penido NO, Borin A, Iha LC, et al. Intracranial complications of otitis media: 15 years of experience in 33 patients. Otolaryngol Head Neck Surg 2005;132(1):37–42

95. Kombogiorgas D, Seth R, Athwal R, Modha J, Singh J. Suppurative intracranial complications of sinusitis in adolescence: single institute experience and review of literature. Br J Neurosurg 2007; 21(6):603–609

96. Osman Farah J, Kandasamy J, May P, Buxton N, Mallucci C. Subdural empyema secondary to sinus infection in children. Childs Nerv Syst 2009;25(2):199–205

97. Ziai WC, Lewin JJ III. Update in the diagnosis and management of central nervous system infections. Neurol Clin 2008;26(2):427–468, viii

98. Yoshikawa TT, Chow AW, Guze LB. Role of anaerobic bacteria in subdural empyema: report of four cases and review of 327 cases from the English literature. Am J Med 1975;58(1):99–104

99. Armstrong W, Boulis N, McGillicuddy I. Infections of the central nervous system. In: Crockard AH, Hoff J, eds. Neurosurgery: The Scientific Basis of Clinical Practice. Vol 2. 3rd ed. Oxford: Blackwell Science; 2000:757–783

100. Tsai YD, Chang WN, Shen CC, et al. Intracranial suppuration: a clinical comparison of subdural empyemas and epidural abscesses. Surg Neurol 2003;59(3):191–196, discussion 196

101. Foerster BR, Thurnher MM, Malani PN, Petrou M, Carets-Zumelzu F, Sundgren PC. Intracranial infections: clinical and imaging characteristics. Acta Radiol 2007;48(8):875–893

102. Zimmerman RD, Weingarten K. Neuroimaging of cerebral abscesses. Neuroimaging Clin N Am 1991;1:1–16

103. Bradley PJ, Shaw MDM. Subdural empyema management of the primary source. Br J Clin Pract 1984;38(3):85–88

104. Mauser HW, Ravijst RA, Elderson A, van Gijn J, Tulleken CA. Nonsurgical treatment of subdural empyema: case report. J Neurosurg 1985;63(1):128–130

105. Pathak A, Sharma BS, Mathuriya SN, Khosla VK, Khandelwal N, Kak VK. Controversies in the management of subdural empyema: a study of 41 cases with review of literature. Acta Neurochir (Wien) 1990;102(1–2):25–32

106. Venkatesh MS, Pandey P, Devi BI, et al. Pediatric infratentorial subdural empyema: analysis of 14 cases. J Neurosurg 2006;105 (5, Suppl):370–377

107. Bhandari YS, Sarkari NBS. Subdural empyema: a review of 37 cases. J Neurosurg 1970;32(1):35–39

108. Bannister G, Williams B, Smith S. Treatment of subdural empyema. J Neurosurg 1981;55(1):82–88

109. Feuerman T, Wackym PA, Gade GF, Dubrow T. Craniotomy improves outcome in subdural empyema. Surg Neurol 1989;32(2):105–110

110. Hockley AD, Williams B. Surgical management of subdural empyema. Childs Brain 1983;10(5):294–300

111. Legg NJ, Gupta PC, Scott DF. Epilepsy following cerebral abscess: a clinical and EEG study of 70 patients. Brain 1973;96(2):259–268

112. Buonaguro A, Colangelo M, Daniele B, Cantone G, Ambrosio A. Neurological and behavioral sequelae in children operated on for brain abscess. Childs Nerv Syst 1989;5(3):153–155

113. Erşahin Y, Mutluer S, Güzelbağ E. Brain abscess in infants and children. Childs Nerv Syst 1994;10(3):185–189

114. Enzmann DR, Britt RH, Yeager AS. Experimental brain abscess evolution: computed tomographic and neuropathologic correlation. Radiology 1979;133(1):113–122

115. Britt RH, Enzmann DR, Yeager AS. Neuropathological and computerized tomographic findings in experimental brain abscess. J Neurosurg 1981;55(4):590–603

116. Haimes AB, Zimmerman RD, Morgello S, et al. MR imaging of brain abscesses. AJR Am J Roentgenol 1989;152(5):1073–1085

117. Epstein F, Whelan M. Cerebritis masquerading as brain abscess: case report. Neurosurgery 1982;10(6 Pt 1):757–759

118. Theophilo F, Burnett A, Jucá Filho G, et al. Ultrasound-guided brain abscess aspiration in neonates. Childs Nerv Syst 1987;3(6):371–374

119. Mangano FT, Limbrick DD Jr, Leonard JR, Park TS, Smyth MD. Simultaneous image-guided and endoscopic navigation without rigid cranial fixation: application in infants—technical case report. Neurosurgery 2006;58(4)377–338

120. Longatti P, Perin A, Ettorre F, Fiorindi A, Baratto V. Endoscopic treatment of brain abscesses. Childs Nerv Syst 2006;22(11):1447–1450

121. Mathisen GE, Johnson JP. Brain abscess. Clin Infect Dis 1997;25(4):763–779, quiz 780–781

122. Carpenter J, Stapleton S, Holliman R. Retrospective analysis of 49 cases of brain abscess and review of the literature. Eur J Clin Microbiol Infect Dis 2007;26(1):1–11

123. Agrawal D, Suri A, Mahapatra AK. Primary excision of pediatric posterior fossa abscesses—towards zero mortality? A series of nine cases and review. Pediatr Neurosurg 2003;38(2):63–67

124. Kombogiorgas D, Solanki GA. The Pott puffy tumor revisited: neurosurgical implications of this unforgotten entity. Case report and review of the literature. J Neurosurg 2006;105(2, Suppl):143–149

125. Fountas KN, Duwayri Y, Kapsalaki E, et al. Epidural intracranial abscess as a complication of frontal sinusitis: case report and review of the literature. South Med J 2004;97(3):279–282, quiz 283

126. Wenig BL, Goldstein MN, Abramson AL. Frontal sinusitis and its intracranial complications. Int J Pediatr Otorhinolaryngol 1983; 5(3):285–302

127. Chang KH, Han MH, Roh JK, et al. Gd-DTPA enhanced MR imaging in intracranial tuberculosis. Neuroradiology 1990;32(1): 19–25

128. Heran NS, Steinbok P, Cochrane DD. Conservative neurosurgical management of intracranial epidural abscesses in children. Neurosurgery 2003;53(4):893–897, discussion 897–898

129. Heran NS, Steinbok P, Cochrane DD. Conservative neurosurgical management of intracranial epidural abscesses in children. Neurosurgery 2003;53(4):893–897, discussion 897–898

12 Chiari Malformations

◆ Decompression with Duraplasty

Chan Roonprapunt, Paolo Bolognese, and Thomas H. Milhorat

In this era of prevalent magnetic resonance imaging (MRI), Chiari malformations and syringomyelia are being diagnosed with increasing frequency. Although tonsillar ectopia appears to be a unifying anatomical marker, it is important to recognize that Chiari malformations are heterogeneous conditions with different pathophysiologic mechanisms, which can often cause overlapping symptoms. To treat these patients, each patient's tonsillar descent must be evaluated in the setting of morphometric analysis of the posterior fossa and stability of the craniovertebral junction. Tonsillar herniation may arise from congenital causes with small posterior cranial fossae (classic Chiari I malformations and craniosynostotic syndromes) and acquired causes with normal posterior cranial fossae (hydrocephalus, Paget disease, posterior fossa tumors, and spinal hypotension). Because of the varied manifestations for Chiari malformations, there have been differences in treatments and surgical outcomes. Therein lies the controversy. Ultimately, successful management depends on appropriate patient selection, tailoring the surgical intervention to treat the underlying anatomical disorder, and complication avoidance.

Diagnosis

The anatomical factors that need to be assessed are the level of cerebellar tonsillar descent, degree of cervical-medullary compression and foramen magnum impaction, presence of skeletal anomalies (basilar impression, platybasia, odontoid alignment, pannus formation, joint hypermobility, and craniocervical instability), and disturbance of cerebrospinal fluid (CSF) circulation (hydrocephalus or syringomyelia). To evaluate all these variables, we routinely perform an extensive imaging work-up. For each new patient, at least one full neuraxis brain and spine MRI is performed. In selected cases, a gadolinium-enhanced study is performed to exclude the presence of any malignancies. A three-dimensional computed tomography (CT) scan is also obtained, which is particularly useful for revision surgery.

Occasionally, this CT will also reveal bony variations, such as an incomplete bifid C1 lamina or C1-occipital assimilation, and aberrant vertebral artery anatomy.

Patients develop symptoms related to Chiari malformations from two primary mechanisms: direct brainstem compression and disturbance of CSF flow.[1] The most common symptom is the suboccipital headache that may radiate to the vertex, behind the eyes, or to the shoulders and neck. Cranial nerve signs may include impaired gag reflexes, facial sensory loss, and vocal cord paralysis. Ocular, otoneurologic, and cerebellar disturbances are also varied and common. Pediatric patients may demonstrate different clinical manifestations. The youngest patients may present with poor Karnofsky scores related to failure to thrive, because of poor oral intake. Other pediatric patients may have vague behavioral problems before they are diagnosed. Some adolescent patients may present after having had orthopedic repair of scoliosis with unrecognized syringomyelia. Finally, an incidental Chiari malformation may be found after a traumatic event. These patients are first given conservative treatment, which often involves pain management and clinical monitoring of the syrinx if present.

Surgical Indications

After conservative remedies have been exhausted, the three main indicators for surgical interventions are poor Karnofsky score ($\leq$ 70), new-onset or progression of syringomyelia (particularly syrinxes occupying > 75% transverse diameter), and severe neurologic deficit.

Surgical Goals

The goals of Chiari surgery are fourfold:

1. Adequate decompression of the cervicomedullary junction, which includes neural structures and relief of CSF block

2. Creation of a normal-sized cisterna magna and retro-cerebellar spaces
3. Establishment of optimal CSF flow between cranial and spinal compartments
4. Stabilization of the craniocervical junction if there is excessive joint hypermobility

Surgical Approach to Decompression with Duraplasty

Since the first posterior fossa decompression procedure performed by Penfield and Coburn in 1938, there has been significant improvement in surgical morbidity and mortality for the treatment of Chiari malformations. The traditional surgical approach includes bony posterior fossa decompression. In surveys sent to international pediatric neurosurgeons (2004)[2] and American pediatric neurosurgeons (1998),[3] suboccipital decompression was considered the standard surgical procedure. The majority of respondents favored routine dural opening at surgery and closure with a pericranial or synthetic patch graft. This technique has been adopted by many surgeons, because it definitively improves the flow of CSF at the level of the foramen magnum. Current surgical debate primarily rests on whether or not to perform a duraplasty.

The majority of published large case series support the overall benefits of duraplasty in achieving definitive surgical treatment.[4–13] The controversy arises from a higher associated morbidity with duraplasty and intradural manipulations. As a result, some surgeons are advocating bony decompression only, as there appears to be a subset of patients who do respond to this intervention.[14–17] In effect, the surgeon's decision is often determined by balancing the risk of a complication (**Fig. 12.1**) versus the risk of undertreatment, necessitating a return to the operating room (**Fig. 12.2**).

Duraplasty and intradural manipulations have been associated with higher morbidity in certain series. When the arachnoid is opened, there is increased risk for bleeding and adhesion formation, which can lead to arachnoiditis, pseudomeningoceles, hydrocephalus, and persistent syringomyelia. In turn, these conditions may cause persistence in symptoms or new posterior fossa syndrome complaints. The advantage of opening the dura is that it provides the necessary exposure to allow for internal decompression. The effect of chronic severe foramen magnum impaction by the cerebellar tonsils is the formation of arachnoidal adhesions, which may be the primary pathologic focus. The adhesions may be quite pervasive involving the brainstem, posteroinferior cerebellar artery, and spinal cord. Microlysis of the adhesions is an important part of the internal decompression. Additionally, we advocate tonsillar reduction if the obex area is closed and there is no evidence of pulsatile flow of CSF from the fourth ventricle. At the end of the operation, the tonsils are ideally positioned slightly above the level of the putative foramen magnum. Those

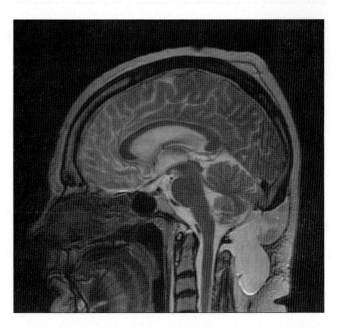

Fig. 12.1 Sagittal magnetic resonance imaging (MRI). Postoperative pseudomeningocele formation from an outside institution requiring reoperation for cerebrospinal fluid leak.

surgeons who elect not to open the dura may not address the potential significant impact of arachnoidal scarring.

Most surgeons have moved away from various intradural techniques, including posterior fossa stenting, catheters, and plugging of the obex, which have not been associated with improved outcomes.[18] The one popular exception is tonsillar shrinkage or complete tonsillar amputation. Some have argued that neural tissue should be preserved whenever possible.[19] Reduction of the cerebellar tonsils appears to be well tolerated. At the time of surgery, cystic changes are often apparent as a consequence of chronic compression and ischemia.[20] There is evidence that the cerebellar tonsils have no neurologic function, and bilateral tonsillectomy is not associated with neurologic deficits.

Although the majority of surgeons who perform duraplasties close the dura, there have been some reports, with good outcomes, supporting leaving the dura opened[12] or stitched laterally to the muscles.[21] According to the authors, it is important to preserve the arachnoid plane. Postoperative complications were related to arachnoidal violations. Limonadi et al reported that a dura-splitting decompression compared with duraplasty can result in reduced operative time, hospital stay, and cost with equivalent early outcome.[22] The counterargument is that one return to the operating room for incomplete decompression would significantly tip the cost-effective analysis in favor of duraplasty.

Duraplasty material provides another variable for surgeons to choose. Duraplasties can include autologous versus nonautologous graft materials. Autologous grafts may be

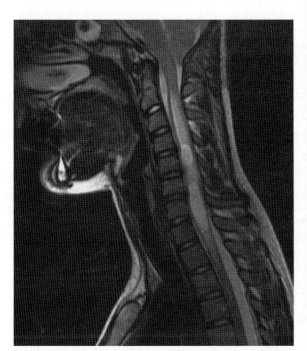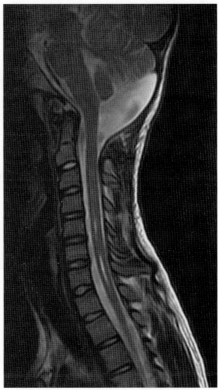

Fig. 12.2 **(A)** Sagittal MRI. **(B)** Initial treatment from an outside institution with only posterior fossa bony decompression resulted in persistent syrinx and symptoms. Subsequent revision employing expansile duraplasty reveals syrinx change within 3 months.

harvested from fascia lata, ligamentum nuchae, and pericranium. Nonautologous materials include, in decreasing order of use, bovine pericardium, cadaveric dura, and synthetics. These products may be favorable because they decrease operative time. We prefer autologous pericranium because of the decreased incidence of inflammatory reactions and CSF leaks.[23,24]

Among these variables, perhaps the central question is what is necessary and sufficient in an operation to achieve our surgical goals. To help answer this, we have adopted the use of the color Doppler ultrasound to guide us intraoperatively. Many of the technical decisions are patient specific. The particular variables in our practice include size of craniectomy, levels of laminectomy, degree of tonsillar reduction, and size of duraplasty. The color Doppler ultrasound is an important tool because it allows us real-time feedback and intraoperative confirmation of the restoration of CSF flow before we leave the operating room.[4] Some surgeons have reported that an intraoperative ultrasound may help in deciding whether to remove bone only or perform a craniectomy with duraplasty.[9] In our experience, the most effective procedure with minimal complications has been a tailored osseous decompression of the craniocervical junction, duraplasty employing autologous pericranium, and

additional intradural steps (microlysis of arachnoidal adhesions, tonsillar shrinkage) as determined by intraoperative color Doppler ultrasonography.

Complications and Revision Surgery

In balancing risks versus benefits for any procedure, it is often useful to review those complications that may lead to additional surgery. There are several pathophysiologic mechanisms for development of problems after surgery for Chiari malformations. First, there may be complications directly related to the index procedure, including transcutaneous CSF leaks, pseudomeningoceles (**Fig. 12.1**), defective duraplasties, meningoceles, cerebellar prolapse, infection, extensive adhesions, cranial settling, and craniocervical instability. Second, there may have been a failure to achieve the original goals (i.e., persistent tonsillar herniation, persistent impaction of the CSF spaces and neuroanatomical structures at the foramen magnum, and persistent and enlarging syringomyelia cavities). Third, there may have been previously unrecognized pathology not treated at the time of decompression (e.g., hydrocephalus, pseudotumor cerebri, basilar invagination, and cranial settling). These complications provide an impetus for further understanding of this complex disorder.

Surgery for Chiari malformations continues to evolve with better understanding of the pathophysiologic mechanisms and improvement in surgical techniques. In pediatric neurosurgery, new intriguing procedures are being introduced, such as tonsillectomy without craniectomy for the management of infantile Chiari I malformation.[25] More information will be required before the value of this procedure, or any new procedure, can be evaluated thoroughly. It is likely that future advances in the management of Chiari malformations will come from prospective multicenter clinical trials that provide class II evidence of long-term surgical outcomes.

♦ Decompression without Duraplasty

Frank J. Attenello, Matthew J. McGirt, and Benjamin S. Carson

Management of Chiari I malformation must consider the wide variability of the disease. The definitive caudal displacement of tonsils first described by Hans Chiari[26] often occurs with multiple associated pathologies, including syringomyelia in 35 to 70%,[26–28] scoliosis in 25 to 85%,[29,30] neurofibromatosis type 1 in 6%,[31] Klippel-Feil anomaly in 5%,[31] basilar invagination in 4%,[31] and other associated skeletal anomalies, such as platybasia and cranial settling. The degree of tonsillar herniation varies widely as well, with radiographic studies using MRI reporting herniation in symptomatic patients ranging from 3 to 29 mm below to the foramen magnum. Dynamic MRI studies suggest that decreased CSF flow occurs at the foramen magnum and may occur with a wide variety of flow abnormalities independent of the degree of tonsil herniation.[27,32,33] It remains debatable whether the anatomical degree of tonsillar hindbrain crowding or the degree of CSF flow pathology plays a greater role in the etiology of this disease.[34] The heterogeneity of Chiari I–associated pathologic conditions, variations in the degree of tonsillar ectopia, and the multifactorial pathogenesis of this disease can often make patient selection and surgical treatment a challenge for its effective management.

As would be expected, patients with Chiari I malformation are a heterogeneous group with respect to symptomatology. Chiari I malformation most commonly presents with headache and/or neck pain, exacerbated by neck movement or physical exertion.[35] Multiple other signs and symptoms of cerebellar, brainstem, and spinal cord pathology also occur with this malformation.[31,36,37] Dyste et al showed that patients with length of symptoms longer than 24 months, ataxia, nystagmus, scoliosis, and trigeminal atrophy demonstrate a decreased response to hindbrain decompression.[38] Tubbs et al found that patients with headache/neck pain and scoliosis were least likely to show symptom relief.[31] Our own series of 279 patients found that patients with subjective headaches alone are twice as likely to experience symptom recurrence as compared with more objective cranial nerve or long tract findings. Of particular note are the differences in presentation and outcome between Chiari I patients with and without syringomyelia. Our own series has shown a delayed response, both clinically and radiographically, in patients with Chiari-associated syringomyelia that in some cases may remain refractory to hindbrain decompression. These variations in Chiari-associated copathologies highlight the importance of approaching each patient individually with a treatment algorithm and plan for surgery.

Surgical Treatments

Independent of these comorbid pathologies, the definitive treatment of Chiari I malformation remains surgical posterior fossa decompression.[39] Although surgical hindbrain decompression remains the standard of care for Chiari I, tremendous variability in surgical approach exists. Variations in surgical treatment for this disease have included posterior fossa craniectomy alone, addition of C1 or more cervical laminectomies, duraplasty, a widely expanded duraplasty, dural scoring, tonsillar coagulation, obex plugging, and fourth ventricle stenting.[40] Considerable debate, however, exists specifically regarding the relative benefit of degree and type of decompression necessary in this procedure. Multiple surveys to define current strategies have been conducted, both by the Pediatric Section of the American Association of Neurological Surgeons (AANS) in 2000 and the International Society for Pediatric Neurosurgery, in 2004.[41,42] Among the International Society for Pediatric Neurosurgery responders, 95% of surgeons perform suboccipital craniectomy, and 5% perform only cervical laminectomy. Seventy-six percent of surgeons always perform duraplasty, 20% perform duraplasty based on patient characteristics, and 1% never open dura.[42] In the AANS survey for the treatment of symptomatic Chiari I, 20% of surgeons recommend only bony decompression, 30% recomme duraplasty, 25% suggest dissecting intradural adhesions in addition to duraplasty, and 30% recommend additional tonsillar coagulation.[41] The results of these two surveys, as well as favorable outcomes in therapeutically diverging studies, highlight the vast variability in treatment options of this heterogeneous disease. Of these surgical options, the greatest debate exists as to the necessity of duraplasty in hindbrain decompression.

Decompression without Duraplasty

Authors who advocate decompression without duraplasty show variation in technique, with most surgeons advocating suboccipital craniectomy, additional C1 laminectomy, and occasionally C2 laminectomy in cases of severe ectopia.[43–45] Caldarelli et al reported successful results without duraplasty and highlighted the need to also resect the thick fibrous band often encountered at the foramen magnum.[46] Also commonly employed is scoring of the outer layer of dura to theoretically enlarge the hindbrain dural covering.[43–45,47]

Authors employing these techniques will often perform intraoperative ultrasound to examine the craniocervical junction after dural scoring, ensuring adequate CSF flow, as seen by tonsillar pulsations.[48] Summation of reported outcomes associated with these various nonduraplasty techniques for the treatment of Chiari I malformation in children and young adults shows resolution of symptoms in 78% of cases (**Table 12.1**). In addition, the reported literature shows a low complication rate after nonduraplasty decompression, with 1.0% wound infection, 0.2% bacterial meningitis, and 0% CSF leak (**Table 12.1**).

Table 12.1 Summary of Reported Outcomes after Hindbrain Decompression with or without Duraplasty*

Nonduraplasty

Author	Year	#	Mean Follow-up (Months)	% Syrinx (No. of Patients)	% Improved (No. of Patients)	Infection	Meningitis	CSF Leak
Hida et al[52]	1995	12	60	100 (12)	92 (11)	0	0	0
Yundt et al[53]	1996	3	10	0 (0)	100 (3)	0	0	0
Gambardella et al[54]	1998	8	24	100 (8)	88 (7)	0	0	0
Genitori et al[44]	2000	26	21	38 (10)	92 (24)	2	0	0
Goel and Desai[55]	2000	31	38	100 (31)	90 (28)	NA	NA	NA
Munshi et al[43]	2000	11	9–96	64 (7)	73(8)	1	0	0
James and Brant[56]	2002	4	108	25 (1)	100 (4)	0	0	0
Ventureyra et al[34]	2003	8	36	50 (4)	75 (6)	NA	NA	NA
Limonadi et al[57]	2004	12	16	0 (0)	100 (12)	0	0	0
Navarro[49]	2004	71	28	34 (24)	72 (51)	0	1	0
Yeh et al[48]	2006	40	20	15 (6)	90 (36)	0	0	0
Caldarelli et al[46]	2007	31	56	42 (13)	94 (29)	0	0	0
Galarza et al[45]	2007	19	21	37 (7)	47 (9)	0	0	0
Carson[69]	2007	128	25	11 (10)	70 (89)	1	0	0
Totals		404		33 (133)	78 (317)	1.0 (4)	0.2 (1)	0 (0)

Duraplasty

Author	Year	#	Mean Follow-up (Months)	% Syrinx (No. of Patients)	% Improved (No. of Patients)	Infection	Meningitis	CSF Leak
Logue and Edwards[58]	1981	25	48	100 (25)	36 (9)	1	0	0
Hoffman et al[59]	1987	2	24	100 (2)	0 (0)	NA	NA	NA
Dyste et al[38]	1989	6	NA	0 (0)	66 (4)	NA	NA	NA
Armonda et al[27]	1994	8	13	50 (4)	100 (8)	0	0	0
Oldfield et al[60]	1994	7	21	100 (7)	100 (7)	NA	NA	NA
Fischer[61]	1995	7	27	86 (6)	71 (5)	0	0	0
Hida[52]	1995	21	60	100 (21)	90 (19)	0	2	0
Guyotat[62]	1998	45	37	100 (58)	71 (32)	0	1	0
Feldstein and Choudri[63]	1999	7	30	100 (7)	100 (7)	0	0	0
Krieger et al[64]	1999	26	46	100 (26)	88 (23)	0	0	3
Sakamoto et al[65]	1999	20	48	100 (20)	100 (20)	0	0	0
Goel and Desai[55]	2000	21	38	100 (21)	81 (17)	NA	NA	NA
Munshi et al[43]	2000	22	9–96	55 (12)	91 (20)	3	0	2

(Continued on page 146)

Table 12.1 (*Continued*)

Duraplasty								
Author	Year	#	Mean Follow-up (Months)	% Syrinx (No. of Patients)	% Improved (No. of Patients)	Infection	Meningitis	CSF Leak
Alzate et al[66]	2001	66	24	52 (34)	100 (66)	1	0	4
Lazareff et al[67]	2002	15	7	53 (8)	87 (13)	0	0	1
Greenlee et al[68]	2002	20	48	60 (12)	90 (18)	2	0	0
Ventureyra et al[34]	2003	8	36	38 (3)	100 (8)	NA	NA	NA
Tubbs et al[31]	2003	130	50	58 (75)	83 (108)	0	0	0
Limonadi and Selden[57]	2004	12	15	100 (12)	100 (12)	0	0	0
Navarro et al[49]	2004	38	28	63 (24)	66 (25)	0	1	1
Yeh et al[48]	2006	85	20	24 (20)	98 (83)	2	2	5
Galarza et al[45]	2007	41	21	41 (17)	80 (33)	0	0	NA
Guo et al[50]	2007	16	36	100 (16)	81 (13)	0	0	1
Carson[69]	2007	151	28	56 (69)	82 (124)	3	0	2
Totals		817		61 (499)	82 (674)	1.5 (12)	0.7 (6)	2.3 (19)

*Nonduraplasty patients include those with bony decompression and/or dural scoring. Duraplasty patients include those with additional tonsillar reduction in some cases. Mean follow-up is recorded in all series as a range when mean is unavailable.

Abbreviations: CSF, cerebrospinal fluid; NA, data unavailable.

Duraplasty

Duraplasty is also commonly employed, with an incision across both layers of the dura, usually in a Y-shaped manner, allowing exposure of neural contents and expansion of the dural covering of the hindbrain.[31,45,49,50] Reported duraplasty techniques vary from large Y-shaped opening to a small linear incision limited to the cranial–cervical junction. Most surgeons have advocated tailoring the degree of duraplasty to the degree of tonsillar herniation. Surgeons report an expansile closure of the dural opening with several different substances, including the pericranium, bovine pericardium, and synthetic dural substitutes.[51] A proven advantage of a particular dural graft is lacking. Authors employing duraplasty have shown an overall symptom improvement rate of 82% by our meta-analysis (**Table 12.1**). Furthermore, the summation of reported complication rates after duraplasty suggests wound infection in 1.5%, bacterial meningitis in 0.7%, and CSF leak in 2.3% of cases (**Table 12.1**).

Discussion: Argument for Nonduraplasty Decompression

Hindbrain decompression without duraplasty can achieve symptomatic improvement in a high percentage of patients with Chiari I malformations, with a reported incidence rate of symptomatic relief ranging from 47 to 100% (mean 78%; **Table 12.1**). Inherent to these reports of favorable outcome after nonduraplasty decompression are the authors' selection criteria for not performing duraplasty. Variability in

patient characteristics, differences in surgical treatment algorithms, and nonstandardized outcome measures make direct comparisons between duraplasty and nonduraplasty studies difficult. However, it is clear from the literature that favorable outcomes can be achieved with both surgical modalities based on current practice patterns. Given the very mild increased incidence of CSF leak reported with duraplasty, it may be advantageous to identify patients who can benefit from bony decompression alone.

We have experienced good results with suboccipital decompression and C1 laminectomy alone without duraplasty. In our series of 128 patients with Chiari I malformations undergoing hindbrain decompression without duraplasty, surgery has resulted in a sustained resolution of brainstem and cranial nerve symptoms in 100 (80%) patients and a sustained resolution of headache in 95 (75%) at a mean of 2 years after surgery. The majority of the 35 patients who did not have complete resolution of symptoms experienced some degree of improvement. In fact, only 11 (8%) patients undergoing bony decompression alone have required subsequent revision decompression with duraplasty, a failure rate consistent with prior reports of duraplasty outcomes (89% success rate; **Table 12.1**). Nevertheless, we do not advocate nonduraplasty decompression for all of our patients. We have found that patients with significant tonsillar herniation (to C2 or below) or with syringomyelia fare better with duraplasty. In our series of 79 patients with Chiari-associated syringomyelia, 10 were treated without duraplasty, and 69 received duraplasty. Symptoms persisted in 40% of patients undergoing bony decompression alone for syrinx versus only 17% of patients receiving duraplasty. Likewise, in patients with tonsillar ectopia below C2, we have observed a twofold increase in the risk of symptom recurrence in non-duraplasty versus duraplasty cases.

In cases of Chiari I without syringomyelia or without marked tonsillar ectopia, we use intraoperative ultrasonography to determine the need for duraplasty as reported in similar studies.[48] Over the past 10 years we have used this methodology in 279 consecutive cases, resulting in bony decompression alone in 128 (46%) patients. In each of these cases, ultrasound immediately after bony decompression demonstrated marked loss of normal cerebellar and tonsillar systolic pulsation due to tonsillar compression and hindbrain crowding. Often, pathologic pistonlike and cyclical herniations of the distalmost tonsils can be seen despite being trapped and relative immobility at the rostralmost aspect of the tonsil. Following bony decompression, we reassess with ultrasonography. In nearly half of our cases

(46%), normal systolic pulsations of the tonsils were observed after suboccipital and C1 bony decompression alone. Furthermore, expansion of subarachnoid spaces was often observed both dorsal and ventral to the tonsils (between the brainstem and tonsils). In cases demonstrating improvement in both of these features on ultrasonography after bony decompression alone, we perform nonduraplasty decompression. In cases where persistent loss of systolic pulsation and compression of the subarachnoid spaces ventral and dorsal to the tonsils remain despite suboccipital and C1 bone removal, we perform duraplasty.

In both our experience and that reported in the literature, hindbrain decompression without duraplasty can achieve excellent results when applied to the appropriate patient. Although further investigation is needed into more objective clinical and radiographic selection criteria, duraplasty may be unnecessary in many patients with symptomatic Chiari I without syringomyelia.

◆ Lessons Learned

The management of Chiari malformation and the appropriate surgical techniques to achieve the treatment goals in this condition are the perennial subject of discussion among pediatric neurosurgeons.

Are we any further in our understanding of this condition and the impact of different variants of treatment than we were 2 decades ago? There is probably some further evidence, and there is certainly more experience.

The authors of the present discussion have outlined the important issues, and indeed, there is progress in our understanding of the treatments and their impact in spite of the lack of hard, prospectively studied evidence.

Both contributions to this chapter, in particular that by Roonprapunt et al, stress the importance of individualizing the management approach. What is appropriate for one patient is not necessarily appropriate for others. Carson et al

remind those of us who are believers in the duraplasty technique that a not so small subgroup of patients with Chiari I malformations do well with a limited exposure and may have a smaller risk for complications. Even though their tabular comparison between the duraplasty and nonduraplasty publications is the exemplified selection bias of retrospective investigations, it does support the concept of individualization. Also, it allows identifying circumstances that do not render themselves to a craniectomy-only treatment. This is the presence of a syrinx, cerebellar tonsils being displaced beyond C2, and the lack of pulsation on intraoperative ultrasound.

So we are in fact smarter than in the past. And perhaps ongoing discussions will lead to the larger interinstitutional trials needed to study the evidence behind the experience.

References

1. Milhorat TH, Chou MW, Trinidad EM, et al. Chiari I malformation redefined: clinical and radiographic findings for 364 symptomatic patients. Neurosurgery 1999;44(5):1005–1017
2. Schijman E, Steinbok P. International survey on the management of Chiari I malformation and syringomyelia. Childs Nerv Syst 2004;20(5):341–348
3. Haroun RI, Guarnieri M, Meadow JJ, Kraut M, Carson BS. Current opinions for the treatment of syringomyelia and chiari malformations: survey of the Pediatric Section of the American Association of Neurological Surgeons. Pediatr Neurosurg 2000;33(6):311–317
4. Milhorat TH, Bolognese PA. Tailored operative technique for Chiari type I malformation using intraoperative color Doppler ultrasonography. Neurosurgery 2003;53(4):899–905, discussion 905–906

5. Alzate JC, Kothbauer KF, Jallo GI, Epstein FJ. Treatment of Chiari I malformation in patients with and without syringomyelia: a consecutive series of 66 cases. Neurosurg Focus 2001;11(1):E3
6. Tubbs RS, McGirt MJ, Oakes WJ. Surgical experience in 130 pediatric patients with Chiari I malformations. J Neurosurg 2003;99(2):291–296
7. Klekamp J, Batzdorf U, Samii M, Bothe HW. The surgical treatment of Chiari I malformation. Acta Neurochir (Wien) 1996;138(7):788–801
8. Guyotat J, Bret P, Jouanneau E, Ricci AC, Lapras C. Syringomyelia associated with type I Chiari malformation: a 21-year retrospective study on 75 cases treated by foramen magnum decompression with a special emphasis on the value of tonsils resection. Acta Neurochir (Wien) 1998;140(8):745–754

9. Yeh DD, Koch B, Crone KR. Intraoperative ultrasonography used to determine the extent of surgery necessary during posterior fossa decompression in children with Chiari malformation type I. J Neurosurg 2006; 105(1, Suppl):26–32

10. Sindou M, Chávez-Machuca J, Hashish H. Cranio-cervical decompression for Chiari type I malformation, adding extreme lateral foramen magnum opening and expansile duraplasty with arachnoid preservation: technique and long-term functional results in 44 consecutive adult cases—comparison with literature data. Acta Neurochir (Wien) 2002;144(10):1005–1019

11. Galarza M, Sood S, Ham S. Relevance of surgical strategies for the management of pediatric Chiari type I malformation. Childs Nerv Syst 2007;23(6):691–696

12. Krieger MD, McComb JG, Levy ML. Toward a simpler surgical management of Chiari I malformation in a pediatric population. Pediatr Neurosurg 1999;30(3):113–121

13. Ellenbogen RG, Armonda RA, Shaw DW, Winn HR. Toward a rational treatment of Chiari I malformation and syringomyelia. Neurosurg Focus 2000;8(3):E6

14. Anderson RC, Emerson RG, Dowling KC, Feldstein NA. Improvement in brainstem auditory evoked potentials after suboccipital decompression in patients with Chiari I malformations. J Neurosurg 2003;98(3):459–464

15. Munshi I, Frim D, Stine-Reyes R, Weir BK, Hekmatpanah J, Brown F. Effects of posterior fossa decompression with and without duraplasty on Chiari malformation-associated hydromyelia. Neurosurgery 2000;46(6):1384–1389, discussion 1389–1390

16. Yundt KD, Park TS, Tantuwaya VS, Kaufman BA. Posterior fossa decompression without duraplasty in infants and young children for treatment of Chiari malformation and achondroplasia. Pediatr Neurosurg 1996;25(5):221–226

17. Navarro R, Olavarria G, Seshadri R, Gonzales-Portillo G, McLone DG, Tomita T. Surgical results of posterior fossa decompression for patients with Chiari I malformation. Childs Nerv Syst 2004;20(5):349–356

18. Levy WJ, Mason L, Hahn JF. Chiari malformation presenting in adults: a surgical experience in 127 cases. Neurosurgery 1983; 12(4):377–390

19. Oldfield EH. Cerebellar tonsils and syringomyelia. J Neurosurg 2002;97(5):1009–1010, discussion 1010

20. Pueyrredon F, Spaho N, Arroyave I, Vinters H, Lazareff J. Histological findings in cerebellar tonsils of patients with Chiari type I malformation. Childs Nerv Syst 2007;23(4):427–429

21. Perrini P, Benedetto N, Tenenbaum R, Di Lorenzo N. Extra-arachnoidal cranio-cervical decompression for syringomyelia associated with Chiari I malformation in adults: technique assessment. Acta Neurochir (Wien) 2007;149(10):1015–1022

22. Limonadi FM, Selden NR. Dura-splitting decompression of the craniocervical junction: reduced operative time, hospital stay, and cost with equivalent early outcome. J Neurosurg 2004;101(2, Suppl): 184–188

23. Rosen DS, Wollman R, Frim DM. Recurrence of symptoms after Chiari decompression and duraplasty with nonautologous graft material. Pediatr Neurosurg 2003;38(4):186–190

24. Vanaclocha V, Saiz-Sapena N. Duraplasty with freeze-dried cadaveric dura versus occipital pericranium for Chiari type I malformation: comparative study. Acta Neurochir (Wien) 1997;139(2):112–119

25. Lazareff JA, Galarza M, Gravori T, Spinks TJ. Tonsillectomy without craniectomy for the management of infantile Chiari I malformation. J Neurosurg 2002;97(5):1018–1022

26. Chiari H. Uber Veranderungen des Kleinhirns infolge von Hydrocephalie des Grosshirns (Concerning changes in the cerebellum due to hydrocephalus of the cerebrum). Dtsch Med Wochenshr 1891;17:1172–1175

27. Armonda RA, Citrin CM, Foley KT, Ellenbogen RG. Quantitative cine-mode magnetic resonance imaging of Chiari I malformations: an analysis of cerebrospinal fluid dynamics. Neurosurgery 1994;35(2): 214–223, discussion 223–224

28. McGirt MJ, Nimjee SM, Fuchs HE, George TM. Relationship of cine phase-contrast magnetic resonance imaging with outcome after decompression for Chiari I malformations. Neurosurgery 2006; 59(1):140–146, discussion 140–146

29. Fischbein NJ, Dillon WP, Cobbs C, Weinstein PR. The "presyrinx" state: a reversible myelopathic condition that may precede syringomyelia. AJNR Am J Neuroradiol 1999;20(1):7–20

30. Ghanem IB, Londono C, Delalande O, Dubousset JF. Chiari I malformation associated with syringomyelia and scoliosis. Spine (Phila Pa 1976) 1997;22(12):1313–1317, discussion 1318

31. Tubbs RS, McGirt MJ, Oakes WJ. Surgical experience in 130 pediatric patients with Chiari I malformations. J Neurosurg 2003;99(2): 291–296

32. Bhadelia RA, Bogdan AR, Wolpert SM, Lev S, Appignani BA, Heilman CB. Cerebrospinal fluid flow waveforms: analysis in patients with Chiari I malformation by means of gated phase-contrast MR imaging velocity measurements. Radiology 1995;196(1):195–202

33. Barkovich AJ, Wippold FJ, Sherman JL, Citrin CM. Significance of cerebellar tonsillar position on MR. AJNR Am J Neuroradiol 1986; 7(5):795–799

34. Ventureyra EC, Aziz HA, Vassilyadi M. The role of cine flow MRI in children with Chiari I malformation. Childs Nerv Syst 2003; 19(2): 109–113

35. Elster AD, Chen MY. Chiari I malformations: clinical and radiologic reappraisal. Radiology 1992;183(2):347–353

36. Milhorat TH, Chou MW, Trinidad EM, et al. Chiari I malformation redefined: clinical and radiographic findings for 364 symptomatic patients. Neurosurgery 1999;44(5):1005–1017

37. Weinberg JS, Freed DL, Sadock J, Handler M, Wisoff JH, Epstein FJ. Headache and Chiari I malformation in the pediatric population. Pediatr Neurosurg 1998;29(1):14–18

38. Dyste GN, Menezes AH, VanGilder JC. Symptomatic Chiari malformations: an analysis of presentation, management, and long-term outcome. J Neurosurg 1989;71(2):159–168

39. Bindal AK, Dunsker SB, Tew JM Jr. Chiari I malformation: classification and management. Neurosurgery 1995;37(6):1069–1074

40. Alden TD, Ojemann JG, Park TS. Surgical treatment of Chiari I malformation: indications and approaches. Neurosurg Focus 2001;11(1):E2

41. Haroun RI, Guarnieri M, Meadow JJ, Kraut M, Carson BS. Current opinions for the treatment of syringomyelia and chiari malformations: survey of the Pediatric Section of the American Association of Neurological Surgeons. Pediatr Neurosurg 2000;33(6):311–317

42. Schijman E, Steinbok P. International survey on the management of Chiari I malformation and syringomyelia. Childs Nerv Syst 2004; 20(5):341–348

43. Munshi I, Frim D, Stine-Reyes R, Weir BK, Hekmatpanah J, Brown F. Effects of posterior fossa decompression with and without duraplasty on Chiari malformation-associated hydromyelia. Neurosurgery 2000; 46(6):1384–1389, discussion 1389–1390

44. Genitori L, Peretta P, Nurisso C, Macinante L, Mussa F. Chiari type I anomalies in children and adolescents: minimally invasive

management in a series of 53 cases. Childs Nerv Syst 2000;16(10–11): 707–718

45. Galarza M, Sood S, Ham S. Relevance of surgical strategies for the management of pediatric Chiari type I malformation. Childs Nerv Syst 2007;23(6):691–696

46. Caldarelli M, Novegno F, Vassimi L, Romani R, Tamburrini G, Di Rocco C. The role of limited posterior fossa craniectomy in the surgical treatment of Chiari malformation type I: experience with a pediatric series. J Neurosurg 2007;106(3, Suppl):187–195

47. Isu T, Sasaki H, Takamura H, Kobayashi N. Foramen magnum decompression with removal of the outer layer of the dura as treatment for syringomyelia occurring with Chiari I malformation. Neurosurgery 1993;33(5):844–849, discussion 849–850

48. Yeh DD, Koch B, Crone KR. Intraoperative ultrasonography used to determine the extent of surgery necessary during posterior fossa decompression in children with Chiari malformation type I. J Neurosurg 2006;105(1, Suppl):26–32

49. Navarro R, Olavarria G, Seshadri R, Gonzales-Portillo G, McLone DG, Tomita T. Surgical results of posterior fossa decompression for patients with Chiari I malformation. Childs Nerv Syst 2004;20(5): 349–356

50. Guo F, Wang M, Long J, et al. Surgical management of Chiari malformation: analysis of 128 cases. Pediatr Neurosurg 2007;43(5): 375–381

51. Danish SF, Samdani A, Hanna A, Storm P, Sutton L. Experience with acellular human dura and bovine collagen matrix for duraplasty after posterior fossa decompression for Chiari malformations. J Neurosurg 2006;104(1, Suppl):16–20

52. Hida K, Iwasaki Y, Koyanagi I, Sawamura Y, Abe H. Surgical indication and results of foramen magnum decompression versus syringosubarachnoid shunting for syringomyelia associated with Chiari I malformation. Neurosurgery 1995;37(4):673–678, discussion 678–679

53. Yundt KD, Park TS, Tantuwaya VS, Kaufman BA. Posterior fossa decompression without duraplasty in infants and young children for treatment of Chiari malformation and achondroplasia. Pediatr Neurosurg 1996;25(5):221–226

54. Gambardella G, Caruso G, Caffo M, Germanò A, La Rosa G, Tomasello F. Transverse microincisions of the outer layer of the dura mater combined with foramen magnum decompression as treatment for syringomyelia with Chiari I malformation. Acta Neurochir (Wien) 1998;140(2):134–139

55. Goel A, Desai K. Surgery for syringomyelia: an analysis based on 163 surgical cases. Acta Neurochir (Wien) 2000;142(3):293–301, discussion 301–302

56. James HE, Brant A. Treatment of the Chiari malformation with bone decompression without durotomy in children and young adults. Childs Nerv Syst 2002;18(5):202–206

57. Limonadi FM, Selden NR. Dura-splitting decompression of the craniocervical junction: reduced operative time, hospital stay, and cost with equivalent early outcome. J Neurosurg 2004;101(2, Suppl):184–188

58. Logue V, Edwards MR. Syringomyelia and its surgical treatment—an analysis of 75 patients. J Neurol Neurosurg Psychiatry 1981;44(4): 273–284

59. Hoffman HJ, Neill J, Crone KR, Hendrick EB, Humphreys RP. Hydrosyringomyelia and its management in childhood. Neurosurgery 1987;21(3):347–351

60. Oldfield EH, Muraszko K, Shawker TH, Patronas NJ. Pathophysiology of syringomyelia associated with Chiari I malformation of the cerebellar tonsils: implications for diagnosis and treatment. J Neurosurg 1994;80(1):3–15

61. Fischer EG. Posterior fossa decompression for Chiari I deformity, including resection of the cerebellar tonsils. Childs Nerv Syst 1995;11(11):625–629

62. Guyotat J, Bret P, Jouanneau E, Ricci AC, Lapras C. Syringomyelia associated with type I Chiari malformation: a 21-year retrospective study on 75 cases treated by foramen magnum decompression with a special emphasis on the value of tonsils resection. Acta Neurochir (Wien) 1998;140(8):745–754

63. Feldstein NA, Choudhri TF. Management of Chiari I malformations with holocord syringohydromyelia. Pediatr Neurosurg 1999;31(3): 143–149

64. Krieger MD, McComb JG, Levy ML. Toward a simpler surgical management of Chiari I malformation in a pediatric population. Pediatr Neurosurg 1999;30(3):113–121

65. Sakamoto H, Nishikawa M, Hakuba A, et al. Expansive suboccipital cranioplasty for the treatment of syringomyelia associated with Chiari malformation. Acta Neurochir (Wien) 1999;141(9):949–960, discussion 960–961

66. Alzate JC, Kothbauer KF, Jallo GI, Epstein FJ. Treatment of Chiari I malformation in patients with and without syringomyelia: a consecutive series of 66 cases. Neurosurg Focus 2001;11(1):E3

67. Lazareff JA, Galarza M, Gravori T, Spinks TJ. Tonsillectomy without craniectomy for the management of infantile Chiari I malformation. J Neurosurg 2002;97(5):1018–1022

68. Greenlee JD, Donovan KA, Hasan DM, Menezes AH. Chiari I malformation in the very young child: the spectrum of presentations and experience in 31 children under age 6 years. Pediatrics 2002; 110(6):1212–1219

69. McGirt MJ, Atlenello FJ, Datoo G, Gathinji M, Atiba A, Weingart JD, Carson B, Jallo GI. Intraoperative ultrasonography as a guide to patient selection for duraplasty after suboccipital decompression in children with Chairi malformation Type 1. J Neurosurg Pediatr 2008;2(1):52–57

13 Intractable Epilepsy

♦ Vagus Nerve Stimulation

Sudesh J. Ebenezer and Anthony M. Avellino

Vagus nerve stimulation (VNS), as delivered by the VNS Therapy System (Cyberonics, Inc., Houston, Texas), is indicated for use as an adjunctive therapy in reducing the frequency of seizures in adults and adolescents over 12 years of age with partial onset seizures that are refractory to antiepileptic medications.[1] VNS is not a cure for epilepsy; therefore, patients should consult their physicians before engaging in unsupervised activities.[1] It is a good treatment choice for patients who have not experienced success with conventional antiepileptic drugs. VNS does not cause adverse cognitive effects. Furthermore, it can be administered concurrently with antiepileptic drugs, but without additional sedative or behavioral side effects.[2,3] Because no formal clinical trials have been conducted in children younger than 12 years when the systems were implanted, the U.S. Food and Drug Administration (FDA) has not approved the use of the device in this age group.[4] Although use of VNS for children younger than 12 years is consequently considered "off label," some physicians do treat patients in this age group with VNS, and such use is according to the individual physician's judgment. Most often, VNS is prescribed for preadolescent children with partial epilepsy refractory to antiepileptic medications who are not candidates for resective surgery.

Contraindications and Precautions

The safety and efficacy of VNS has not been established for use in patients with arrhythmias, respiratory conditions, preexisting swallowing difficulty, ulcers, vasovagal syncope, only one vagus nerve, other concurrent forms of brain stimulation, preexisting hoarseness, age younger than 12 years, primary generalized seizures, or pregnancy. VNS could affect the operation of a cardiac pacemaker or implanted defibrillator. VNS cannot be used in patients after a bilateral or left cervical vagotomy.[1]

Special precautions must be taken when a patient undergoes magnetic resonance imaging (MRI). MRI should not be performed with a magnetic resonance body coil in the transmit mode on persons implanted with VNS. The heat induced in the lead by an MRI body scan can cause injury. If an MRI needs to be done, use only a transmit-and-receive type of head coil. Magnetic and radio frequency (RF) fields produced by MRI may change the pulse generator settings or activate the device. The following pulse generator and MRI procedures can be used safely without adverse events:[1]

- Pulse generator output programmed to 0 mA for the MRI procedure
- Head coil type: transmit-and-receive only
- Static magnetic field strength: ≤2.0 tesla
- Specific absorption rate (SAR): <1.3 W/kg
- Time-varying intensity: <10 tesla/sec

Pathophysiology

The mechanism of anticonvulsant action is not precisely known. It is believed that the VNS disrupts the abnormal pattern of neuronal epileptogenic discharge, increases the threshold of seizures, excites inhibitor pathways, and releases inhibitory neurotransmitters.[5] In animal models, VNS prevented seizures or seizure spread in these models: maximum electroshock, pentylenetetrazol (PTZ), 3-mercaptopropionic acid (3-MPA), alumina gel, potassium penicillin, strychnine, and kindling. Localization of vagus-initiated activity in the brain has been observed through animal studies of Fos immunoreactivity, regional brain glucose metabolism, and positron emission tomography (PET) imaging in human patients.[1]

In a $[^{15}O]H_2O$ PET study of 10 patients receiving VNS, increases in blood flow were seen in the rostral medulla, right thalamus, right anterior parietal cortex, bilateral hypothalamus, anterior insula, and inferior cerebellum.[6] In the same study, blood flow was decreased bilaterally in the hippocampus, amygdala, and posterior cingulate gyrus. Henry et al[6] suggested that VNS brought about acute increases in the synaptic activity of the structures that are directly innervated by the central vagal structures, as well as the areas that process left-sided somatosensory information. In addition, VNS seems to alter synaptic activity in the bilateral multiple limbic system structures. The altered synaptic activities at these sites of VNS-induced cerebral blood flow (CBF) changes may indicate areas of therapeutic VNS activity.[6]

Other studies have shown that VNS can reduce the onset or propagation of seizures. These studies also showed that VNS can cause inhibition of the hippocampus/amygdala, leading to long-term clinical effectiveness.[7,8]

The electrodes of the VNS device are coiled around the left, rather than the right, vagal nerve because efferent innervations seem to be asymmetrical. The sinoatrial node is innervated by the right vagus nerve, and the left vagus nerve supplies the atrioventricular node. Stimulation of the right vagus nerve therefore has the potential to produce greater cardiac slowing than similar stimulation of the left vagus nerve.[9]

Operative Procedure

Preoperative antibiotics are given 30 to 60 minutes before skin incision, depending on antibiotic type. The patient's neck and chest are prepped and draped in the usual standard sterile fashion (**Fig. 13.1**). The left carotid sheath is exposed, as it extends along the anterior border of the sternocleidomastoid muscle, and then the left vagus nerve is identified. An exposure of >3 cm of the vagus nerve facilitates placement of the electrodes on the nerve. It is preferable to choose a 3 cm section of nerve halfway up between the clavicle and the mastoid process, where it is clear of nerve branches (**Fig. 13.2**). Above this area, superior and inferior cervical cardiac branches separate from the vagus nerve. Stimulation of these branches during the system diagnostics (lead test) may cause bradycardia and/or asystole. The nerve usually lies in a posterior groove between

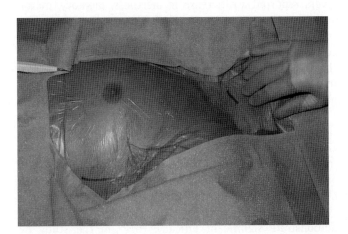

Fig. 13.1 The skin incisions are marked. (From Cyberonics, Inc., Houston, Texas. Reprinted with permission.)

the carotid artery and the internal jugular vein.[1] A pocket is then created in the left upper chest below the clavicle for the pulse generator. In small children, this preaxillary incision can be made posterior to the lateral border of the pectoralis major to avoid the pulse generator from placing pressure on the incision line.[10] A subpectoral implantation may allow better coverage with soft tissue, especially in children with minimal subcutaneous fat, and it may reduce the likelihood of the skin breaking down and damage to the generator.[11] The lead is tunneled subcutaneously from the neck to the pulse generator pocket in the chest, and the two electrodes (three helixes) are wrapped around the left vagus nerve. A strain relief bend and loop are then formed (i.e., the lead body is curled around and secured to the fascia with Silastic tie-downs to allow for some movement), and the lead is connected to the pulse generator. System diagnostics (i.e., testing of lead) is then performed. We then place the pulse generator in the chest pocket, with the extra coiled lead next to the pulse generator, and repeat the system diagnostics. Both incisions are closed in the standard fashion.[1] **Figure 13.3** shows the hardware that is implanted.

Patient Follow-up

During the 7 to 14 days after implantation, the patient should be seen to confirm wound healing and proper operation of the pulse generator. The pulse generator's output current for both the magnet and the programmed stimulation should be set at 0.0 mA for the first 14 days after implantation to allow for healing. Because VNS is an adjunctive therapy to existing antiepileptic medications, we generally keep all antiepileptic medications stable for the first 3 months of stimulation before we attempt to reduce or change a patient's medication.

During initial programming, the output current should be programmed to start at nominal parameters (0.0 mA) and then be slowly increased in 0.25 mA increments until the patient feels the stimulation at a comfortable level. Patients who are receiving replacement generators should also be started at nominal parameters, with 0.25 mA-step increases to allow reaccommodation. The average output current used during the clinical studies was ~1.0 mA. Other standard treatment settings were 30 Hz, 500 μsec pulse width, 30 second on time, and 5 minute off time. There is no proven correlation between high output current (mA) and device effectiveness, nor is there a standard treatment level that should be achieved during treatment ramping. Excessive stimulation at an excessive duty cycle has resulted in degenerative nerve damage in laboratory animals.[1]

Results

Several studies have featured VNS in the pediatric population. Many have reported benefit in children with a variety of epilepsy syndromes.[12–15] Results from several small

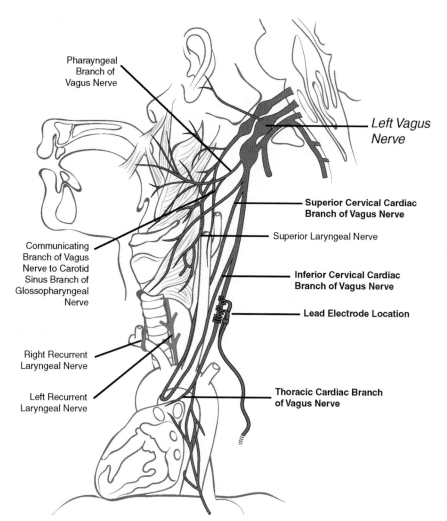

Pharayngeal
Branch of
Vagus Nerve

*Left Vagus
Nerve*

**Superior Cervical Cardiac
Branch of Vagus Nerve**

Superior Laryngeal Nerve

Communicating
Branch of Vagus
Nerve to Carotid
Sinus Branch of
Glossopharyngeal
Nerve

**Inferior Cervical Cardiac
Branch of Vagus Nerve**

Lead Electrode Location

Right Recurrent
Laryngeal Nerve

Left Recurrent
Laryngeal Nerve

**Thoracic Cardiac Branch
of Vagus Nerve**

Fig. 13.2 Branches of the vagus nerve. The three helixes should be placed around the vagus nerve below the level of the inferior cervical cardiac branch. (From Cyberonics, Inc., Houston, Texas. Reprinted with permission.)

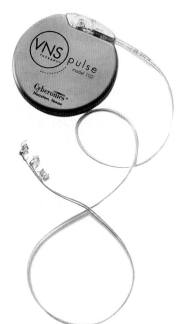

Fig. 13.3 Hardware showing pulse generator and lead. (From Cyberonics, Inc., Houston, Texas. Reprinted with permission.)

observational studies suggest that the therapeutic effect of VNS is better in children than in adults, and the benefit in children is achieved more rapidly.[3,9,12,16–26] Parents and caregivers reported an increase in alertness, memory, motor, verbal, and cognitive function.[19,20,27,28]

Three VNS studies did not note any negative effects on cognition in adults or in children.[29–31] Studies have shown that VNS is effective in preadolescent patients.[12,15,25,27,28,32,33] In one study, response was more favorable in the younger group compared with children older than 12 years.[4]

Studies have suggested that children with highly medication-resistant seizures, such as children with Lennox-Gastaut syndrome (LGS), may derive significant benefit from VNS.[3,18,21,22,28] A study of 16 children with LGS showed an overall seizure reduction of 26.9% following VNS.[21] With LGS, some studies indicate that VNS can produce satisfactory seizure control, whereas other studies have failed to demonstrate significant efficacy.[3,18,20,34] In the study by Rychlicki et al, the clinical effectiveness of the VNS seemed greater in the group of patients with partial epilepsy and drop attacks than in the group of patients with LGS.[34] In a series of patients with autism and Landau-Kleffner syndrome, improvements in quality of life were seen in up to 76% of pediatric patients at 12 months of follow-up.[35] In a series of children with epileptic encephalopathies, a >50% decrease in seizure frequency was seen in 72% of patients at 12 months and in 50% of patients at 18 months.[36]

We present highlights of several studies' findings here, in chronological order:

1. Study E04, an open-label safety study done during the preapproval period, included patients 12 years old and younger. Sixteen patients under age 12, ranging from 3.6 to 12.0 years old, were evaluated. These patients experienced a 17.9% median reduction in seizures, and 31% of the patients experienced a >50% seizure reduction.[1]

2. Murphy et al reported a reduction of >90% in the frequency of seizures in 3 out of 12 children with intractable epilepsy.[27] In a study of 19 children, 6 (32%) had a >90% reduction in the number of seizures, and 10 other patients (52.6%) had a >50% seizure reduction. This study had a follow-up period ranging from 2 to 30 months.[3] Murphy et al described the results of at least 3 months of VNS treatment in 60 patients (<18 years of age) enrolled in three different multicenter trails. A median reduction in seizure frequency of 23% at 3 months, 31% at 6 months, 34% at 12 months, and 42% at 18 months was observed. This study included 16 children younger than 12 years of age, enrolled in a compassionate use uncontrolled preapproval trial. These younger children appeared to derive a benefit similar to that of the entire group.[12]

3. Patwardhan et al's 2000 retrospective study of 38 consecutive pediatric patients, at a median follow-up period of 12 months, seizure reduction >50% was achieved in 26 of 38 patients (68%). There was no difference in the response observed in the younger (<12 years at implantation; n = 28) as compared with the older pediatric patients. The quality of life was improved in the majority of patients in this study.[25]

4. Farooqui et al reported six patients with ages ranging from 7 to 18 years, one of whom underwent VNS explantation because of a self-inflicted wound that was secondary to persistent trauma at the site of implantation. The remaining five patients had an average of 73 seizures per month. After an average follow-up time of 6.5 months with VNS, these patients had an average of 14 seizures per month, a 78% reduction.[37]

5. Helmers et al published a six-center retrospective series in 125 patients younger than 18 years of age who had been treated with VNS for 3 months to 1 year. Average seizure reduction was 36.1% at 3 months and 44.7% at 6 months. The authors did not observe any difference in seizure reduction among the group of 41 patients younger than 12 years at the time of VNS implantation.[28] Zamponi et al reported a seizure reduction rate in children >50% in 10 of 13 patients.[23]

6. Murphy et al examined outcome in the first 100 patients implanted at a single pediatric epilepsy center. Twelve patients were older than 18 years at the time of implantation. At a mean follow-up of 2.7 years, seizure reduction >50% was achieved in 45% of patients. At their last follow-up, 18% of the patients had been seizure free for 6 months. The percentage of seizure-frequency reduction in younger (6–11 years; n = 50) and older (12–18 years at the time of VNS implantation; n = 34) patients was similar in the two groups.[38]

7. In a study of 13 patients ranging in age from 6 to 28 years, Buoni et al reported 38.4% of patients obtained a >50% reduction in seizure frequency.[26] In the Hallbook et al study, 6 of 15 children showed a 50% or more reduction in seizure frequency, 12 showed an improvement in quality of life, and 11 improved in seizure severity and mood. Behavior, mood, and depressive parameters tended to improve over time.[39]

8. Blount et al studied VNS in six patients younger than 5 years, of whom 83% had a significant decrease in the frequency of their seizures. Two became seizure free (33%), three improved (50%), and one (17%) had no change in seizure status. Age at implantation did not seem to correlate with patient success.[32]

9. Alexopoulos et al compared the efficacy in children younger than 12 years at the time of VNS implantation versus adolescent children older than 12 years. They studied 46 children (ages 2.3–17.9 years); 21 patients (45.6%) were younger than 12 years at the time of surgery. Median seizure-frequency reduction was 56% at 3 months, 50% at 6 months, 63% at 12 months, 83% at 24 months, and 74% at 36 months. A total of 24 patients experienced a seizure-frequency reduction of >75%, and 19 patients experienced no response (increase in seizures or <50% reduction). Finally, five patients (10.1%) experienced no seizures for >6 months at the time of their last follow-up. Response was more favorable in the younger group.[4]

10. In the Rychlicki et al study of pediatric patients, ~55% of patients showed a reduction in seizure frequency of at least 50%. Efficacy progressively improved with the duration of treatment up to 24 months postoperatively. Among study patients with partial epilepsy, a small number experienced long-term seizure freedom. The authors noted that during seizure freedom, patients may function better during daily activities and achieve improvements in quality of life and neuropsychological performances.[34]

11. Large studies of children have described multicenter[28] and company database series.[13] Most single-center studies range from 1 to 28 patients.[12,20,25,26,40] Many studies have not separated younger (<12 years) from older (>12 years) children in their analysis.

12. Saneto et al studied 43 children younger than 12 years. Overall median seizure reduction was 55%, and 37% had at least 90% reduction. VNS was effective in children with generalized, mixed, and partial medically refractory seizures, indicating that VNS may be effective in multiple seizure types and across age ranges.[15]

Pulse Generator and Lead Replacement

Generators eventually require surgical replacement due to battery depletion. Projected battery life decreases as lead impedance increases. Battery life also depends on the pulse generator model, parameter settings, and the frequency of magnet use. In our experience, a battery can last ~5 years. Generator replacement does not, of itself, require lead replacement unless a lead fracture is suspected. Fractures can happen but are infrequent and can often be revealed when performing diagnostic testing. A lead's lifetime is undetermined at this time, but it can easily outlast adolescent growth spurts and several battery lives. Events that can shorten the life expectancy of the lead are blunt trauma to an area of the body beneath which the lead is implanted and twisting or picking at the lead or generator. Improper surgical implantation of the VNS device, such as inadequate strain relief, suturing directly on the lead or to muscle, and not using tie-downs, can also decrease life expectancy of the lead.[1]

Complications

Hoarseness, the most common complication in all patients, can be caused by device malfunction, nerve fatigue, or vocal cord dysfunction due to trauma at the implantation site. Adverse events reported also include voice alteration (hoarseness), increased coughing, pharyngitis, paresthesias, dyspnea, dyspepsia, nausea and vomiting, laryngismus, ataxia, hypesthesia, infection, and insomnia.[1] It has been reported that 54% of pediatric patients have hoarseness, 14% have cough, and 9% have dysphagia.[25]

During the clinical trials (N = 454 persons ages 12 years and older except for E04, which was a compassionate use trial and included some children), 1.1% of the patients developed infections that required explantation of the device, and 1.8% developed infections that did not require explantation.[41] Wound infection has been reported as <3% by DeGiorgio et al.[42] The risk of infection in pediatric patients may be higher. Studies of VNS in children[10,25,43,44] report infection rates from 2.9 to 12.5%. In the study by

Kirse et al, infections seemed to occur more commonly with the axillary incision compared with the cervical incision.[10] Kirse et al also found the most common surgical complication leading to generator explantation is skin breakdown and infection at the implantation sites.[10] The pediatric population poses particular challenges with regard to this complication because they may tamper with the wound or may experience trauma to the wound or generator.[43,45] Manipulation of the pulse generator or lead through the skin may damage or disconnect the lead from the pulse generator and/or possibly cause damage to the vagus nerve.[1] One developmentally disabled child in the study by Smyth et al caused a lead fracture by rotation of the device in the subcutaneous pocket.[43] Vassilyadi and Strawsburg suggested that infections requiring explantation may be more common in younger children, especially those with mental retardation.[46]

Although device implantation in children can sometimes be risky, VNS is usually not associated with adverse effects that can limit the use of antiepileptic drugs. Adverse effects can include dizziness, ataxia, insomnia, cognitive impairment, and weight gain.[4]

The VNS discontinuation rate in one study[4] was 21.7% (10/46 patients) and primarily reflected the absence of clinical response after 12 months or more of intermittent VNS. Five patients developed a wound infection around the generator, which necessitated device removal in four.[4] In our experience, when a child has an infection around the electrodes and requires explantation, help from an experienced otolaryngology surgeon is invaluable for the challenging neck dissection.

Conclusion

Although reported numbers are small, in children younger than 12 years, ~40 to 60% exhibit a 40 to 50% seizure reduction, which improves over 6 to 18 months of stimulation.[12,13,15,20,26,28] These results seem to be at least similar to or even better than the results in the two randomized, blinded, active control trials[17,29] (E03 and E05, participants ages 12 years and older). In these original studies based on 114 and 196 patients, respectively, there was a 24% and 28% mean reduction in seizures per day. In study E03, 23.4% of patients and in study E05, 35% of patients had >50% response.[17,29] Response to VNS seems more robust among younger children with a lesser duration of epilepsy than other children.[47] VNS is an effective treatment for LGS[22] and can be considered the first surgical option for treatment of LGS and related syndromes because it is less invasive, reversible, and has few serious side effects.

Most studies in adolescents and preadolescents have limitations related to their retrospective and uncontrolled design. Patient assessment has not always been blinded. Seizure frequency data many times have been based on reporting by patients and/or their families. Without randomized, controlled trials (i.e., without a nonstimulated control group) and without examining long-term outcomes, it is difficult to speculate on the net benefit of VNS.[4] VNS studies in pediatric populations are often heterogeneous and include patients with different epileptic syndromes. Because each study has so few participants, it is not yet feasible to perform a stratification to form a more homogeneous group. Also, follow-up periods and drug regimen changes are frequently not specified.[12,18–21,25,28]

The use of VNS in children merits further investigation in a randomized, controlled fashion, but at the same time, the limited available evidence supports its continued use in preadolescent and adolescent children. Future research using economic decision analysis could help determine whether the potential benefits are worth the additional cost (i.e., removal of an infected generator and the need for battery changes) in a pediatric population. Such research would be even more useful if compared with the results of long-term studies of VNS in larger, more homogeneous populations to determine optimal stimulation parameters and

determine which patients achieve the best response rates.[34] In the meantime, empirical evidence suggests that VNS is suitable as an adjunctive treatment for medically refractory seizures in pediatric and adolescent patients who are not suitable candidates for resective surgery.[26] VNS may be suitable for children younger than 12 years, as studies have shown that they may respond as well as or even better than adolescents with medically refractory seizures.[4] VNS can be applicable for a variety of seizure types across ages.[15] Brain plasticity or earlier use of VNS may account for the apparent greater efficacy of VNS in children younger than 12 years.[4,48]

Acknowledgments The authors thank Timothy Peoples, who was compensated by Cyberonics, Inc., manufacturer of the VNS Therapy System, and Susan E. Siefert, ELS, CBC, an employee and stockholder of Cyberonics, Inc., for editing the article. We also thank Jennifer Stitzel, senior VNS therapeutic consultant for Cyberonics, Inc., for providing us the VNS *Physician's Manual*. The authors used information from the VNS *Physician's Manual*, which is referenced in the text. The authors have no financial or commercial interest in the VNS Therapy System or Cyberonics, Inc.

◆ Corpus Callosotomy

Oğuz Çataltepe

Corpus callosotomy is one of the oldest surgical techniques used in patients with medically intractable epilepsy to alleviate the seizures.[49] Although resective surgical interventions are always preferable in the surgical treatment of intractable epilepsy, many patients are not candidates for resective surgery because of the location, extent, or multifocality of the seizure onset zones, and corpus callosotomy constitutes an alternative surgical option for this patient group. Corpus callosotomy is a palliative procedure that is also associated with well-documented cognitive and behavioral side effects. Corpus callosotomy enjoyed a revival as an epilepsy surgery technique in the 1970s and had a widespread application during the 1980s.[50–54] However, the number of patients that underwent a corpus callosotomy procedure was dramatically decreased in parallel to the increasing popularity of vagal nerve stimulator placement procedures during the following decades. Nevertheless, corpus callosotomy is still a viable option to control seizures in certain cases.

History

Historically, the corpus callosotomy technique underwent considerable modifications since its first application, including the extent of the sectioning and the number of commissures that were divided.[55,56] The application of

corpus callosotomy in the treatment of intractable epilepsy was first reported by Van Wagenen and Herren[49] in 1940. Van Wagenen operated on 10 patients with intractable epilepsy and performed a partial or full corpus callosotomy by approaching the corpus callosum through a large right frontoparietal craniotomy and frequently by dividing the sagittal sinus and anterior falx as well. Thereafter, Bogen et al[57] published their experience with a series of articles in the 1960s. They divided the anterior commissure, hippocampal commissure, and, in some cases, massa intermedia along the corpus callosum. Luessenhop et al[52] and Wilson et al[50,51] reported their experiences in several articles published in the 1970s. Luessenhop et al[52] exposed the full length of the callosum with a single large frontoparietal craniotomy and divided the corpus callosum and anterior commissure, and frequently the right fornix as well. Thereafter, Wilson et al,[50,51] who are largely responsible for the revival and subsequent popularity of the procedure, published several articles and also introduced the operating microscope to this procedure. They initially performed the procedure by dividing the corpus callosum, hippocampal and anterior commissures, and one-sided fornix. They modified this approach in the mid-1970s because of the high rate of complications, such as ventriculitis and hydrocephalus. Wilson et al limited the sectioning with the corpus callosum and hippocampal commissure only and did not divide the anterior commissure and fornix to leave the ependymal lining intact to avoid exposing ventricles. They further modified this technique by defining the two-stage sectioning of the corpus callosum with 2-month intervals to reduce the postoperative sequelae.[50,51] In the 1980s, staged callosotomy became more popular. The first step of staged callosotomy was the two-thirds anterior callosotomy; it was followed by a second craniotomy for complete callosotomy only if the seizure control was not satisfactory. Thereafter, an increasing number of articles were published on the subject with more details about postoperative complications and outcome-related issues.[58-64] Although the early series had high morbidity and mortality rates, corpus callosotomy became a safe, effective, and well-established procedure with the introduction and refinement of modern microsurgical techniques.[56,65-67]

Anatomy and Physiology

The corpus callosum is the largest commissure and principal anatomical and neurophysiologic connection pathway between the two hemispheres. It mostly links homotopic areas together in corresponding locations of the large portions of the two hemispheres, but it also connects heterotopic areas. Although the corpus callosum is the largest midline commissure, there are some other midline commissural structures, such as the anterior commissure, posterior commissure, hippocampal commissure, and massa intermedia. The corpus callosum consists of 180 million to 200 million axons, with a mean area of 622 mm^2, mean length of 74 mm, and mean thickness of 12 mm (at the genu and splenium) and 6 mm (at the body).[56,68,69] It can be divided into four parts: the rostrum, genu, body, and splenium. The anterior half of the corpus callosum includes the rostrum, genu, and anterior half of the body of the corpus callosum and includes fibers from premotor, motor, anterior insular, and anterior cingulate cortical areas. The anterior half of the corpus callosum is thus essential for the generalization of tonic and tonic-clonic seizures and atonic drop attacks. The posterior half of the callosum includes the splenium and the posterior half of the body and connects fibers from the parietal, temporal, posterior insular, and primary auditory areas and caudal portions of the parahippocampal gyrus and occipital lobes and transfers somatosensory and auditory information.[63,70] The corpus callosum is the most critical commissure in propagation, crossing, and generalization of the epileptogenic discharges to the contralateral hemisphere. Bilateral synchronization of epileptiform discharges occurs primarily via the corpus callosum. Therefore, sectioning of the corpus callosum inhibits seizure generalization because generalized or secondarily generalized seizures are dependent on synchronization via the corpus callosum.[71]

Surgical Indications and Presurgical Assessment

Despite being one of the oldest surgical techniques in epilepsy surgery, there is still not a general consensus on indications of corpus callosotomy. In general, it has been accepted as a palliative surgical intervention used in patients with severe, medically refractive generalized seizures who are not candidates for resective procedures. In particular, patients with drop attacks and those with secondary rapid generalized seizures are accepted as ideal candidates for corpus callosotomy. Other indications include infantile spasms, LGS, and generalized tonic-clonic and partial seizures with frontal lobe onset and without clear-cut lateralization.[66] Among these, LGS is the most responsive epilepsy syndrome to callosotomy and is considered one of the main indications for this procedure. Another group of patients who may benefit from corpus callosotomy are those with bilateral, diffuse malformations of cortical development who exhibit generalized seizures.[72] Corpus callosotomy might also have a diagnostic utility in patients who may have independent epileptogenic foci in either hemisphere with an undetermined epileptogenic zone.[60] In these patients, defining the seizure focus may be challenging due to rapid secondary generalization, and corpus callosotomy may be helpful to determine the focus of ictal onset and thus provide the opportunity for resective surgeries to achieve better seizure control. Some authors consider mixed or crossed cerebral dominance as a relative contraindication because of worsening lateralized deficits that have been noted in this patient group.[61]

Surgical Technique

The most common callosotomy technique practiced today is anterior two-thirds corpus callosotomy as the initial procedure, followed by complete callosotomy if the patient does not benefit from the initial procedure. Corpus callosotomy is performed by placing the patient in a Mayfield pin head holder in a supine position. A right-sided approach is used unless the patient has a pathology on the left hemisphere or has a right hemispheric dominance. The neck is flexed 20 degrees and tilted to slightly to the right side to use gravity to decrease the need for retraction during the procedure. A 6 cm lazy-S incision is marked 2 cm anterior and parallel to the coronal suture. Two cm of the incision crosses the midline to the left side. Two bur holes are placed over the sagittal sinus ~2 cm anterior and 3 cm posterior to the coronal suture, and one bur hole is placed over the coronal suture ~4 cm lateral to the midline. A triangular craniotomy flap with rounded anterior and posterior edges is removed after dissecting the dura and sagittal sinus gently. The sagittal sinus is covered with Surgifoam and cottonoids. Epidural spaces are also filled with Surgifoam before tenting the dura to drill holes on the bone edges. Intravenous mannitol can be administered at this point if the dura is tight. We do not use a lumbar drain routinely in these cases. The dura is opened in a U shape and reflected over the sagittal sinus. An MR venogram should be obtained preoperatively and reviewed carefully before surgery to avoid injuring large bridging veins and venous dural lakes. The interhemispheric fissure and falx are exposed by dissecting the arachnoid granulations gently from the dura and sagittal sinus wall, and cottonoid pledgets are placed over the exposed cortex. At this stage, a surgical microscope is brought into the field, and the remaining part of the surgery is continued under the microscope. If there are major bridging veins entering the sagittal sinus, their arachnoid sleeves can be dissected as far lateral as possible to minimize their stretch during the retraction. It is exceptionally rare to have a major bridging vein anterior to the coronal suture. If large bridging veins are noted, the surgical procedure can be performed between the veins using separate surgical corridors anterior and posterior to the major veins. Division of larger veins posterior to the bregma should be strictly avoided. After preparing the surgical corridor, the cortex is gently retracted away from the falx, and a single retractor blade with a tapered end attached to a self-retaining retractor holder is placed on the mesial frontal cortex. The orientation of the surgical corridor is determined, and a cottonoid is placed onto the mesial surface of the superior frontal gyrus along the planned surgical corridor. The retractor blade is then gently slid downward until the cingular gyrus is seen. At this stage, two moderate-sized cotton balls are placed into the interhemispheric fissure anterior and posterior to the surgical corridor to keep the mesial frontal gyrus separated from the falx and to minimize the necessity of the retraction as much as possible. Some arachnoid adhesions extending from the cortex to the sagittal sinus or falx can be seen at this stage and can be easily separated with bipolar and microscissors while sliding the retractor blade lower. The inferior edge of the falx also can be seen at this stage. The arachnoid membrane over the mesial frontal cortex in the interhemispheric fissure is opened at a few separate points using a fine bipolar forceps, and CSF is drained by suctioning it through the cotton balls for a few minutes. This maneuver provides a much relaxed exposure, and the retractor can be removed briefly to avoid unnecessary pressure over the cortex. Subsequently, the tip of the retractor blade is placed again on the cottonoids and advanced downward to expose the cingulate gyri. Dissection of the cingulate gyri from each other can be quite difficult in some cases because of arachnoid adhesions. The ideal point to start dissecting the cingulate gyri should be determined by exploring the exposed area anteriorly and posteriorly. When a relatively free part is found, dissection of the cingulate gyri can be performed easily using bipolar forceps tips and a Penfield no. 4 dissector. At this point, the supracallosal

cistern is opened, and the underlying glistening white corpus callosum is encountered. The corpus callosum has a very distinctive appearance and consistency. Next, the cortical ribbon is repositioned, and further CSF drainage is obtained through the supracallosal cistern. Then cotton balls are replaced downward toward the corpus callosum to keep the cingulate gyri separated and to expose the corpus callosum better. At this stage, pericallosal arteries are also exposed. They frequently travel very close to each other, and even some tiny bridging vessels can be encountered. These vessels need to be mobilized and separated to have a wider exposure of the corpus callosum. Although, rarely, more than one retractor ribbon is needed throughout this stage if brain relaxation is not sufficient, and a second ribbon may be placed on the falx to provide a better exposure. The corpus callosum is then divided longitudinally using microdissectors and bipolar forceps. When the division of the corpus callosum is deepened, the grayish color of the ependymal lining can be easily appreciated. It is preferable not to enter the ventricle by opening the ependyma to avoid the risk of chemical meningitis. The division of the corpus callosum is continued around the genu until the visualization of the anterior commissure between the fornices. Exposure of the anterior commissure indicates the end of the anterior part of the division procedure. The anterior commissure should be left intact. The ribbon is readjusted posteriorly, and dissection continues on the rostrum and anterior body of the corpus callosum by sweeping the dissector through the corpus callosum. If the goal is an anterior two-thirds callosotomy, then one challenge at this stage is translating the planned length of the callosotomy onto the surgical field. The length of the planned callosotomy can be measured preoperatively using midsagittal MR images. This measurement can be translated to the surgical field using a ruler or by calculating the thickness of the ribbon as a measuring tool. Another practical and reliable tool is the neuronavigator. Using the frameless neuronavigator, the preplanned two-thirds distance can be easily determined and marked with a probe on the corpus callosum. After reaching the posterior end of the division, the ribbon is relaxed to see if there is any bleeding and then removed once meticulous hemostasis is obtained. The dura is closed primarily. Then the bone flap is fixated with microplates, and scalp layers are closed appropriately.

If the goal is posterior callosotomy or completing the anterior two-thirds craniotomy to a complete callosotomy, the patient is placed in a prone position with a 20-degree retroflexion of the neck for better exposure of the splenium. The head is placed in a Mayfield pin head holder, and a lazy-S incision is placed at the vertex level. The incision crosses the midline 2 cm to the left, and the surgical field is exposed with two small self-retaining retractors. The anterior point of the exposed area is 4 cm anterior to the lambda, and the posterior end of the incision is just over 1 cm behind the lambda. The bur holes in the midline are placed on the sagittal sinus, and the lateral bur hole is placed 4 cm lateral to the midline; a free bone flap is then removed. Using the same surgical technique as described above, the dura is opened, and the dissection is continued toward the posterior body of the callosum and splenium by following the midline. It is very critical to stay on the midline during this part of the procedure to avoid any injury to the fornices. A neuronavigator can be used to achieve this goal. The division of the corpus callosum continues toward the splenium and ends with the exposure of the arachnoid covering the vein of Galen beneath the splenium. Division of the hippocampal commissure is not necessary and should be avoided.

If the plan is to perform a complete callosotomy in one session, then we use a 10 cm S-incision located on the midline and parallel to the sagittal suture. Four centimeters of the incision is placed anterior to the coronal suture, and 6 cm of the incision is placed posterior to the coronal suture. Next, we place three midline bur holes over the sagittal suture and three lateral bur holes ~5 cm lateral to the midline. This way, we remove a larger free bone flap to determine the most appropriate surgical corridors to stay away from major draining veins and also to use multiple surgical corridors if needed. The remaining part of the procedure proceeds as described above.

Several advanced techniques aimed at achieving a better exposure with minimally invasive surgical approaches have been described and have shown to benefit some cases. These techniques include preoperative planning with sophisticated MRI software, use of intraoperative frameless neuronavigator guidance, and neuroendoscopic-assisted microsurgery and radiosurgery.[73]

Complications and Side Effects

Surgery-related complication rates have been reported as 3 to 10% and include cerebral edema, infarction, meningitis (septic/aseptic), hydrocephalus, ischemia, and bleeding, such as subdural/epidural hematomas originating from parasagittal veins.[66] The side effects of corpus callosotomy are well defined, and disconnection-related syndromes have been categorized based on the extent of the callosotomy. An anterior two-thirds callosotomy may cause decreased spontaneity of speech lasting for a few days to weeks. This might be seen in a range from mild speech disturbance to complete mutism. Acute disconnection syndrome is also well known and is seen in the early postoperative period in the majority of the patients. It includes mutism, transient reduction in spontaneity of speech, difficulty of initiating speech, stuttering, left-sided neglect, apraxia, various degrees of left leg paresis, hemiparesis, left-sided or bilateral forced grasp reflexes, bilateral extensor plantar responses, and urgency incontinence.[63,65,66] Speech difficulties with protected writing skills have been reported in right-handed

patients with right-sided language dominance. In addition, dysraphia with retained speech has been observed in left-handed individuals with left-sided speech dominance.[55,56,61] This syndrome might be related to retraction and brain edema on the nondominant parasagittal cortex, supplementary motor area, or premotor cortex. Symptoms typically improve over days to weeks.

A posterior callosotomy causes interhemispheric somatosensory, auditory, and visual disconnection syndromes. These are frequently temporary findings, but permanent interhemispheric sensory disconnection can also develop. Sectioning of the splenium can result in two types of posterior disconnection syndromes: visual disconnection and sensory disconnection. These are detected as an inability to describe the objects presented visually or tactilely on the nondominant side. The patient may recognize an object by sight or touch but cannot name it.[55,56,61,63]

Side effects of a complete corpus callosotomy include both anterior and posterior callosotomy-related findings and loss of one hemisphere's access to the other. A complete corpus callosotomy may also, though infrequently, cause interhemispheric antagonism. Split-brain syndrome can develop after a complete callosotomy and involves language impairment, hemisphere competition, and disordered attention–memory sequencing. These findings generally improve with time. Hemisphere competition refers to unresponsiveness of the nondominant hand (alien hand) to verbal commands. The dominant hemisphere no longer has access to the nondominant hemisphere to perform skilled distal movements in these patients. However, owing to the presence of the ipsilateral uncrossed motor pathways, each hemisphere is still able to control some proximal movements of the ipsilateral limb.[56]

Outcome

One of the largest reviews on the subject includes 563 patients who had corpus callosotomies at multiple centers.[53] This study reported that only 7.6% of the patients had seizure-free outcome, and 31.4% had no improvement. However, 60.9% of the patients had worthwhile improvement with rare seizures. In another study, Spencer et al[54] reported that corpus callosotomies resulted in a significant improvement in >70% of patients with atonic seizures. In another series, Wong et al[63] reported that of the 74 patients who underwent corpus callosotomy,18.9% were seizure-free, and 66.2% had a >50% reduction in seizure frequency.

Outcomes of corpus callosotomies have been reviewed based on the callosotomy technique (complete callosotomy vs two-thirds anterior callosotomy), and controversial results have been reported.[58,60,62,65,67] Some authors reported better outcomes in patients who underwent complete callosotomy. Spencer et al[54] reported that, although 80% of patients with complete corpus callosotomy became seizure-free or had significant improvement, this rate was only 50% in partial callosotomy cases. Roberts and Siegel[65] reported that 38% of patients with anterior two-thirds callosotomies had significant improvement (>80% seizure reduction), but this rate became 81% when they completed the callosotomy in second-stage surgeries. Other authors also reported better outcome results with complete corpus callosotomy in comparison with partial corpus callosotomy.[62,64,67] Fuiks et al,[58] however, did not find any significant difference between the two approaches.

The outcome assessments based on seizure type also attracted a significant interest among the authors and was reviewed in several series. Roberts and Siegel[65] published a detailed outcome analysis based on seizure types. They reported that atonic seizures responded best to corpus callosotomy, with a 72% significant improvement rate, 21% of them being seizure-free. These authors observed 34% seizure freedom and 24% significant improvement (>50% reduction in seizure frequency) in patients with generalized major motor seizures and 42% seizure freedom and 20% significant improvements in patients with complex partial seizures. The worst outcome was seen in the focal motor seizure group. Pinard et al[67] reported that the best outcomes were associated with drop attacks that either completely resolved or dramatically reduced in frequency in 90% of the children. Kawai et al[72] also reported 10 patients with bihemispheric malformations of cortical development who underwent corpus callosotomy. The drop attacks resolved completely in 8 of 10 patients in this series.

Nei et al[74] compared the responses to corpus callosotomy and placement of a vagal nerve stimulator in a series of 50 patients. They reported that 79.5% of patients who underwent corpus callosotomy had >50% decrease in seizure frequency, and 60% had >80% decrease in seizure frequency. These rates were 50% and 33%, respectively, in the vagal nerve stimulator group (n = 21). The complication rates were 21% (3.8% permanent) and 8% (transient) for corpus callosotomy and vagal nerve stimulator groups, respectively. As a result, Nei et al concluded that callosotomy is associated with greater efficacy but higher risk for complications, although mostly transient. In another study, You et al[75] found that the efficacy and safety of corpus callosotomy and VNS were comparable in children with LGS.

Conclusion

Corpus callosotomy is a palliative surgical treatment option for certain types of seizures and is associated with a low rate of seizure freedom but a high rate of improvement. Anterior two-thirds corpus callosotomy is the most commonly used technique and provides very satisfactory results in the majority of patients. Corpus callosotomy should be considered as a treatment option especially in patients with disabling drop attacks and generalized seizures. Although VNS has comparable results in controlling drop attacks, corpus callosotomy is a viable option in patients who did not respond well to VNS. Corpus callosotomy can also be used as a diagnostic tool in determining surgical candidacy for subsequent resective procedures.

◆ Lessons Learned

Every seizure is a hurricane moving over the brain. Intractable frequent seizures may make patients just as desperate as their caregivers and treating physicians. There may be less controversy between the advocates of invasive and destructive surgery such as callosotomy and those of the presumably less invasive technique of VNS. Many aspects, also outlined in this chapters, may in fact show that both techniques have their place in individual patient circumstances.

The contribution by Cataltepe nicely outlines the history of this well-known technique and cites the classic literature up to Gazzaniga's work, which showed the split-brain neurocognitive pathology. The present-day practice is clearly outlined, as one would primarily perform the surgery in a two-stage method, with an anterior two-thirds callosotomy first, sparing the splenium. The concept includes a possible second surgery if the seizure activity warrants it. None of the smaller commissures would be divided. There is a fairly robust understanding of the role of the corpus callosum in

the generalization of seizure activity, and thus the pathophysiologic thinking behind the surgery is rather clear. We learn also the neuropsychological sequelae of the procedure, as well as its complications and downsides. It appears that drop attacks and LGS, as well as rapidly generalized intractable seizure, are the best indications for this procedure.

Improvement rates are around two thirds, with one fifth of patients having a chance of becoming seizure free. This comes at a price, as one study is cited with 20% transient and 4% permanent complications. This was compared with 8% transient complications in a comparison to VNS, although the latter therapy did not achieve a comparable benefit.

This is probably the most clear-cut difference between the two: the "big" surgery (callosotomy) appears to have a higher seizure control rate, however inhomogeneous any study population may be, but a significant complication rate. The "small" surgery (if there is such a thing as "small" surgery) of implantation of a VNS has much less morbidity, but the seizure control rates are also not as good. We learn that a small fraction of patients become seizure free, about one third to one half benefit significantly, such as a ≥50% seizure frequency reduction. There appears to be a peculiar increase in effect over time. The authors detail the available study literature. Still, very little is understood about the physiology of VNS; in fact, we have little idea about how this stimulation works. An important aspect discussed is the fact that at this time, the FDA has not approved VNS for children younger than age 12. Nonetheless, off-label use has shown that children appear to benefit even more from this treatment than adults. The best indications clearly overlap with callosotomy: drop attacks, generalized seizures not amenable to resective procedures, and LGS. The authors make a convincing case for the use of this treatment modality in otherwise untreatable circumstances for children, in spite of the fact that the formal FDA requirements have not been met.

Both contributions to this chapter provide a fine overview of two highly developed and probably somewhat complementary techniques of epilepsy surgery.

References

1. Physician's Manual: VNS Therapy™ Pulse Model 102 Generator and VNS Therapy™ Pulse Duo Model 102R Generator. Houston: Cyberonics; 2005
2. Shields WD. Management of epilepsy in mentally retarded children using the newer antiepileptic drugs, vagus nerve stimulation, and surgery. J Child Neurol 2004;19(Suppl 1):S58–S64
3. Hornig GW, Murphy JV, Schallert G, Tilton C. Left vagus nerve stimulation in children with refractory epilepsy: an update. South Med J 1997;90(5):484–488
4. Alexopoulos AV, Kotagal P, Loddenkemper T, Hammel J, Bingaman WE. Long-term results with vagus nerve stimulation in children with pharmacoresistant epilepsy. Seizure 2006;7(15):491–503
5. Uthman BM, Wilder BJ, Penry JK, et al. Treatment of epilepsy by stimulation of the vagus nerve. Neurology 1993;43(7):1338–1345
6. Henry TR, Votaw JR, Bakay RA, et al. Vagus nerve stimulation-induced cerebral blood flow changes differ in acute and chronic therapy of complex partial seizures. Epilepsia 1998;39(Suppl 6):92
7. Van Laere K, Vonck K, Boon P, Brans B, Vandekerckhove T, Dierckx R. Vagus nerve stimulation in refractory epilepsy: SPECT activation study. J Nucl Med 2000;41(7):1145–1154
8. Van Laere K, Vonck K, Boon P, Versijpt J, Dierckx R. Perfusion SPECT changes after acute and chronic vagus nerve stimulation in relation to prestimulus condition and long-term clinical efficacy. J Nucl Med 2002;43(6):733–744
9. Amar AP, Heck CN, Levy ML, et al. An institutional experience with cervical vagus nerve trunk stimulation for medically refractory epilepsy: rationale, technique, and outcome. Neurosurgery 1998;43(6):1265–1276, discussion 1276–1280
10. Kirse DJ, Werle AH, Murphy JV, et al. Vagus nerve stimulator implantation in children. Arch Otolaryngol Head Neck Surg 2002;128(11):1263–1268
11. Bauman JA, Ridgway EB, Devinsky O, Doyle WK. Subpectoral implantation of the vagus nerve stimulator. Neurosurgery 2006;58(4, Suppl 2):ONS-322–ONS-325
12. Murphy JV; the Pediatric VNS Study Group. Left vagal nerve stimulation in children with medically refractory epilepsy. J Pediatr 1999;134(5):563–566
13. Wheless JW, Maggio V. Vagus nerve stimulation therapy in patients younger than 18 years. Neurology 2002;59(6, Suppl 4):S21–S25
14. Wakai S, Kotagal P. Vagus nerve stimulation for children and adolescents with intractable epilepsies. Pediatr Int 2001;43(1):61–65
15. Saneto RP, Sotero de Menezes MA, Ojemann JG, et al. Vagus nerve stimulation for intractable seizures in children. Pediatr Neurol 2006;35(5):323–326
16. Aldenkamp AP, Van de Veerdonk SH, Majoie HJ, et al. Effects of 6 months of treatment with vagus nerve stimulation on behavior in children with Lennox-Gastaut syndrome in an open clinical and nonrandomized study. Epilepsy Behav 2001;2(4):343–350
17. DeGiorgio CM, Schachter SC, Handforth A, et al. Prospective long-term study of vagus nerve stimulation for the treatment of refractory seizures. Epilepsia 2000;41(9):1195–1200
18. Labar D. Vagus nerve stimulation for intractable epilepsy in children. Dev Med Child Neurol 2000;42(7):496–499
19. Lundgren J, Amark P, Blennow G, Strömblad LG, Wallstedt L. Vagus nerve stimulation in 16 children with refractory epilepsy. Epilepsia 1998;39(8):809–813
20. Parker AP, Polkey CE, Binnie CD, Madigan C, Ferrie CD, Robinson RO. Vagal nerve stimulation in epileptic encephalopathies. Pediatrics 1999;103(4 Pt 1):778–782
21. Majoie HJ, Berfelo MW, Aldenkamp AP, Evers SM, Kessels AG, Renier WO. Vagus nerve stimulation in children with therapy-resistant epilepsy diagnosed as Lennox-Gastaut syndrome: clinical results, neuropsychological effects, and cost-effectiveness. J Clin Neurophysiol 2001;18(5):419–428
22. Frost M, Gates J, Helmers SL, et al. Vagus nerve stimulation in children with refractory seizures associated with Lennox-Gastaut syndrome. Epilepsia 2001;42(9):1148–1152
23. Zamponi N, Rychlicki F, Cardinali C, Luchetti A, Trignani R, Ducati A. Intermittent vagal nerve stimulation in paediatric patients: 1-year follow-up. Childs Nerv Syst 2002;18(1–2):61–66
24. Hosain S, Nikalov B, Harden C, Li M, Fraser R, Labar D. Vagus nerve stimulation treatment for Lennox-Gastaut syndrome. J Child Neurol 2000;15(8):509–512
25. Patwardhan RV, Stong B, Bebin EM, Mathisen J, Grabb PA. Efficacy of vagal nerve stimulation in children with medically refractory epilepsy. Neurosurgery 2000;47(6):1353–1357, discussion 1357–1358
26. Buoni S, Mariottini A, Pieri S, et al. Vagus nerve stimulation for drug-resistant epilepsy in children and young adults. Brain Dev 2004;26(3):158–163
27. Murphy JV, Hornig G, Schallert G. Left vagal nerve stimulation in children with refractory epilepsy: preliminary observations. Arch Neurol 1995;52(9):886–889
28. Helmers SL, Wheless JW, Frost M, et al. Vagus nerve stimulation therapy in pediatric patients with refractory epilepsy: retrospective study. J Child Neurol 2001;16(11):843–848
29. Handforth A, DeGiorgio CM, Schachter SC, et al. Vagus nerve stimulation therapy for partial-onset seizures: a randomized active-control trial. Neurology 1998;51(1):48–55

30. Dodrill CB, Morris GL. Effects of vagal nerve stimulation on cognition and quality of life in epilepsy. Epilepsy Behav 2001;2(1):46–53

31. Elger G, Hoppe C, Falkai P, Rush AJ, Elger CE. Vagus nerve stimulation is associated with mood improvements in epilepsy patients. Epilepsy Res 2000;42(2–3):203–210

32. Blount JP, Tubbs RS, Kankirawatana P, et al. Vagus nerve stimulation in children less than 5 years old. Childs Nerv Syst 2006;22(9):1167–1169

33. Labar D. Vagal nerve stimulation: effects on seizures. In: Luders HO, ed. Deep Brain Stimulation and Epilepsy. London: Martin Dunitz; 2004:255–262

34. Rychlicki F, Zamponi N, Trignani R, Ricciuti RA, Iacoangeli M, Scerrati M. Vagus nerve stimulation: clinical experience in drug-resistant pediatric epileptic patients. Seizure 2006;15(7):483–490

35. Park YD. The effects of vagus nerve stimulation therapy on patients with intractable seizures and either Landau-Kleffner syndrome or autism. Epilepsy Behav 2003;4(3):286–290

36. Disabato RD, Barnhurst R, Levisohn PM. Efficacy of vagus nerve stimulation in young children with generalized epilepsies. Epilepsia 2001;42:171

37. Farooqui S, Boswell W, Hemphill JM, Pearlman E. Vagus nerve stimulation in pediatric patients with intractable epilepsy: case series and operative technique. Am Surg 2001;67(2):119–121

38. Murphy JV, Torkelson R, Dowler I, Simon S, Hudson S. Vagal nerve stimulation in refractory epilepsy: the first 100 patients receiving vagal nerve stimulation at a pediatric epilepsy center. Arch Pediatr Adolesc Med 2003;157(6):560–564

39. Hallböök T, Lundgren J, Stjernqvist K, Blennow G, Strömblad LG, Rosén I. Vagus nerve stimulation in 15 children with therapy resistant epilepsy: its impact on cognition, quality of life, behaviour and mood. Seizure 2005;14(7):504–513

40. Nagarajan L, Walsh P, Gregory P, Lee M. VNS therapy in clinical practice in children with refractory epilepsy. Acta Neurol Scand 2002;105(1):13–17

41. Cyberonics. Data on file. 2004

42. DeGiorgio CM, Amar A, Apuzzo ML. Surgical anatomy, implantation technique, and operative complications. In: Schachter SC, Schmidt D, eds. Vagus Nerve Stimulation. London: Martin Dunitz; 2001:35–50

43. Smyth MD, Tubbs RS, Bebin EM, Grabb PA, Blount JP. Complications of chronic vagus nerve stimulation for epilepsy in children. J Neurosurg 2003;99(3):500–503

44. Murphy JV, Hornig GW, Schallert GS, Tilton CL. Adverse events in children receiving intermittent left vagal nerve stimulation. Pediatr Neurol 1998;19(1):42–44

45. Le H, Chico M, Hecox K, Frim D. Interscapular placement of a vagal nerve stimulator pulse generator for prevention of wound tampering: technical note. Pediatr Neurosurg 2002;36(3):164–166

46. Vassilyadi M, Strawsburg RH. Delayed onset of vocal cord paralysis after explantation of a vagus nerve stimulator in a child. Childs Nerv Syst 2003;19(4):261–263

47. Helmers SL, Griesemer DA, Dean JC, et al. Observations on the use of vagus nerve stimulation earlier in the course of pharmacoresistant epilepsy: patients with seizures for six years or less. Neurologist 2003;9(3):160–164

48. Renfroe JB, Wheless JW. Earlier use of adjunctive vagus nerve stimulation therapy for refractory epilepsy. Neurology 2002;59(6, Suppl 4): S26–S30

49. Van Wagenen WP, Herren RY. Surgical division of the commissural pathways in the corpus callosum: relation to spread of an epileptic attack. Arch Neurol Psychiatry 1940;44:740–759

50. Wilson DH, Reeves A, Gazzaniga M. Division of the corpus callosum for uncontrollable epilepsy. Neurology 1978;28(7):649–653

51. Wilson DH, Reeves AG, Gazzaniga MS. "Central" commissurotomy for intractable generalized epilepsy: series 2. Neurology 1982; 32(7):687–697

52. Luessenhop AJ, Dela Cruz TC, Fenichel GM. Surgical disconnection of the cerebral hemispheres for intractable seizures: results in infancy and childhood. JAMA 1970;213(10):1630–1636

53. Engel J, Van Ness PJ, Rasmussen TB, Ojemann LM. Outcome with respect to epileptic seizures. In: Engel J, ed. Surgical Treatment of the Epilepsies. 2nd ed. New York: Raven Press; 1993:609–621

54. Spencer SS, Spencer DD, Sass KJ, Westerveld M, Katz A, Mattson R. Anterior, total, and two-stage corpus callosum section: differential and incremental seizure responses. Epilepsia 1993;34(3):561–567

55. Spencer SS, Gates JR, Reeves AR, Spencer DD, Maxwell RE, Roberts D. Corpus callosum section. In: Engel J, ed. Surgical Treatment of Epilepsies. New York: Raven Press; 1987:425–444

56. Zentner J. Surgical aspects of corpus callosum section. In: Tuxhorn I, Holthausen H, Boenigk H, eds. Pediatric Epilepsy Syndromes and Their Surgical Treatment. London: John Libbey; 1997:830–849

57. Bogen JE, Sperry RW, Vogel PJ. Commissural section and propagation of seizures. In: Jasper HH, Ward AA, Pope A, eds. Basic Mechanism of the Epilepsies. Boston: Little, Brown; 1969:439–440

58. Fuiks KS, Wyler AR, Hermann BP, Somes G. Seizure outcome from anterior and complete corpus callosotomy. J Neurosurg 1991;74(4): 573–578

59. Maehara T, Shimizu H. Surgical outcome of corpus callosotomy in patients with drop attacks. Epilepsia 2001;42(1):67–71

60. Clarke DF, Wheless JW, Chacon MM, et al. Corpus callosotomy: a palliative therapeutic technique may help identify resectable epileptogenic foci. Seizure 2007;16(6):545–553

61. Sass KJ, Novelly RA, Spencer DD, Spencer SS. Postcallosotomy language impairments in patients with crossed cerebral dominance. J Neurosurg 1990;72(1):85–90

62. Rahimi SY, Park YD, Witcher MR, Lee KH, Marrufo M, Lee MR. Corpus callosotomy for treatment of pediatric epilepsy in the modern era. Pediatr Neurosurg 2007;43(3):202–208

63. Wong TT, Kwan SY, Chang KP, et al. Corpus callosotomy in children. Childs Nerv Syst 2006;22(8):999–1011

64. Maehara T, Shimizu H. Surgical outcome of corpus callosotomy in patients with drop attacks. Epilepsia 2001;42(1):67–71

65. Roberts D, Siegel A. Section of corpus callosum for epilepsy. In: Schmideck HH, Sweet WH, eds. Operative Neurosurgical Techniques. 4th ed. Philadelphia: WB Saunders; 2000:1490–1498

66. Menezes MS. Indications for corpus callosum section. In: Miller JW, Silbergerd DL, eds. Epilepsy Surgery: Principles and Controversies. New York/London: Taylor & Francis; 2006:556–562

67. Pinard JM, Delalande O, Chiron C, et al. Callosotomy for epilepsy after West syndrome. Epilepsia 1999;40(12):1727–1734

68. Tomasch J. Size, distribution, and number of fibres in the human corpus callosum. Anat Rec 1954;119(1):119–135

69. Gazzaniga M, Ivry RB, Mangun GR. Cerebral lateralization and specialization. In: Cognitive Neuroscience: The Biology of the Mind. 2nd ed. New York: WW Norton; 2002:405–410

70. Funnell MG, Corballis PM, Gazzaniga MS. Cortical and subcortical interhemispheric interactions following partial and complete callosotomy. Arch Neurol 2000;57(2):185–189

71. Jenssen S, Sperling MR, Tracy JI, et al. Corpus callosotomy in refractory idiopathic generalized epilepsy. Seizure 2006;15(8):621–629

72. Kawai K, Shimizu H, Yagishita A, Maehara T, Tamagawa K. Clinical outcomes after corpus callosotomy in patients with bihemispheric malformations of cortical development. J Neurosurg 2004;101(1, Suppl): 7–15

73. Eder HG, Feichtinger M, Pieper T, Kurschel S, Schroettner O. Gamma Knife radiosurgery for callosotomy in children with drug-resistant epilepsy. Childs Nerv Syst 2006;22(8):1012–1017

74. Nei M, O'Connor M, Liporace J, Sperling MR. Refractory generalized seizures: response to corpus callosotomy and vagal nerve stimulation. Epilepsia 2006;47(1):115–122

75. You SJ, Kang HC, Ko TS, et al. Comparison of corpus callosotomy and vagus nerve stimulation in children with Lennox-Gastaut syndrome. Brain Dev 2008;30(3):195–199

14 Moyamoya Disease

♦ Pial Synangiosis: Encephaloduroarteriosynangiosis–Encephalomyosynangiosis

Ronald T. Grondin, Edward R. Smith, and R. Michael Scott

Moyamoya syndrome is a vasculopathy characterized by chronic progressive stenosis to occlusion at the distal portions of the intracranial internal carotid arteries, including the proximal anterior cerebral arteries (ACAs) and middle cerebral arteries (MCAs). It is associated with ~6% of childhood strokes.[1,2] As progressive stenosis occurs, characteristic arterial collateral vessels develop at the base of the brain. These collateral vessels, when visualized on angiography, have been likened to the appearance of "something hazy, like a puff of cigarette smoke drifting in the air," which translates as *moyamoya* in Japanese.

Some authors have distinguished between moyamoya disease, the idiopathic form of moyamoya, and moyamoya syndrome, defined as the vasculopathy found in conjunction with systemic conditions such as heart disease, sickle cell disease, and Down syndrome.[3,4] In both moyamoya disease and moyamoya syndrome, treatment strategies are directed toward improving the cerebral blood supply. Medical management is an important adjunct in improving the outcomes of patients with moyamoya, but definitive treatment of the disease appears to require cerebral revascularization. Here, we review the diagnosis and management of moyamoya, with a particular focus on the utilization of a specific method of "indirect" (not directly anastomosing two vessels together) cerebral revascularization–pial synangiosis.

Clinical Presentation and Natural History

Adults with moyamoya often present with hemorrhage, leading to rapid diagnosis. In contrast, children usually present with recurrent transient ischemic attacks (TIAs), stroke, seizures, or headaches; only ~3% of pediatric patients in the Children's Hospital, Boston series had an intracerebral hemorrhage as their first symptom.[3]

The natural history of moyamoya syndrome is variable, ranging from slow progression, with rare, intermittent events, to rapid progression with fulminant neurologic decline.[3,5] At the time of their initial presentation, almost all children have bilateral involvement by arteriography, and the majority of remaining patients presenting with unilateral disease will go on to develop disease in the contralateral hemisphere.[3] It has also been estimated that up to 66% of patients with moyamoya have progression of the disease with poor outcomes if left untreated.[6–8] This number contrasts strikingly to an estimated rate of only 2.6% of symptomatic disease progression in a meta-analysis of 1156 surgically treated pediatric patients.[9] A more recent review of asymptomatic patients reported an annual stroke rate of 3.2% and reported radiographic progression of disease in 80%.[10] The experience of Children's Hospital, Boston has been that ~67% of patients will demonstrate radiographic progression of disease within a 5-year period.

The overall prognosis of patients with moyamoya syndrome depends on the rapidity and extent of vascular occlusion, the patient's ability to develop effective collateral circulation, the age at onset of symptoms, the severity of presenting neurologic deficits and degree of disability, and the extent of infarction seen on computed tomography (CT) or magnetic resonance imaging (MRI) studies at the time of initial presentation.[11] In general, neurologic status at the time of treatment, more so than the age of the patient, predicts long-term outcome.[3,12]

Importantly, individual patients have an excellent prognosis if surgical revascularization is performed prior to disabling infarction, even if severe angiographic changes are already present.[3] Even in asymptomatic patients, surgical revascularization has been reported to protect against infarction.[10] However, if left untreated, both the angiographic process and the clinical syndrome invariably progress, producing clinical deterioration with potentially irreversible neurologic deficits over time.[13]

Diagnostic Investigations

Moyamoya syndrome should be considered and diagnostic evaluation begun in any child who presents with symptoms of cerebral ischemia (e.g., a TIA manifesting as episodes of hemiparesis, speech disturbance, sensory impairment, involuntary movement, and/or visual disturbance), especially if the symptoms are precipitated by physical exertion, hyperventilation, or crying. The diagnosis of moyamoya is confirmed by radiographic studies. Radiographic evaluation of a given patient suspected of having moyamoya usually proceeds through several studies.

On CT, small areas of hypodensity suggestive of stroke are commonly observed in cortical watershed zones, basal ganglia, deep white matter, or periventricular regions.[14,15] Hemorrhage from moyamoya vessels can be readily diagnosed on head CT.

CT findings often lead to an MRI study, with acute infarcts seen using diffusion weighted imaging (DWI) and chronic infarcts visualized with T1 and T2 imaging. Ongoing cortical ischemia may be inferred from fluid attenuation inversion recovery (FLAIR) sequences that demonstrate linear high signal following a sulcal pattern, felt to represent slow flow in poorly perfused cortical circulation (the so-called ivy sign).[15,16] The most diagnostic MRI findings in moyamoya disease are diminished flow voids in the internal carotid and middle and anterior cerebral arteries coupled with prominent collateral flow voids in the basal ganglia and thalamus.[15,17–21]

Cerebral angiography is the gold standard for the diagnosis of moyamoya disease. Angiographic studies should include selective injection of both internal and external carotid arteries and vertebral arteries. External carotid imaging is essential to identify preexisting collateral vessels, so that surgery, if performed, will not disrupt them. Aneurysms or arteriovenous malformations (AVMs), known to be associated with some cases of moyamoya, can also be best detected by conventional angiography.

Cerebral Perfusion Studies and Follow-up Imaging

Cerebral blood flow studies can be helpful in the diagnostic evaluation of patients with moyamoya disease and assist in treatment decisions. Techniques include transcranial Doppler (TCD) ultrasonography, xenon-enhanced CT, positron emission tomography (PET), and single-photon emission computed tomography (SPECT) with acetazolamide challenge.

Although each of these studies has the potential to add information on the diagnosis and management of moyamoya, not all are routinely used in the United States. MRI/MR angiography (MRA) and conventional angiography are the standard diagnostic tools used for most patients with moyamoya. Following treatment, an angiogram and an MRI/MRA are often obtained 1 year after surgery and, depending on the age of the patient, yearly MRI thereafter.

Surgical Treatment

Once a major stroke or hemorrhage has occurred, children with moyamoya disease frequently are left with permanent neurologic impairment.[5,22] Therefore, early diagnosis and prompt treatment of this disorder are of utmost importance to prevent additional neurologic deficits. Despite this urgency, there is no agreed-upon method of treatment for patients with this chronic occlusive cerebrovascular disorder. There are reports of some patients who stabilize clinically without intervention, but this typically occurs after they have experienced significant, debilitating neurologic disability.

The majority of data available supports the use of surgical revascularization as a first-line therapy for the treatment of moyamoya syndrome, particularly for patients with recurrent or progressive symptoms.[9] Some studies have suggested that there may be differences in the effectiveness of surgery for the treatment of moyamoya depending on the type of presentation of the patient—hemorrhagic or ischemic.[6] These studies suggest that revascularization procedures prevent recurrent ischemic attacks, an important finding given that the majority of pediatric patients with moyamoya present with ischemic symptoms. Two relatively large studies with long-term follow-up have demonstrated a good safety profile for surgical treatment of moyamoya (4% risk of stroke within 30 days of surgery per hemisphere), with a 96% probability of remaining stroke-free over a 5-year follow-up period.[3,6] These data suggest that surgical therapy of moyamoya confers an effective, durable treatment for the disease.

Advantages and Disadvantages of Direct Revascularization Procedures Relative to Indirect Revascularization Procedures

Surgical treatments designed to increase perfusion of ischemic neural tissue in patients with moyamoya can be classified as direct, in which a healthy vessel is transected and anastomosed end to side to a cortical vessel distal to the site of moyamoya stenosis, or indirect, in which vascularized tissue, including muscle, dura, and scalp vessels, are put into contact with the brain and serve as a new source of collateral vessel development over time.

Direct anastomosis procedures, most commonly superficial temporal artery (STA)–to–MCA bypasses, may achieve instant improvement in focal cerebral perfusion, but these procedures are technically difficult to perform because pediatric patients often do not have a large enough donor scalp artery or recipient MCA to allow for an anastomosis large enough to supply a significant amount of additional collateral blood supply. Because of proximal stenoses, new blood supply provided to a single MCA branch may not allow wide redistribution of the newly available collateral. Temporary occlusion of a middle cerebral branch during the anastomosis may interfere with leptomeningeal collateral pathways already present and lead to an increased incidence of perioperative stroke. Furthermore, there is a paucity of reported series documenting the effectiveness of STA-MCA bypass in children in the United States. There is however, extensive evidence, including long-term follow-up, substantiating the efficacy of indirect revascularization procedures, such as pial synangiosis.[3]

Indirect Revascularization Procedures

A variety of indirect anastomotic procedures have been described: encephaloduroarteriosynangiosis (EDAS), whereby the STA is dissected free over a course of several inches and then sutured to the cut edges of the opened dura; encephalomyosynangiosis (EMS), in which the temporalis muscle is dissected and placed onto the surface of the brain to encourage collateral vessel development; and the combination of both, encephalomyoarteriosynangiosis (EMAS).[23–25] There are multiple variations of these procedures, including solely drilling bur holes, without vessel anastomosis,[26,27] and craniotomy with inversion of the dura in hopes of enhancing new dural revascularization of the brain.[28] Cervical sympathectomy,[29] omental transplantation,[30–32] and omental pedicle grafting[33–35] have also been described, although sympathectomy has largely been abandoned due to its ineffectiveness.[36] Finally, several groups have reported improved results in the use of combined direct and indirect anastomoses.[23,37–39] A modification of the EDAS procedure has been described to treat moyamoya syndrome in both children and adults, termed *pial synangiosis* (described below), which leads to the induction of new collateral vessels in the patient with chronic ischemia due to moyamoya. The efficacy and durability of this specific variant of indirect revascularization have been validated by the largest surgical series of children with moyamoya reported in North America.[3]

Direct versus Indirect Procedures

One major consideration in the treatment of patients with moyamoya is the decision of which surgical technique to employ. A meta-analysis of 1156 pediatric patients treated with surgery concluded that 87% (1003 patients) derived symptomatic benefit from surgical revascularization (complete disappearance or reduction in symptomatic cerebral ischemia), but that there was no significant difference between the indirect and direct/combined groups.[9] Guidelines from Japan's Ministry of Health and Welfare regarding indications for the surgical treatment of moyamoya syndrome (in both children and adults) discuss only direct

bypass surgery for revascularization, a technique that is often not feasible in young children due to the small caliber of their vessels.[40] A review of pediatric patients with moyamoya has proposed that children under the age of 8 years should all receive indirect revascularization surgery, whereas older children could potentially receive both direct and indirect revascularization (if feasible).[39] The Children's Hospital, Boston series strongly supports the utilization and long-term effectiveness of indirect revascularization with pial synangiosis in children of all ages. Although proponents of direct surgery often cite the primary benefit of immediate increases in perfusion, there is substantial evidence supporting the premise that indirect procedures, such as pial synangiosis, provide similar or improved long-term outcomes when compared with direct procedures in children. In addition, pial synangiosis is technically less demanding than direct bypass procedures, is less likely to fail, and does not present the risk of hyperperfusion injury.

Surgical Technique of Pial Synangiosis

The posterior (parietal) branch of the STA is identified by a pencil Doppler probe, and the artery is traced from its base above the zygomatic arch to the parietal convexity. Its course is accurately marked on the skin with an 18- or 21-gauge needle. We attempt to mark out at least 10 cm of vessel in most patients, but in young children, often only 6 to 7 cm can be identified. Although the parietal branch of the STA is most frequently used because the skin incision can be kept behind the hairline and the majority of the MCA circulation lies beneath that branch of the artery, the frontal branch can be used if necessary. Prior to draping, bilateral electroencephalography (EEG) electrodes are applied to the scalp so that continuous EEG monitoring can be performed throughout the case. Standard skin prep and draping can then be performed.

Skin Incision

We use the microscope right from the beginning of the artery dissection, finding it particularly helpful in very young children because of the fragility and small size of the STA and in young adults because of the frequent tortuosity of the vessel and its branches. A small skin incision down to subcutaneous tissue is made directly over the vessel at its most distal marked point with a no. 15 scalpel. The artery is identified by scalp retraction with toothed forceps and dissected using a delicate curved pediatric hemostat. A linear incision following the course of the artery is then performed, using the hemostat to dissect and then protect the STA as the assistant incises the skin overlying it. The skin edges rarely require coagulation, and most scalp edge bleeding will stop spontaneously, despite preoperative daily aspirin therapy, which is maintained throughout the peri- and postoperative period.

Synangiosis Procedure

After the artery is exposed, we use a needle-tip cautery ("Colorado needle") at a low setting to separate the artery with its subjacent galea strip from the galea on either side. The artery pedicle is then encircled with a vessel loop distally and elevated and separated from the underlying periosteum and temporalis fascia using standard monopolar cautery, attempting to preserve as much adventitia and loose areolar tissue beneath the vessel as possible.

Anterior and posterior scalp flaps are then developed with electrocautery dissection to minimize bleeding, and disposable fishhook-type retractors are used to maintain scalp retraction. The artery pedicle is retracted out of the field as needed using the vessel loop, and the temporalis muscle is incised with the electrocautery into four equal quadrants, which are retracted widely using the previously placed skin hooks. Generous bur holes are drilled inferiorly and superiorly in the exposure, and as large a craniotomy as possible is turned using power equipment. The dura is then opened vertically along the exposure and cut into six separate flaps that are retracted on sutures; care is taken to preserve any significant middle meningeal collateral observed on the preoperative arteriogram, and the dura is opened around or between such vessels. Under high-power microscope, the arachnoid is incised linearly over the exposed cortex using a disposable arachnoid knife and jeweler's forceps, beginning inferiorly over the temporal lobe in a sulcus and when possible laterally toward the crown of the adjacent gyri. Vannas ophthalmic scissors are helpful in making long, continuous arachnoid openings over MCA branches in certain patients. The pial vasculature will be profuse and tortuous in patients with advanced disease, and these areas of the pia should be avoided when the arachnoid is opened. Bleeding that occurs from the pial surface or from small vessels within the sulci usually stops after a few moments of irrigation with a microirrigator or the application of a minuscule pledget of Gelfoam soaked in saline. After completion of the arachnoid opening through as much of the length of the exposure as possible, the STA with its galea investiture is brought down onto the surface of the brain, placing the vessel over areas of opened arachnoid. Using jeweler's forceps and a Castroviejo needle holder, the vessel is fixed to the cortical surface by placing three to six interrupted 10–0 nylon sutures through the vessel adventitia and the outermost layer of the pial-cortical surface (**Fig. 14.1**). At the completion of the pial synangiosis, the donor vessel is affixed to the cortical surface (**Fig. 14.2**). This tight pial approximation leads to a more satisfactory postoperative result then simply placing the vessel on the brain or suturing the vessel into the dura.

The dura is then laid loosely on the brain surface and not sutured, as collateralization of the underlying brain will also occur from the cut edges of the dura. A large piece of

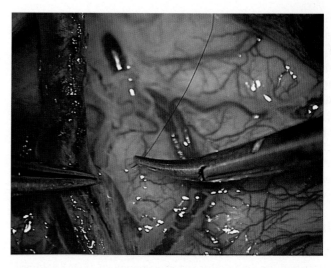

Fig. 14.1 Photomicrograph illustrating suture (10–0 nylon) passed though the adventitia of a donor vessel prior to a pial stitch.

DuraGen or Gelfoam soaked in saline and trimmed to the size of the bony opening is placed over the entire exposure, and the bone flap is repositioned using three to four miniplates. The bur hole openings at either end of the flap should be enlarged if necessary prior to its repositioning to ensure that the artery is not compressed when the flap is replaced. The temporalis muscle is approximated only from inferior to superior so that the superficial temporal artery is not compressed. The scalp is closed in two layers, using 3–0 or 4–0 Vicryl suture on the galea followed by 4–0 or 5–0 monofilament Vicryl Rapide to approximate the skin edges. A sterile Telfa-over-Xeroform gauze dressing is applied, but the head is not wrapped tightly to avoid compressing the scalp arteries. Patients are extubated and sent to the intensive care unit for 24 hours following the procedure.

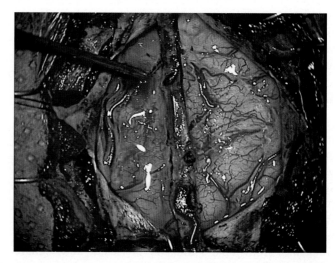

Fig. 14.2 Photograph of a donor artery after pial synangiosis demonstrating attachment to the cortical surface and wide arachnoid opening.

Postoperative Management

The patient's head is slightly elevated to assist in venous return and to avoid cerebrospinal fluid accumulations under the skin flaps. The patient is given sufficient pain medication so that there is a minimum of crying and hyperventilation. Antibiotics are given postoperatively for 24 hours. Patients are mobilized as tolerated and kept well hydrated. Blood loss with the procedure should be well under 100 cc, and transfusions should be avoided if at all possible because of the rheologic problems that can be created by a high hematocrit. Postoperative seizure medication is continued on an individualized basis, and aspirin is begun 24 hours after surgery. Postoperative hypertension is rarely treated unless significant elevations occur, and care must be taken if treatment is required to avoid rebound hypotension.

Results and Complications

The clinical and radiographic results following indirect revascularization with pial synangiosis are excellent. Postoperative angiograms or MRI/MRA studies obtained 12 months after surgery typically demonstrate MCA collateralization from both the donor STA and the meningeal arteries (**Fig. 14.3**).[3,39] A review of 143 children with moyamoya syndrome treated with pial synangiosis demonstrated marked reductions in stroke frequency after surgery, especially after the first year postoperatively.[3] In this group, only 3.2% of patients had strokes after at least 1 year of follow-up, compared with 67% preoperatively and 7.7% in the perioperative period. After a minimum of 5 years of follow-up, the overall stroke rate was 4.3% (2 of 46). This finding supports the premise that surgical treatment of moyamoya with an indirect procedure such as pial synangiosis provides a significant protective effect against new strokes in this patient population.

The most significant postoperative complication in our series has been stroke, which in a consecutive series of 143 patients occurred at ~4% per operated hemisphere. Patients at greatest risk appear to be those with neurologic instability around the time of surgery, those who have suffered a stroke within 2 months of the operation, and those with certain angiographic risk factors, such as moyamoya disease in the posterior circulation. These risks would also be present—and perhaps magnified—in a patient undergoing STA-MCA bypass. We feel that the argument that a rapid increase in cerebral blood flow following a direct bypass is better for the patient is specious: the small size of the anastomosed vessels and the presence of significant proximal stenoses due to the moyamoya prevent the bypass from supplying much blood to the operated hemisphere initially, and patients who are unstable neurologically are at greatest risk following such procedures, as the cerebral bypass data have demonstrated in the past. The excellent follow-up angiographic results from pial synangiosis procedures have been well documented in the literature, whereas there is a paucity of similar data in the pediatric neurosurgical literature demonstrating angiographic results following bypass. In fact, the site of the bypass is often difficult to detect on postoperative angiograms, with much of the new collateral to the brain coming from dural and scalp vessels, as in a synangiosis procedure. Chronic subdural hematomas developed in 3 of 143 patients (2%). Two of the chronic subdural hematomas required evacuation via a bur hole, but there was no permanent hematoma-related morbidity in any of these cases.[3] This complication probably related to preexisting brain atrophy and chronic antiplatelet therapy and might have occurred regardless of which surgical technique had been used for revascularization.

Conclusion

Moyamoya disease is a chronic vasculopathy that, if left untreated, results in progressive stenosis in the cerebral vasculature and symptomatic ischemic insult to the brain. Surgical treatment consists of revascularization of affected hemispheres through a variety of direct and indirect techniques. Indirect revascularization techniques, such as pial synangiosis, provide excellent long-term protection from new or recurrent ischemic events with a low risk of perioperative complications and should be strongly considered as the primary treatment of choice in the pediatric population.

◆ Extracranial-Intracranial Bypass Surgery

Nadia Khan and Yasuhiro Yonekawa

The spontaneous occlusion of the circle of Willis was first described in 1957 by Takeuchi and Shimizu.[41] Their first case demonstrated a peculiar angiographic presentation consisting of bilateral stenosis of the intracranial internal carotid arteries (ICAs) beginning at the terminal portion with formation of an abnormal vascular network of collaterals in the basal ganglia resembling "a puff of smoke drifting in the air," or *moyamoya* in the Japanese language, the term commonly used for this angiopathy.

The presence of these angiographic findings in combination with other rare congenital or acquired systemic diseases is termed *moyamoya syndrome.* Moyamoya

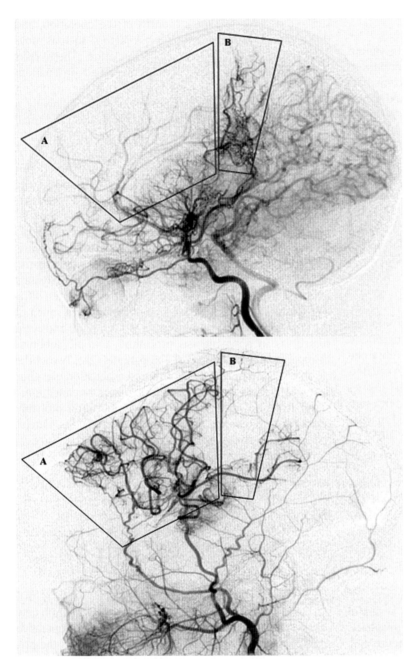

Fig. 14.3 Preoperative (*top*) and postoperative (*bottom*) angiograms in a patient managed with pial synangiosis. The top image demonstrates an internal carotid injection of a hemisphere with Suzuki (stage 3?) moyamoya disease. Angiography of the external carotid artery at 12 months postsurgery demonstrates Matsushima grade A revascularization. Box labeled **A** demonstrates the area that underwent revascularization through the external carotid circulation. Box labeled **B** shows the area of the cortex that maintained its blood supply from the internal carotid circulation.

angiopathy is referred to here as both moyamoya disease and the moyamoya syndrome form of presentation.[42,43] Two clinical manifestations can be distinguished: childhood or juvenile moyamoya (peak age at presentation 5–10 years) and adult moyamoya (peak age at presentation 30–40 years). Patients with moyamoya become symptomatic due to episodes of recurrent cerebral ischemia or complete stroke. The clinical symptoms can vary from headaches to recurrent TIAs, epileptic seizures, and disturbances of speech and/or cognition. In cases of recurrent and even chronic frontal ischemia, retardation of normal mental development may result. Ischemic symptoms are most common in the juvenile form of moyamoya and are more often seen in Caucasian adult patients, whereas the primary manifestation in Asian adults is cerebral hemorrhage arising from the region of the network of collateral vessels. Mortality can range from 2% in the acute infarct phase to 16% with intracranial intracerebral hemorrhage.

The natural history of the disease is not known. The juvenile form appears to progress into puberty, thereafter stabilizing spontaneously.[43] Eighty percent of patients have a rather benign course in terms of life expectancy with or without surgery but have to expect significant neurologic dysfunction. At the other end of the spectrum, children presenting with the disease prior to the age of 5 may suffer from significant impairment in normal psychomotor development. Therefore, early detection and early surgical management to augment cerebral perfusion by surgical revascularization procedures are essential. Moyamoya angiopathy occurs primarily in Japan and the Southeast Asian countries. It was first recognized in Europe in the late 1960s. The last epidemiological survey was performed in 1996, when a total of 168 patients were reported with peaks in the 0 to 9 years and 20 to 29 years age groups.[44]

Methodology

A systematic presurgical work-up protocol is important to determine the optimal revascularization procedure and timing of surgery.

The presurgical assessment includes a clinical and neuropsychological evaluation, TCD MRI scans to demonstrate ischemia or infarcts, and hemodynamic studies to evaluate regional perfusion reserves deficits. Depending on the available expertise, this may include perfusion MRI, xenon CT, hexamethylpropyleneamine oxime (HMPAO)-SPECT, or $H_2^{15}O$-PET with a Diamox challenge.[45,46]

In addition to these noninvasive investigations, a conventional cerebral angiography is essential to determine the anatomy of the affected vasculature and the extent and anatomy of already existing collateral vessels, as well as the caliber of potential bypass vessels. The choice of the number and location of revascularization is based anatomically on the severity and extent of disease, as demonstrated by the angiogram, and functionally on the regional vascular perfusion reserve, as demonstrated by the Diamox challenge studies (**Figs. 14.4** and **14.5**).

Patients

Over a period of 10 years, 65 patients underwent surgical revascularization for moyamoya angiopathy at the University Hospital of Zurich, Switzerland. Sixty-six percent (42/65) were children between 4 months and 15 years of age. Moyamoya syndrome was seen in 17 patients. Their associated conditions were neurofibromatosis in six, optic glioma in one, compound hemoglobinopathy in one, G6P dehydrogenase deficiency in one, protein S deficiency in one, trisomy 21 in two, "morning glory" optic disk anomaly in one, factor V deficiency with compensated cardiac valvular defect in one, pupillary sphincter dysplasia in two, and Grange syndrome in one. Presenting symptoms at the time of surgery were TIAs (unilateral in 21, bilateral in 21); 11 patients had previous watershed strokes with moderate to good recovery of neurologic function. Accompanying headaches were seen in six patients, and seizures occurred in four. One child had visual symptoms, two children had an attention deficit and hyperkinetic disorder, and eight children with an average age of 7 years presented with developmental delay.

Clinical and neuropsychological assessment
Angiographic confirmation and staging
Preoperative transcranial Doppler

Preoperative SPECT/$H_2^{15}O$ PET Diamox challenge
Regional differences of cerebral perfusion reserves

⬇

Direct EC-IC bypass
MCA (parietotemporal)   ACA (frontal)   PCA (occipital)

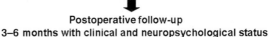

STA-MCA   STA-ACA   OA-PCA

⬇

Indirect dura- or arteriorsynangiosis
(when donor or recipient vessel not available)

⬇   ⬇   ⬇

Parietal branch of STA   Frontal branch of STA   Occipital artery

⬇

Postoperative follow-up
3–6 months with clinical and neuropsychological status
TCD, angiography, neuropsychology, PET

Fig. 14.4 Algorithm of management of moyamoya patients from their preoperative diagnosis, choice of revascularization procedures, to a follow-up plan. ACA, anterior cerebral artery; EC, extracranial; IC, intracranial; MCA, middle cerebral artery; OA, occipital artery; PCA, posterior cerebral artery; PET, positron emission tomography; SPECT, single-photon emission computed tomography; STA, superficial temporal artery; TCD, transcranial Doppler.

Choice of Revascularization

Depending on the severity of the clinical symptoms, the extent of disease (unilateral vs bilateral) on angiography, and the perfusion reserve deficits observed after a Diamox challenge on $H_2^{15}O$-PET, a variety of revascularization procedures were performed in this group of children. Thirty-four children underwent bilateral STA-MCA bypass; in 4 patients an STA-MCA bypass was performed on only one side.

In 20 patients where a decrease in the frontal perfusion reserve deficit was seen, a unilateral STA–ACA; 16 patients bypass and a bilateral STA-ACA bypass (4 patients) were performed. In addition, indirect revascularization was performed in the frontal region unilaterally using bur holes in 14 patients and bilaterally in 6 patients. Placement of a bur hole in the occipital region was performed in one child, and arteriosynangiosis using the occipital artery (OA) was performed in two patients. The temporalis muscle was used unilaterally in two patients to provide for indirect revascularization in the MCA region. Furthermore, a posterior

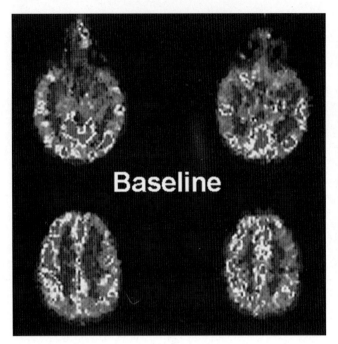
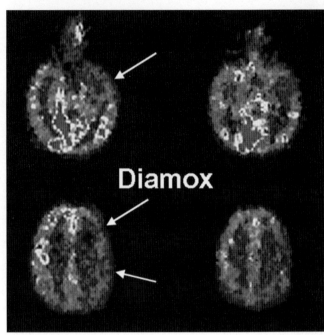

A

B

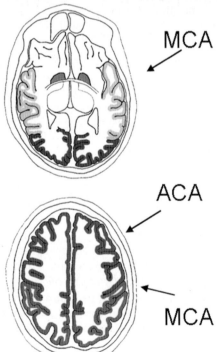

C

Fig. 14.5 H$_2$^{15}O-PET scans, **(A)** baseline and **(B)** with Diamox challenge, showing perfusion reserve deficits (*arrows*) in the frontal (ACA) and parietotemporal (MCA) arterial distribution areas. **(C)** Schematic showing the same deficits in the ACA and MCA.

temporal craniotomy with a large dural inversion was performed in the temporo-occipital region in one patient who had posterior cerebral artery (PCA) stenosis and clear preoperative perfusion deficits on Diamox-PET in this region. Frontal arteriosynangiosis using the frontal branch of the STA was performed unilaterally in two patients and bilaterally in one patient. One patient was not operated and just followed up for 3 years.

We advocate cerebral revascularization with a direct extracranial-intracranial (EC-IC) bypass as the gold standard in the management of moyamoya angiopathy in children. Direct microsurgical vessel-to-vessel EC-IC bypass anastomosis, if necessary at more than one site, and even bilaterally, should be offered whenever technically possible.

Neovascularization after indirect vessel transfer of bur hole placement takes longer to establish and therefore comes with a delay in efficacy, which may not be demonstrable at 3 months' follow-up.

The cerebral perfusion status in the frontal region needs special attention. Moyamoya in children younger than 5 years with recurrent and chronic frontal ischemia can be devastating to mental and cognitive development. Prevention of severe mental retardation therefore justifies early surgical revascularization, particularly on the dominant side. This has led us to perform frontal bypass procedures with anastomosis between the distal STA and a branch of the ACA. In the American and Japanese literature,[47-51] STA-MCA bypass procedures are reported frequently for moyamoya angiopathy, but comparatively little attention is paid to frontal brain reperfusion; thus, only a small number of STA-ACA bypasses[49-52] are being performed, especially in children. The reason is the considerable technical difficulty of such a procedure. Therefore, most surgeons prefer indirect revascularization in younger children because this is less demanding to perform. This is an issue of specialized training and referral of patients to specialized centers with the required expertise. This also emphasizes the importance of interdisciplinary cooperation among caregivers and specialists.

Only when a direct bypass is technically impossible (unavailability of or too small a donor or cortical vessel caliber) are indirect revascularization procedures such as durasynangiosis and arteriosynangiosis used.

and PET hemodynamic analysis showed no evidence of further strokes in any child. Repeat angiography at 6 months demonstrated patency of grafts in all patients (**Fig. 14.6**). The $H_2^{15}O$ PET Diamox challenge testing showed improvement in perfusion reserves in the majority of cases.

Both the clinical stabilization and the improvement of functional hemodynamic parameters confirm the concept of compromised cerebral perfusion, which may be at risk of decompensating, and its reversal by early surgical revascularization.[53,54] The efficacy of multiple direct vessel-to-vessel bypass procedures even performed bilaterally in one sitting could be demonstrated in the majority of our patients. In addition to hemodynamic tests, the postoperative angiography demonstrated an increase in the focal perfusion in the region of the bypass (**Fig. 14.6**). Because moyamoya angiopathy is a bilateral disease, surgical revascularization may be required not only for multiple vascular territories but also bilaterally.

Clinical follow-up alone, without a full set of noninvasive tests, is currently available for a postoperative period of as long as 2 to 5 years. No patient had recurrence of TIAs or strokes.

Improvement in cognitive function and school performance in the majority of children has been observed by parents and caregivers. This aspect is currently investigated with extensive objective neuropsychological evaluation.

Outcome

Long-term follow-up of these patients continues. The postoperative follow-up of 6 months with clinical, angiographic,

Complications

Immediate postoperative complications resulting from perioperative ischemia were observed in only two patients.

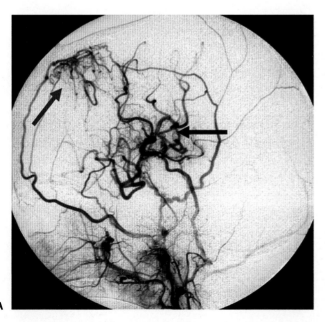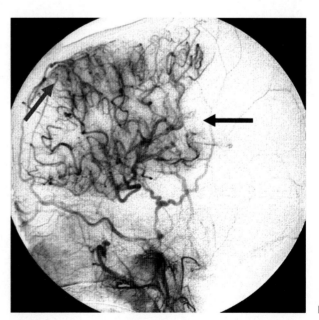

A   B

Fig. 14.6 (A,B) Lateral projections of a postoperative angiography demonstrating the functioning STA-MCA and STA-ACA bypasses and their territorial blush in the frontal and parietotemporal regions (*arrows*).

In one patient a reversible postoperative ischemia of the operated frontoparietal side was seen that recovered completely at 3 months' follow-up. One patient died 1 day after surgery due to massive MCA infarction of the nonoperated side.

Surgical Techniques

Multiple Direct Extracranial-Intracranial Bypass

Depending on the angiographic findings demonstrating the anatomical severity of disease (stenosis or occlusion of unilateral or bilateral ICA, MCA, ACA, or PCA) and the hemodynamic reserve tested after a Diamox challenge in the distribution/perfusion territories of the MCA, ACA, or PCA, the number of bypass procedures can be planned. The aim is always to perform multiple direct anastomoses in the regions most affected by hypoperfusion (STA-MCA, STA-ACA, and OA-PCA).

Superficial Temporal Artery–Middle Cerebral Artery Bypass

Anastomosis of the extracranial STA and to a branch of the intracranial MCA involves the following (**Figs. 14.6** and **14.7**):

A linear incision over the parietal branch of the STA is made with dissection of the artery (8–10 cm of dissection and free preparation). This is followed by a small craniotomy (2.5 cm in diameter) corresponding to the end of the sylvian fissure. After locating a suitable MCA branch, a direct anastomosis between the parietal branch of the STA and the branch of the MCA is performed. Preoperative external carotid angiographies, as well as immediate preoperative TCD Doppler scans, are used to evaluate the presence of suitable donor vessels. In cases where the STA is hypoplastic, the OA or the posterior auricular artery can be used. In cases where the frontal branch of the STA is not long enough, the parietal branch of the STA is used as an interposition graft. The choices of cortical branches that can be used as recipient vessels are angular, posterior temporal, posterior parietal, rolandic, and prerolandic. In case the craniotomy has to be extended due to the nonavailability of a suitable branch, the craniotomy can be extended anterior to the classic location to use the operculofrontal or candelabra group of branches for a direct anastomosis. Attention must be paid to cut the dura carefully without sacrificing already developed transdural arterial collateral vasculature. This can be done by avoiding a single large flap of dura and limiting dural coagulation and by using dural clips in case of bleeding. Sometimes in cases where further revascularization of the frontoparietal region is desired, double anastomoses can be performed. This can be achieved by preparing a frontoparietal skin flap, dissecting both the parietal and the frontal branches of the STA, and using them individually for the anastomosis in the frontal-opercular and frontoparietal regions, respectively.

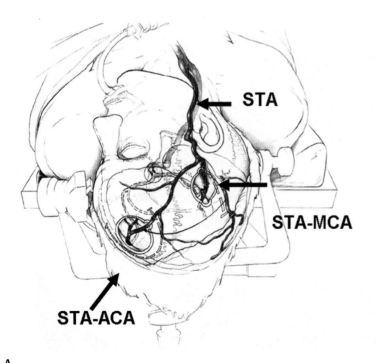

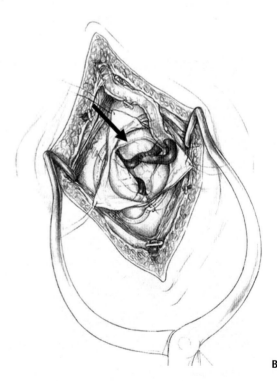

Fig. 14.7 (A) Patient positioning and the two bypass procedures (*arrows*) using the STA, parietal and frontal branches, for the STA-MCA and STA-ACA bypasses, respectively. **(B)** End-to-side anastomosis (*arrow*).

Superficial Temporal Artery–Anterior Cerebral Artery Bypass

If there is severe perfusion deficit in the medial frontal region, an additional STA-ACA bypass from the frontal branch of the STA to the middle internal frontal branch of the ACA can be constructed (**Figs. 14.6** and **14.7**).

The frontal branch of the STA is dissected using a frontal skin flap. A small craniotomy (2.5 cm in diameter) is then placed just in front of the coronal suture medially extending to the midline. After locating a branch of the middle internal frontal artery of the ACA, along the brain convexity, an end-to-side anastomosis to the already dissected and prepared STA frontal branch is performed. In cases where the frontal branch is not long enough, the parietal branch of the STA can be prepared and part of it used as an interposition graft.

Occipital Artery–Posterior Cerebral Artery Bypass

Moyamoya angiopathy with stenosis/occlusion in the posterior circulation appears to be particularly frequent, though less symptomatic, in children, but little attention has been paid to this aspect in the literature to date. Revascularization of the posterior circulation can be achieved via the supracerebellar transtentorial approach in the sitting position by a direct bypass between the OA and the PCA,[55] although this has rarely been reported. This procedure is technically demanding, especially in children. Therefore, in rare cases where a posterior revascularization is required, dural carpeting after an occipital craniotomy or an arteriosynangiosis using the OA is a more frequently used option.

Multiple Direct Extracranial-Intracranial Bypasses Combined with Indirect Revascularization

STA-MCA bypass with indirect frontal arteriosynangiosis or frontal dural carpeting or STA-MCA bypass combined with indirect occipital arteriosynangiosis or occipital dural carpeting can be performed.

Dural Carpeting, Arteriosynangiosis

Larger craniotomies are performed with inversion of several flaps of vascularized dura onto the surface of the brain. This can be done in any region requiring revascularization: frontal, frontotemporal, frontoparietal, or temporal-posterior.

Either the frontal or parietal branch of the STA or the OA can be placed directly on the surface of the brain in an en passant fashion, where the vessel and its surrounding tissue are transposed onto the pia and sutured to the pia. Either a small frontal, temporal, or occipital craniotomy can be used. Neovascularization sprouts from these transposed vessel segments as new vascularity is recruited by the chronically ischemic brain tissue. These techniques can be used in addition to the direct STA-MCA bypass procedures or if there is no suitable recipient vessel available.

Timing of Surgery

A variety of clinical scenarios may be encountered, such as the asymptomatic patient who had imaging for some unrelated cause, or a patient with prior resolved stroke, and, of course, patients with acute stroke and those with recurrent TIAs. This may be seen in the context of unilateral or bilateral disease, not all of which necessarily are symptomatic at a given time.

As a rule, surgery is performed at a time period of clinical stabilization. After a complete ischemic stroke, a minimum interval of 3 to 4 weeks from the onset of stroke to surgery is desirable. Bilateral bypass operations can be performed as one- or two-stage procedures. The time interval between two surgeries can vary in each individual child, sometimes allowing more time for clinical stabilization. Bilateral bypasses as a one-stage operation are now preferred to prevent ischemia of the contralateral side. The side with the more extensive disease and symptoms is operated first, followed by the other, less severely affected side. The one-stage bilateral procedure has been performed without additional anesthesiological or surgical side effects to the patient. Total operative time increases from, on an average, 3 to 4 hours per operation to 8 hours (range 6.0–9.5 hrs). All patients spend the first 24 hours in an intensive care unit and are transferred to a regular floor thereafter. The length of stay in the hospital for a one-stage bilateral bypass operation is similar to that of a unilateral bypass operation. Blood loss is usually minimal, irrespective of a one- or two-stage procedure. No local or systemic complications have been observed. Special attention to neuroanesthesia is essential in surgery for moyamoya angiopathy. Hypovolemia, hypotension, and hyper- or hypocapnia must be avoided. Furthermore, a regime of sufficient preoperative hydration and daily intake of 100 mg of aspirin should be ensured. Postoperative analgesia is important for patient comfort, especially in children, to prevent profuse crying and the resulting hypocapnia/hyperventilation.

Conclusion

Direct extracranial-intracranial microanastomosis for revascularization in moyamoya angiopathy is the method of choice in children with relevant hemodynamic compromise tested after a Diamox challenge. Multiple direct bypass procedures for revascularization even performed bilaterally at the same surgery and anastomoses to a branch of the ACA have proved to be effective in preventing stroke.[51,52,54] Indirect revascularization procedures (arteriosynangiosis and durasynangiosis) are used in combination or as an adjunct or alternative to direct bypass, in cases where the donor or recipient arteries are not available or are of inadequate caliber for the anastomosis. Postoperative follow-up of 2 to 5 years has demonstrated no further stroke in these children. Improvement in cognitive functions in children who demonstrated a preoperative frontal lobe executive functional impairment has been observed.

◆ Lessons Learned

The management of moyamoya in children depends on the secondary vascularization of the ischemic brain areas affected. It is clear from the contributions in this chapter that the disease carries a major morbidity.

One central principle applies to all patients: function that is lost cannot be recovered by later intervention.

Thus, it appears essential to treat patients early, preferably when they are in a stable situation after an initial TIA or even a first stroke. As in many other fields, it seems important to individualize the planned treatment. In particular, a meticulous analysis of the preoperative angiogram, including the selective angiogram of the external carotid artery, is essential. It is important to determine not only the appropriate selection of vessels to bypass (both external carotid branches and intracranial receiving vessels) and areas to graft, but also the presence of existing neovascularization in order to avoid destroying new vessels in the surgical approach.

There is a clear difference between both groups in terms of preference of technical revascularization. From the editor's point of view, it seems reasonable to accept an individual surgeon's preference for vessel-to-vessel bypass if the extraordinary experience required for this delicate surgery is available. For the most part, however, it may be more realistic to follow the Boston group's (Grondin et al) recommendation of not using direct bypass in children under the age of 8 years.

There may also be an overlap of concepts, as stressed by the Boston group: even if a bypass itself is not remaining open in cases of very small vessel diameter, there is still the effect of vessel and stalk transposition amounting to an indirect procedure. Thus, the indirect procedure may still be effective even though a direct bypass was attempted.

There seems to be little controversy about the clinical progression with a stroke rate of 3% per year and an even much higher rate of radiographic progression of about two thirds.

Overall, the results of both the direct and the indirect procedures appear to be good, with a perioperative morbidity of ~4% per hemisphere. Ninety-six percent of patients remain stroke-free after that.

We find it interesting that the authors advocate the continued use of aspirin all the way through surgery and postoperatively. There is more concern about the morbidity following hemorrhage than the morbidity of perioperative stroke.

References

1. Nagaraja D, Verma A, Taly AB, Kumar MV, Jayakumar PN. Cerebrovascular disease in children. Acta Neurol Scand 1994;90(4): 251–255

2. Soriano SG, Sethna NF, Scott RM. Anesthetic management of children with moyamoya syndrome. Anesth Analg 1993;77(5):1066–1070

3. Scott RM, Smith JL, Robertson RL, Madsen JR, Soriano SG, Rockoff MA. Long-term outcome in children with moyamoya syndrome after cranial revascularization by pial synangiosis. J Neurosurg 2004;100(2, Suppl Pediatrics):142–149

4. Jea A, Smith ER, Robertson R, Scott RM. Moyamoya syndrome associated with Down syndrome: outcome after surgical revascularization. Pediatrics 2005;116(5):e694–e701

5. Ohaegbulam C, Magge S, Scott RM. Moyamoya syndrome. In: McLone D, ed. Pediatric Neurosurgery. Philadelphia: WB Saunders; 2001: 1077–1092

6. Choi JU, Kim DS, Kim EY, Lee KC. Natural history of moyamoya disease: comparison of activity of daily living in surgery and non-surgery groups. Clin Neurol Neurosurg 1997;99(Suppl 2):S11–S18

7. Ezura M, Yoshimoto T, Fujiwara S, Takahashi A, Shirane R, Mizoi K. Clinical and angiographic follow-up of childhood-onset moyamoya disease. Childs Nerv Syst 1995;11(10):591–594

8. Kurokawa T, Tomita S, Ueda K, et al. Prognosis of occlusive disease of the circle of Willis (moyamoya disease) in children. Pediatr Neurol 1985;1(5):274–277

9. Fung LW, Thompson D, Ganesan V. Revascularisation surgery for paediatric moyamoya: a review of the literature. Childs Nerv Syst 2005;21(5):358–364

10. Kuroda S, Hashimoto N, Yoshimoto T, Iwasaki Y ; Research Committee on Moyamoya Disease in Japan. Radiological findings, clinical course, and outcome in asymptomatic moyamoya disease: results of multi-center survey in Japan. Stroke 2007;38(5):1430–1435

11. Maki Y, Enomoto T. Moyamoya disease. Childs Nerv Syst 1988;4(4): 204–212

12. Fukuyama Y, Umezu R. Clinical and cerebral angiographic evolutions of idiopathic progressive occlusive disease of the circle of Willis ("moyamoya" disease) in children. Brain Dev 1985;7(1): 21–37

13. Imaizumi T, Hayashi K, Saito K, Osawa M, Fukuyama Y. Long-term outcomes of pediatric moyamoya disease monitored to adulthood. Pediatr Neurol 1998;18(4):321–325

14. Shin IS, Cheng R, Pordell GR. Striking CT scan findings in a case of unilateral moyamoya disease—a case report. Angiology 1991;42(8): 665–671

15. Fujita K, Shirakuni T, Kojima N, Tamaki N, Matsumoto S. [Magnetic resonance imaging in moyamoya disease.] No Shinkei Geka 1986; 14(3, Suppl):324–330

16. Chabbert V, Ranjeva JP, Sevely A, Boetto S, Berry I, Manelfe C. Diffusion- and magnetisation transfer-weighted MRI in childhood moya-moya. Neuroradiology 1998;40(4):267–271

17. Yamada I, Matsushima Y, Suzuki S. Moyamoya disease: diagnosis with three-dimensional time-of-flight MR angiography. Radiology 1992;184(3):773–778

18. Sunaga Y, Fujinaga T, Ohtsuka T. [MRI findings of moyamoya disease in children.] No To Hattatsu 1992;24(4):375–379

19. Brady AP, Stack JP, Ennis JT. Moyamoya disease—imaging with magnetic resonance. Clin Radiol 1990;42(2):138–141

20. Rolak LA. Magnetic resonance imaging in moyamoya disease. Arch Neurol 1989;46(1):14

21. Bruno A, Yuh WT, Biller J, Adams HP Jr, Cornell SH. Magnetic resonance imaging in young adults with cerebral infarction due to moyamoya. Arch Neurol 1988;45(3):303–306

22. Scott RM. Moyamoya syndrome: a surgically treatable cause of stroke in the pediatric patient. Clin Neurosurg 2000;47:378–384

23. Matsushima T, Inoue T, Katsuta T, et al. An indirect revascularization method in the surgical treatment of moyamoya disease—various kinds of indirect procedures and a multiple combined indirect procedure. Neurol Med Chir (Tokyo) 1998;38(Suppl):297–302

24. Houkin K, Kamiyama H, Abe H, Takahashi A, Kuroda S. Surgical therapy for adult moyamoya disease: can surgical revascularization prevent the recurrence of intracerebral hemorrhage? Stroke 1996;27(8):1342–1346

25. Kawaguchi S, Okuno S, Sakaki T. Effect of direct arterial bypass on the prevention of future stroke in patients with the hemorrhagic variety of moyamoya disease. J Neurosurg 2000;93(3):397–401

26. Sencer S, Poyanli A, Kiriş T, Sencer A, Minareci O. Recent experience with moyamoya disease in Turkey. Eur Radiol 2000;10(4):569–572

27. Houkin K, Kuroda S, Nakayama N. Cerebral revascularization for moyamoya disease in children. Neurosurg Clin N Am 2001;12(3):575–584, ix

28. Dauser RC, Tuite GF, McCluggage CW. Dural inversion procedure for moyamoya disease: technical note. J Neurosurg 1997;86(4):719–723

29. Suzuki J, Takaku A, Kodama N, Sato S. An attempt to treat cerebrovascular "moyamoya" disease in children. Childs Brain 1975;1(4):193–206

30. Karasawa J, Kikuchi H, Kawamura J, Sakai T. Intracranial transplantation of the omentum for cerebrovascular moyamoya disease: a two-year follow-up study. Surg Neurol 1980;14(6):444–449

31. Karasawa J, Touho H, Ohnishi H, Miyamoto S, Kikuchi H. Cerebral revascularization using omental transplantation for childhood moyamoya disease. J Neurosurg 1993;79(2):192–196

32. Ohtaki M, Uede T, Morimoto S, Nonaka T, Tanabe S, Hashi K. Intellectual functions and regional cerebral haemodynamics after extensive omental transplantation spread over both frontal lobes in childhood moyamoya disease. Acta Neurochir (Wien) 1998;140(10):1043–1053, discussion 1052–1053

33. Yoshioka N, Tominaga S, Suzuki Y, et al. Cerebral revascularization using omentum and muscle free flap for ischemic cerebrovascular disease. Surg Neurol 1998;49(1):58–65, discussion 65–66

34. Yoshioka N, Tominaga S, Inui T. Cerebral revascularization using omentum and serratus anterior muscle free flap transfer for adult moyamoya disease: case report. Surg Neurol 1996;46(5):430–435, discussion 435–436

35. Havlik RJ, Fried I, Chyatte D, Modlin IM. Encephalo-omental synangiosis in the management of moyamoya disease. Surgery 1992;111(2):156–162

36. Suzuki J, Kodama N. Moyamoya disease—a review. Stroke 1983;14(1):104–109

37. Matsushima Y. [Indirect anastomoses for moyamoya disease.] No Shinkei Geka 1998;26(9):769–786

38. Matsushima T, Inoue T, Ikezaki K, et al. Multiple combined indirect procedure for the surgical treatment of children with moyamoya disease: a comparison with single indirect anastomosis and direct anastomosis. Neurosurg Focus 1998;5(5):e4

39. Ikezaki K. Rational approach to treatment of moyamoya disease in childhood. J Child Neurol 2000;15(5):350–356

40. Fukui M. Guidelines for the diagnosis and treatment of spontaneous occlusion of the circle of Willis ("moyamoya" disease). Research Committee on Spontaneous Occlusion of the Circle of Willis (Moyamoya Disease) of the Ministry of Health and Welfare, Japan. Clin Neurol Neurosurg 1997;99(Suppl 2):S238–S240

41. Takeuchi K, Shimizu K. Hypoplasia of the bilateral internal carotid arteries. Brain Nerve. 1957;9:37–43

42. Yonekawa Y, Taub E. Moyamoya disease: status 1998. Neurologist 1999;5:13–23

43. Khan N, Yonekawa Y. Moyamoya angiopathy in Europe: the Zürich experience. Stroke 2005;9(3):181–188

44. Yonekawa Y, Ogata N, Kaku Y, Taub E, Imhof HG. Moyamoya disease in Europe, past and present status. Clin Neurol Neurosurg 1997;99(Suppl 2):S58–S60

45. Horowitz M, Yonas H, Albright AL. Evaluation of cerebral blood flow and hemodynamic reserve in symptomatic moyamoya disease using stable xenon-CT blood flow. Review Surg Neurol 1995;44(3):251–261, discussion 262

46. Ikezaki K, Matsushima T, Kuwabara Y, Suzuki SO, Nomura T, Fukui M. Cerebral circulation and oxygen metabolism in childhood moyamoya disease: a perioperative positron emission tomography study. J Neurosurg 1994;81(6):843–850

47. Golby AJ, Marks MP, Thompson RC, Steinberg GK. Direct and combined revascularization in pediatric moyamoya disease. Neurosurgery 1999;45(1):50–58, discussion 58–60

48. Matsushima T, Aoyagi M, Suzuki R, Nariai T, Shishido T, Hirakawa K. Dual anastomosis for pediatric moyamoya patients using the anterior and posterior branches of the superficial temporal artery. Nerv Syst Child 1993;18:27–32

49. Iwama T, Hashimoto N, Miyake H, Yonekawa Y. Direct revascularization to the anterior cerebral artery territory in patients with moyamoya disease: report of five cases. Neurosurgery 1998;42(5):1157–1161, discussion 1161–1162

50. Iwama T, Hashimoto N, Tsukahara T, Miyake H. Superficial temporal artery to anterior cerebral artery direct anastomosis in patients with moyamoya disease. Clin Neurol Neurosurg 1997;99:134–136

51. Suzuki Y, Negoro M, Shibuya M, Yoshida J, Negoro T, Watanabe K. Surgical treatment for pediatric moyamoya disease: use of the superficial temporal artery for both areas supplied by the anterior and middle cerebral arteries. Neurosurgery 1997;40(2):324–329, discussion 329–330

52. Khan N, Schuknecht B, Boltshauser E, et al. Moyamoya disease and moyamoya syndrome: experience in Europe; choice of revascularisation procedures. Acta Neurochir (Wien) 2003;145(12):1061–1071, discussion 1071

53. Iwama T, Hashimoto N, Yonekawa Y. The relevance of hemodynamic factors to perioperative ischemic complications in childhood moyamoya disease. Neurosurgery 1996;38(6):1120–1125, discussion 1125–1126

54. Ikezaki K. Rational approach to treatment of moyamoya disease in childhood. Review J Child Neurol 2000;15(5):350–356

55. Yonekawa Y, Imhof HG, Taub E, et al. Supracerebellar transtentorial approach to posterior temporomedial structures. J Neurosurg 2001;94(2):339–345

15 Pediatric Aneurysms

◆ Surgical Management

Sid Chandela and David J. Langer

The first report of aneurysmal subarachnoid hemorrhage (SAH) in a child was published in a German pathology journal in 1871.[1] Here, Eppinger detailed a case of a 15-year-old boy who collapsed while exercising. Autopsy revealed an intracerebral hemorrhage associated with an aneurysm and aortic stenosis.[2] Several authors have referenced an even earlier report, by Biumi of Milan in 1778, of a ruptured intracranial aneurysm in a child.[3,4] This report similarly describes another German youth with aortic coarctation who died suddenly of a ruptured aneurysm while playing football. Interestingly, early thinking associated cerebral aneurysms with a complication of an aortic condition and thus prevented the recognition of the importance of cerebrovascular disease.[1] Since then, our understanding of pediatric intracranial aneurysms and cerebrovascular disease has evolved.

Incidence

Aneurysms in the pediatric population are rare, representing ~0.5 to 4.6% of all aneurysms.[5,6] Only 700 cases have been reported in the literature,[7–17] and these are predominantly case reports. The rarity of pediatric aneurysms was first highlighted by McDonald and Korb in 1939, when they found only 28 pediatric aneurysms out of 1125 (~2.5%) total cases.[3] Later large population-based reviews supported this early finding. The largest published series of pediatric aneurysms, described by Patel and Richardson,[18] included 58 aneurysms in patients younger than 19 years. This summarized the British combined cohort of patients with aneurysms at Queens Square and Atkinson Morley Hospital between 1944 and 1968, when a total of 58 out of 3000 (1.9%) cases of ruptured intracranial aneurysms were recognized in children younger than 19 years. None, however, were younger than 2 years. The rarity of childhood aneurysms is further accentuated when the patients are substratified by age. Rarely have intracranial aneurysms been reported in neonates.[19,20] Thus, the exact incidence of pediatric aneurysms is variable, 0.5 to 4.6%, and is more prevalent in the teenage age range and exceptionally rare in younger children.[1] In adults, there is a female preponderance; in contrast, boys, particularly during the neonatal and infant periods, are more prone to intracranial aneurysms.[14,20–22]

Pathophysiology

Despite the rarity of pediatric intracranial aneurysms, controversy exists regarding their pathophysiologic features. Data on aneurysms in adults suggest that the initial defect is an injury to the internal elastic membrane by hemodynamic forces, which ultimately leads to aneurysm formation.[16,23,24] Arterial bifurcations are the most vulnerable to shearing damage because they accept most of the hemodynamic forces, and pathologic analysis confirms that the greatest amount of fenestrations of the internal elastic membrane is at the apex.[16] This theory explains the presence of saccular aneurysms in adults and even adolescents.[16,22,23] Aneurysms occurring in neonates and children also have vessel wall structural defects; however, these are congenital and related to other disorders. Intracranial aneurysms in children are usually associated with various connective tissue disorders, namely, Ehlers-Danlos syndrome type IV, Marfan syndrome, neurofibromatosis type 1, autosomal dominant polycystic kidney disease, and aortic coarctation, as previously described.[25] Lipper and colleagues suggested a large congenital medial defect as an initiating factor for aneurysm development in neonates and children.[26] An alteration in parietal connective tissue has been postulated by Ostergaard et al.[27,28] Even more, Stehbens and associates observed that an infectious process can also induce fissures in the internal elastic membrane, leading to aneurysm formation.[29] Indeed, the incidence of bacterial infections in the pediatric population is estimated to be ~10%, whereas it is only 2.5% in the general population.[30] Interestingly, along with blunt head trauma, it has been reported that neonatal birth trauma could potentiate aneurysm formation near the tentorial incisura.[31]

Although strong evidence exists associating neonatal aneurysms to a congenital defect secondary to other connective tissue disorders, Stehbens et al add to the controversy by defending the assertion that these aneurysms are degenerative hemodynamically determined lesions in children.[29] A hemodynamic cause is explained by a force of axial stream on the apex of the vessel at the bifurcation followed by sudden dissipation of kinetic energy, resulting in structural fatigue causing aneurysm formation.[16,30] Proust and colleagues observed the preponderance of internal carotid artery (ICA) bifurcation aneurysms in the pediatric population to be 36.4% in their series compared with 2.1% in the adult counterparts. The large ICA bifurcation angle makes it a favorable place for aneurysm formation in children.[16] Therefore, we surmise that the early appearance of aneurysms in children reflects a genetic predisposition to the effects of hemodynamic stresses, possibly combined with anatomical susceptibility.

In adults, most aneurysms are found in the anterior circulation (anterior communicating artery, posterior communicating artery, and middle cerebral artery [MCA]) and are small; 5 to 15% are noted in the posterior circulation. In contrast, carotid bifurcation is the most common site for pediatric intracranial aneurysms, followed by the posterior circulation. These are often large (1.0–2.5 cm), and 16 to 54% are giant (>2.5 cm) aneurysms compared with those found in adults.[21] Posterior circulation aneurysms are more prevalent in children than adults by threefold. Lastly, adults are more prone to multiple aneurysms than children.[32,33]

Presentation

The initial clinical presentation of a child harboring an intracranial aneurysm is SAH between 50 and 75% of the time, according to most reports in the literature.[14,21,34,35] Symptoms of adolescents presenting with SAH are similar to adults with SAH: sudden severe headache, nausea, vomiting, collapse, photophobia, nuchal rigidity, and focal neurologic deficits. Neonates and infants are more likely to present with nonspecific signs, such as irritability, seizures, drowsiness, and vomiting. Generally speaking, the pediatric population with SAH presents in better clinical grades than adults, and the incidence of delayed ischemic deficits secondary to vasospasm is less.[10,36] Because large and giant aneurysms are fairly common in children, they often present with signs and symptoms of mass effect, seizures, and obstruction, especially with posterior fossa lesions.[21] Because of the rarity of pediatric intracranial aneurysms, their diagnosis can be easily missed. Any child with unexplained neurologic symptoms or unexplained sudden headaches should be investigated thoroughly to rule out intracranial aneurysm rupture. The investigation of a child

with a suspected aneurysm or SAH is similar to that for an adult. The work-up is tailored to the patient and could include any combination of computed tomography (CT) scan, magnetic resonance imaging (MRI)/MR angiography (MRA), and lumbar puncture looking for xanthrochromia. Four-vessel cerebral angiography remains the gold standard;[21] however, CT angiography (CTA) has proven to be very safe and efficacious in most settings.[37]

Surgical Treatment

With the recent advancements in diagnostic, microsurgical, and neuroanesthetic techniques, aggressive surgical treatment should always be employed in a pediatric patient with SAH to generate favorable outcome.[14,35,36,38–40] In their review of 48 cases, Choux et al noted that 73% of their surgically treated group had an excellent outcome compared with the 7% in the nonsurgical group.[41] There is a lower incidence of rebleeding in children (7–13%) when compared with adult controls (20–30%).[38,42] Khoo and coworkers espouse early and immediate surgical obliteration of cerebral aneurysm in children with low-grade SAH. Postponement of surgical treatment of high-grade SAH allows for stabilization with respect to edema, hydrocephalus, and vasospasm, thus lowering surgical morbidity.[41] The timing of surgery in patients with high clinical grade SAH must be individualized. The threshold to treat, however, ought to be low in the pediatric patient.

The operative management of saccular aneurysms in children is governed by the same principles as in adults, with added concerns of a smaller physiologic reserve in pediatric patients. Extra appreciation of the smaller anatomy and decreased tolerance of temperature changes, blood loss, and large fluid shifts are warranted intraoperatively.[36,41] Because of the anatomical variability and typically larger aneurysms in children, surgical obliteration is not straightforward. In a review of the literature, it was observed that direct clip ligation of the aneurysmal neck is possible in only 29.5% of cases.[41] Contrary to adults, children often require specialized and innovative techniques to obliterate intracranial aneurysms.[10,18,39,43] These include various combinations of clip ligation, entrapment in giant lesions, tandem clipping, angioplastic clipping, aneurysmectomy, microvascular anastomosis and bypass,[14] direct excision with reanastomosis, ligation of the parent artery with tourniquet,[40] direct ligation of the cervical carotid or vertebral arteries, extracranial-intracranial bypass, and direct excision without bypass.[35] Lansen and associates demonstrated that even giant lesions could be treated effectively with microsurgical techniques. They reviewed 47 cases of giant childhood and adolescent aneurysms; 36 of these lesions were successfully obliterated with surgical occlusion of proximal artery.[41] Of these, 29 were completely thrombosed postoperatively. Trapping (six cases), sac resection followed by extracranial-intracranial bypass (three cases), direct neck clipping (two cases), and exploration (two cases) were used in the remainder of patients. Excellent results were obtained in 36 out of 47 cases, with significant morbidity in 6 cases and 5 deaths.[41] When treating childhood aneurysms, we must often use creative strategies to individualize treatment to gain a favorable outcome. We describe a recent case at our institution where we effectively treated vertebral artery (VA)–posteroinferior cerebellar artery (PICA) aneurysm with an in situ side-to-side PICA–PICA bypass. An 11-year-old boy with a partially coiled enlarging VA–PICA aneurysm presented with brainstem compression. **Figure 15.1** shows the giant aneurysm. Rather than just employing hunterian ligation of the VA and risking a PICA territory infarct in an intact child, we decided to preserve the PICA by revascularization through an in situ side-to-side PICA–PICA bypass due to the lack of an adequate occipital artery donor. **Figure 15.2** shows the bypass intraoperatively, and **Fig. 15.3** demonstrates a postoperative angiogram showing filling of the medullary segment of the PICA territory and obliteration of the aneurysm. The patient remained intact 15 months later.[44]

Despite our overall limited surgical experience with childhood aneurysms, various authors have cited certain surgical observations from their experience. Children evidently tolerate proximal arterial occlusion and hunterian ligation far better than adults.[40] Successful carotid and vertebral artery ligation with a Drake tourniquet is well known.[45,46] Cervical carotid occlusion may be especially effective for control of some carotid-ophthalmic aneurysms or for otherwise untreatable cavernous or petrous aneurysms. Surprisingly, it has also been shown that basilar artery occlusion can be tolerated with few deficits.[45] It is unclear whether this is due to a larger collateral supply or increased plasticity of the child's brain. The rationale for ligation is to reduce the pressure head and filling within the lesion, thereby allowing the sac to thrombose.[46]

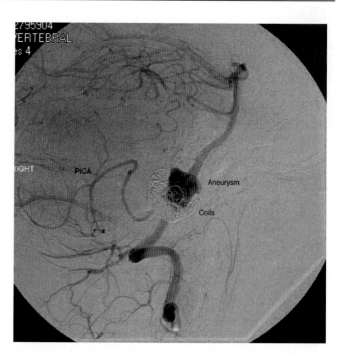

Fig. 15.1 Lateral angiogram of the right vertebral artery revealing a compacted large aneurysm at the vertebral artery–posteroinferior cerebellar artery (PICA) junction.

Aneurysmorrhaphy or evacuation of intraluminal clot in such partially thrombosed aneurysms improves preoperative neural compression syndromes.[39] Every attempt should be made to avoid vessel deconstruction in young patients due to the concern regarding long-term risks of large vessel sacrifice, although recent literature describes sacrifice to be relatively safe.[47]

Endovascular treatment of pediatric intracranial aneurysms cannot be ignored. It is an attractive option for obvious reasons. Compared with microsurgical experience for these lesions, endovascular therapy is still in its nascent stage.

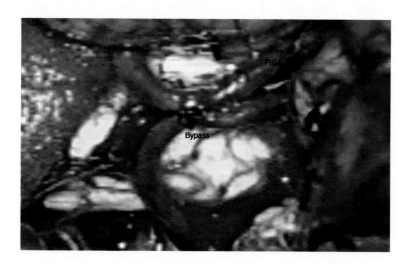

Fig. 15.2 Intraoperative picture of bilateral caudal loops of the PICA in a side-to-side bypass using 9–0 Prolene suture.

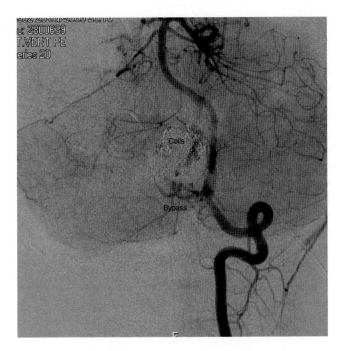

Fig. 15.3 Anteroposterior angiogram of the left vertebral artery revealing filling of the bypass and the distal medullary segment of the PICA. There is no filling of the aneurysm or the vertebral artery.

The long-term outcomes following endovascular treatment are not fully elucidated in the literature. Longer life expectancies and differences in underlying disease in children with aneurysms raise important issues regarding the durability of treatment choice between microsurgical and endovascular therapy. Direct comparisons between endovascular and microsurgical treatment are starting to emerge in the literature. Sanai and colleagues at the University of California, San Francisco reviewed this question (**Table 15.1**).[48] They

retrospectively reviewed a total of 43 pediatric aneurysms treated between 1977 and 2003 at their institution with a focus on treatment durability. Their results show that microsurgical treatment offered a 94.1% aneurysm obliteration rate compared with 81.8% for the endovascular group (**Table 15.2**). The authors concluded that both endovascular and microsurgical treatments are generally successful. Microsurgical therapy, however, is more efficacious in completely eliminating the aneurysm and more durable over the extended lifetime of these patients. Furthermore, the coiling of large aneurysms often results in significant recanalization rates, arguing against their use in pediatric patients.[48]

Outcome

The overall outcome of pediatric aneurysmal disease is good. Krishna et al reported an 82% favorable outcome in surgically treated cases.[49] Children presenting with low clinical grades had 100% favorable outcome. A similar experience has been documented in the literature.[9,14–16] Norris and Wallace argued that children usually present in better clinical grades after SAH compared with adults and that overall surgical outcome is better.[15] According to Ferrante et al, younger patients tolerate surgery better due to greater brain functional capacity and a robust collateral circulation.[16,50] Delayed surgery for higher grades has improved surgical outcome; however, this is at the expense of management morbidity.

Conclusion

The incidence of pediatric aneurysms is rare. Thus, our collective experience in managing these lesions is relatively limited and localized at specialized tertiary institutions. However, the current sophistication of microsurgical technique, various

Table 15.1 Successful Aneurysm Obliteration in Pediatric Series Involving Microsurgical and Endovascular Treatment*

Obliteration Rate					
Study	No. of Patients	Mean Age (Years)	No. of Aneurysms	Microsurgical Treatment	Endovascular Treatment
Storrs et al[32]	29	NR	29	76.0% (16 of 21)	NA
Herman et al[10]	16	8	20	94.7% (18 of 19)	NA
Yazbak et al (1995)	7	9	7	100.0% (7 of 7)	NA
Ter Brugge[98]	21	10	25	88.9% (8 of 9)	100.0% (6 of 6)
Proust et al[16]	22	13	25	95.0% (19 of 20)	100.0% (4 of 4)
Huang et al[11]	19	10	19	100.0% (13 of 13)	100.0% (3 of 3)
Present series	32	12	43	94.1% (16 of 17)	81.8% (18 of 22)

* Successful obliteration is defined as the absence of the following: residual aneurysm, aneurysm recurrence, and death after initial treatment.

Abbreviations: NA, not applicable; NR, not reported.

Source: Adapted from Sanai N, Quinones-Hinojosa A, Gupta N, Perry V, Sun P, Wilson C, Lawton M. Pediatric intracranial aneurysms: durability of treatment following microsurgical and endovascular management. J Neurosurg 2006;104:82–89.

Table 15.2 Comparison of Data Obtained in Microsurgical and Endovascular Treatment Groups

Treatment Group (%)		
Variable	Microsurgical	Endovascular
No. of patients	13	16
No. of aneurysms	17	23
Complete obliteration	16 (94.1)	18 (81.8)
Recurrence	0 (0)	3 (13.6)
De novo formation	1 (5.9)	3 (18.8)
New neurologic deficits	1 (7.7)	1 (6.3)
Mortality rate	0	0

Source: Adapted from Sanai N, Quinones-Hinojosa A, Gupta N, Perry V, Sun P, Wilson C, Lawton M. Pediatric intracranial aneurysms: durability of treatment following microsurgical and endovascular management. J Neurosurg 2006;104:82–89.

revascularization options, neurophysiologic monitoring, excellent imaging modalities, high-level pediatric intensive care, and neuroanesthetic techniques have made the surgical management of SAH in children very safe. The unique pathophysiologic features, along with size and distribution variability of pediatric aneurysms, require creative and innovative surgical strategies to obliterate these lesions. It is imperative to individualize treatment. Indeed, endovascular techniques have become quite sophisticated, and this treatment modality is very effective in selected cases. Controversy regarding the durability of microsurgical versus endovascular repair exists in the literature, and as we become more advanced, there will be more emerging issues that will continue to fuel the debate. As far as we are concerned, the best and safest way to tackle pediatric aneurysmal disease is a combination of microsurgical and endovascular therapy in highly specialized neurovascular centers.

◆ Endovascular Treatment

Monica S. Pearl, Ingrid M. Burger, and Philippe Gailloud

Pediatric intracranial aneurysms account for <5% of all intracranial aneurysms.[51–55] Morphologically, they differ from aneurysms seen in adults in that they tend to be larger and more dysplastic, have a wide neck, and more often occur in atypical locations. In addition, intracranial aneurysms seen in children are more often associated with etiologic factors such as trauma, congenital disorders, and infection than in the adult population.[52] Intracranial aneurysms may be classified as saccular, fusiform, infectious ("mycotic"), or dissecting aneurysms, each category having its specific natural history, management options, and clinical outcome, as aneurysm morphology is a key factor in regard to the degree of aneurysm obliteration and the rate of recurrence after either microsurgical or endovascular treatment.[56]

Therapeutic options for pediatric intracranial aneurysms include surgical and endovascular techniques, or a combination of these, with a slow but gradual shift noted over the last 15 years in favor of endovascular treatment.[51] This tendency reflects the progresses made in neurointerventional techniques, as well as the promising results observed in the endovascular treatment of adult aneurysms.[51] The International Subarachnoid Aneurysm Trial (ISAT), a randomized controlled trial comparing surgical clipping with endovascular coiling for the treatment of ruptured cerebral aneurysms, has shown better outcomes in the endovascular treatment group.[57,58] It was found in particular that, for ruptured aneurysms felt to be equally treatable by either method, the relative risk of death or significant disability at 1 year for patients treated by coiling was lower than in the surgical group (absolute risk reduction of 7.4%), whereas the risk of late rebleeding was higher in the endovascular group. The study has been criticized in regard to possible selection biases detrimental to the surgical group, as well as to the level of expertise of the neurosurgeons performing the surgical treatments (general rather than vascular neurosurgeons).[59] The ISAT study nonetheless helps support the notion that endovascular therapy is a valid alternative to surgical clipping; although no child was included, it may suggest that embolization could be a safe and effective treatment option for pediatric patients as well. However, endovascular therapy for pediatric intracranial aneurysms, either ruptured or unruptured, requires further evaluation before its exact role can be determined.

Technical Considerations

Endovascular techniques for the treatment of intracranial aneurysms with conservation of the parent artery, also known as constructive therapies, include standard coil embolization, coil embolization with balloon remodeling or stent assistance, and balloon-assisted liquid polymer embolization (**Fig. 15.4A–C**). The use of covered stents (or stent grafts) has been proposed as an option for large fusiform or wide-necked aneurysms, primarily located in the carotid and vertebral arteries, where the risk of occluding functionally important side branches is relatively low (**Fig. 15.4D**). The long-term patency of stent grafts placed in relatively small vessels, such as the ICA, is another potential

Detachable coils

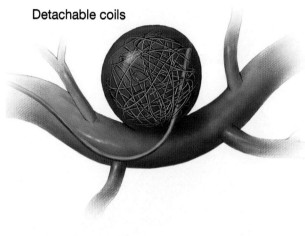

Balloon-assisted coils

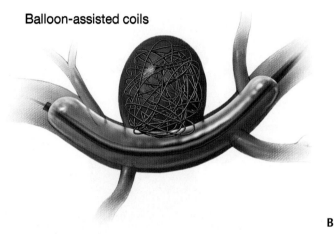

B

Stent-assisted coils

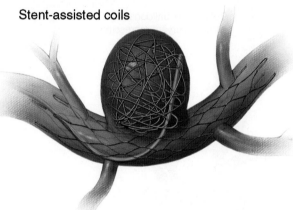

Covered stent

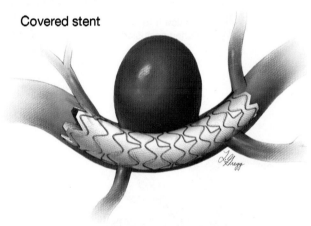

D

Fig. 15.4 Constructive endovascular techniques. **(A)** Coil embolization: the microcatheter is placed within the aneurysmal cavity, which is progressively filled (packed) with detachable microcoils of various nominal diameters, lengths, and geometric configurations (helical, two-dimensional, three-dimensional, etc.). Dense packing resulting in exclusion of the aneurysm from the circulation is obtained with a volume of coil material not exceeding 40% of the total aneurysm volume,[101] the residual space being filled with thrombus. Standard coil embolization requires a favorable aneurysm geometry, particularly in regard to the sac-to-neck ratio. A low ratio (i.e., wide neck) aneurysm will not hold the coils within the aneurysmal cavity, jeopardizing the patency of the parent artery. **(B)** Balloon remodeling: inflation of a compliant microballoon across the aneurysm neck concomitantly to coil deployment allows treating lesions with an unfavorable sac-to-neck ratio. The balloon is sequentially inflated and deflated to assist in the placement of each coil. We believe that there is an increased risk of thromboembolic events related to the wide coil–lumen interface and to the repeated flow interruption caused by balloon inflation. **(C)** Stent-assisted coiling: the deployment of a stent prior to

aneurysm catheterization and coiling offers assistance for wide neck aneurysms without the need for iterative parent artery obliteration, but it leaves a permanent intravascular device that necessitates dual antiplatelet therapy (aspirin and clopidogrel) and carries a still uncharacterized risk of delayed flow impairment (acute or subacute in stent thrombosis, chronic in stent stenosis from endothelial hyperplasia). Stent and balloon remodeling assistance can be combined for the treatment of dysplastic and/or fusiform aneurysms. **(D)** Stent graft: stent grafts can potentially interrupt the flow within the aneurysmal cavity without placement of intra-aneurysmal material. Such an approach would be rapid (low radiation exposure) and solve the mass effect issues sometimes associated with dense packing of aneurysms located in the immediate vicinity of fragile structures, such as the optic nerve. Drawbacks of currently available stent grafts include poor trackability, unknown long-term patency of the parent artery, and, even more importantly for neurovascular applications, the risk of occlusion of side branches. Some of these issues may be addressed by the new generation of stent grafts with a semipermeable architecture currently under development.

drawback of this approach and remains currently unknown.[60] Semipermeable membranes may represent an improvement over conventional stent grafts both in terms of parent artery and side branches patency, and may expand the indications of stent grafting to intracranial lesions in the future. Although promising, these approaches remain

experimental and will not be developed further in this discussion. Parent artery occlusion, also referred to as deconstructive therapy, remains a valid alternative option for nonsurgical candidates whose aneurysms are not amenable to the aforementioned constructive treatment methods (**Fig. 15.5**).

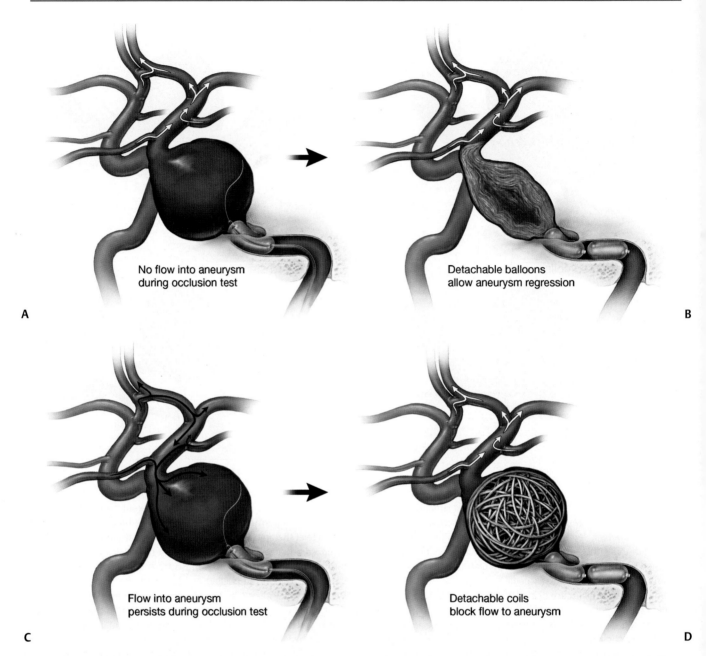

A   No flow into aneurysm during occlusion test

B   Detachable balloons allow aneurysm regression

C   Flow into aneurysm persists during occlusion test

D   Detachable coils block flow to aneurysm

Fig. 15.5 Deconstructive endovascular techniques. **(A)** The balloon occlusion test, performed with a nondetachable balloon, shows adequate collateral flow through the anterior and/or posterior communicating arteries, without flow within the aneurysmal cavity. **(B)** The internal carotid artery can be occluded, for example, with two detachable balloons, without placement of coils within the aneurysm cavity. Advantages of this approach include short procedure duration (low radiation exposure) and minimal foreign material, possibly allowing for secondary aneurysm shrinkage. **(C)** In this situation, the balloon occlusion test still shows adequate collateral flow through the anterior and/or posterior communicating arteries, but the aneurysm is now filled via retrograde flow through the distal internal carotid artery. **(D)** Occlusion of the internal carotid artery alone might result in aneurysm thrombosis and must be combined with coiling of the aneurysmal cavity.

The clinical condition of the patient, the aneurysm location and morphology, particularly the diameter of the neck and its relation to the parent artery, and the presence of branches arising from either the sac or the neck are important considerations when choosing the most appropriate treatment plan. The aneurysm neck, especially its size and relation to the parent artery and potential side branches, is the key feature in determining if coil embolization is an appropriate treatment option. Standard coil embolization is considered feasible for aneurysms with a small neck

(< 4 mm), a dome-to-neck ratio ≥ 2, and in the absence of important branches arising from the sac and/or the neck.[61] Coil embolization is achieved primarily with platinum coils. Advances made in platinum coil technology have tried to address incomplete aneurysm occlusion, which increases the risk of coil compaction and aneurysm recanalization. Reported rates of recanalization are ~21.0% to 28.6%, but they can be as high as 60% for giant aneurysms.[62–64] Recently developed hybrid, or "biologically active," coils are chemically pretreated to enhance their thrombogenicity[52] and try to decrease the recanalization rate.[65] (See the editorial commentary by Cloft about the ambiguities surrounding the "biologically active" coil concept and its regulation.[66]) Currently available modified coils include polyglycolic acid/lactide copolymer (PGLA)–coated coils (Matrix, Boston Scientific Corp., Natick, Massachusetts; Cerecyte, Micrus, Sunnyvale, California; Nexus coils, MicroTherapeutics, Irvine, California) and hydrogel-coated coils (HydroCoil, MicroVention, Aliso Viejo, California).[67] Other types of coated or active devices, such as coils with radioactive components or coils coated with biological material such as collagen or cells, are in the experimental phase. Matrix coils comprise an inner core of platinum covered with a biodegradable polymer (PGLA) designed to accelerate aneurysm fibrosis, neointima formation, and inflammation.[65] The safety of these coils for the treatment of endovascular aneurysms has been shown to be similar to that of bare platinum coils.[68,69] However, higher rates of recanalization (32%,[65] from 26.1% for small aneurysms with small necks to 75% for large aneurysms[70]) and thromboembolic events (up to 20%[71] vs 2.5–11.0%[72]) are now reported with Matrix coils versus bare platinum coils. Progressive resorption of the polymer coat leading to loss of volume and instability is thought to be a possible explanation for the high recurrence rates associated with Matrix coils.[73] HydroCoils are standard platinum coils coated with an expandable hydrogel material that result in delayed progressive coil expansion upon contact with blood.[74] These coils are supposed to provide superior aneurysm volume filling than bare platinum coils[75] and promote healing and endothelialization at the aneurysm neck.[75,76] Despite these features, recanalization rates remain high, up to 27% for large aneurysms.[77] More concerning, however, are reported cases of aseptic meningitis and delayed hydrocephalus,[67,77,78] which seem to be specific to the HydroCoil, as no cases have so far been described with PGLA-coated coils alone,[68] although some have occurred when Matrix coils were used in combination with HydroCoils.[79] Delayed perianeurysmal inflammation with dramatic neurologic dysfunction (bilateral visual loss) has been reported after embolization with HydroCoils.[80] Perianeurysmal inflammation leading to visual loss has also been described in cases of paraclinoid aneurysms treated with either standard platinum or coated coils.[81] The factors leading to these various coil-related

events have not been elucidated yet, and more information is needed regarding the role of coils, clot burden, aneurysm size, and inflammatory mediators in the development of these complications. At this stage, in view of growing safety concerns regarding unexpected complications such as meningitis, delayed inflammatory reaction, and hydrocephalus of unclear mechanisms, although potential benefits when compared with standard platinum coils remain undefined, it seems prudent to avoid using "bioactive" devices in children.

Stent-assisted coiling of intracranial aneurysms with balloon-expandable stents is rarely performed in children.[82] Recent advances in stent technology have led to the development of flexible self-expanding nitinol stents (Neuroform, Boston Scientific Neurovascular, Natick, Massachusetts; Enterprise, Cordis Neurovascular, Miami Lakes, Florida; LEO, Balt, Montmorency, France) dedicated to intracranial aneurysm therapy, specifically for the treatment of complex and wide-necked aneurysms. Advantages of these self-expanding intracranial stents over the balloon-expandable stents previously used for assisted coiling include improved trackability, helping navigate tortuous intracranial vasculature (although this is true only for the latest generation of self-expanding stents), improved deliverability, and decreased vessel injury during deployment.[83] Despite several technical differences in stent design, these devices have been shown to be safe and effective in the treatment of cerebral aneurysms.[84–86] Variations in stent design include open cell (Neuroform)[87] versus closed cell design (Enterprise, LEO),[88,89] low radial force (Neuroform)[87] versus high radial force (LEO)[85] versus low radial force/high compression resistance (Enterprise), and stent recoverability after partial deployment (a characteristic inherent to the closed cell design, with up to 70% of stent length for the Enterprise[83] and up to 90% of the stent length for the Leo[85]). Several case-based series studying the Neuroform,[84,88–92] Enterprise,[83,86] and Leo stents[85] have been published. Of the total of 341 patients treated in these various series, only 2 were children, ages 11 years[84] and 10 years,[89] both of whom were treated with Neuroform stents. Immediate and short-term results within that limited experience are promising, but data about the long-term efficacy and potential side effects specific to the pediatric age group are obviously still lacking. Additionally, the thrombogenic properties of stents mandate long-term anticoagulation, usually involving a dual antiplatelet regimen of clopidogrel and aspirin for at least 4 to 6 weeks after the procedure (with aspirin often continued for life in adult patients).[83,84,86,87,90] Although limited data are currently available, long-term antiplatelet therapy appears safe in children.[93,94] Intracranial stents are very promising, but at this time they should be used primarily, in children as in adults, for aneurysms that have failed or carry a high likelihood of failing conventional endovascular therapy.

Endovascular Aneurysm Therapy

When a deconstructive method is indicated, endovascular occlusion of the parent artery, with or without aneurysm coiling, is clearly the technique of choice. When a constructive method is contemplated, choosing between an endovascular and a surgical approach remains controversial, as neither approach can be deemed superior for all cases of pediatric intracranial aneurysms. As for adult aneurysm management, treatment decisions are therefore best made on an individual basis by a multidisciplinary team.[95]

Constructive endovascular therapy with preservation of the parent artery is the ideal treatment option for saccular aneurysms, but experience currently remains very limited. In a series of 37 aneurysms detected in 33 pediatric patients, only 5 saccular aneurysms out of the 13 treated via an endovascular approach over a 12-year period involved constructive methods.[51] Although the outcome for constructive versus deconstructive was not specifically addressed in that report, 77% (10 of 13) of patients in the endovascular treatment group made a good recovery, and 23% (3 of 13)[11] had a significant neurologic deficit.[51] The outcome appears comparable to that seen in surgical treatment of pediatric saccular aneurysms, with reported favorable outcomes ranging from 60 to 80%.[96,97] Based on their series reflecting a local experience, Agid et al recommended endovascular treatment as the primary option for pediatric aneurysms, stating that it offers better clinical outcomes than surgery.[51]

Among the important factors to be considered when choosing between an endovascular and a surgical approach for children are the immediate efficacy and the expected durability of the treatment. In their experience of 43 aneurysms treated in 32 pediatric patients between 1977 to 2003, Sanai et al noted that microsurgical treatment was associated with higher rates of complete obliteration than endovascular therapy, 94.1% (16 of 17) versus 81.8% (18 of 22), respectively.[64] This contradicts other series in which endovascular treatment was associated with obliteration rates equal to or greater than those of microsurgical treatment: 100% (6 of 6) versus 88.9% (8 of 9),[98] 100% (4 of 4) versus 95% (19 of 20),[55] and 100% (3 of 3) versus 100% (13 of 13).[11] Sanai et al further supported the surgical approach by demonstrating a lower rate of aneurysm recurrence after microsurgical treatment (0%) than in the group treated by endovascular techniques (14%).[64] However, both lower aneurysm obliteration and higher recurrence rates in the endovascular treatment group reported by Sanai et al may be related to the older (and sometimes obsolete) endovascular techniques used during the 25-year period covered in their study, which even includes a case treated by balloon embolization of the aneurysmal cavity. Given the constant advances made in endovascular technology, improvements in efficacy and durability are bound to occur, and series

covering a long time span using a wide range of techniques may be of historical interest only. It is not a surprise that the aneurysm treated by balloon embolization is among the three aneurysms that recurred in the endovascular group.[64] Yet we fully agree with these authors that a "deliberated and individualized approach to treatment selection" is required,[99] a statement that we consider valid for patients in all age categories. The following illustrative case has been chosen as an example of the value placed on multidisciplinary team management at our institution.

Illustrative Case

Right Middle Cerebral Artery Aneurysm in an 18-Month-Old Girl

The patient is an 18-month-old girl who, at the of age 6 months, suffered a right MCA stroke in the setting of preceding viral infection, reactive thrombocytosis, and reduced protein C activity. Initial cerebral MRI and MRA revealed restricted diffusion involving the right putamen and caudate nucleus (**Fig. 15.6**), as well as a severe stenosis involving the right M1 segment, with attenuation of distal right MCA branches (**Fig. 15.7A**). Follow-up MRI 8 months later showed persistent severe stenosis of the M1 segment with an aneurysm at the site of the stenosis (**Fig. 15.7B**). Digital subtraction angiography confirmed the presence of a saccular aneurysm and showed collateral flow from the right anterior cerebral artery to the distal right MCA territory via a complex arterial network located within the sylvian cistern and surrounding the aneurysm (**Fig. 15.8**). Management options were discussed during a weekly multidisciplinary neurovascular conference, and endovascular therapy was considered superior to surgical clipping in view of this particular collateral anatomy.

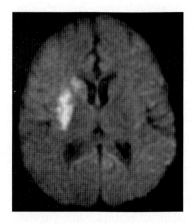

Fig. 15.6 Diffusion-weighted magnetic resonance (MR) image shows hyperintensity in the right putamen and head of the caudate nucleus, indicating acute ischemic injury.

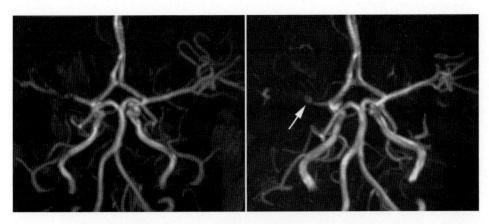

A   B

Fig. 15.7 (A) Three-dimensional time-of-flight MR angiography image obtained at the time of initial presentation. Irregular narrowing of the right middle cerebral artery is observed, with attenuation of distal branches, indicating flow impairment. **(B)** Anteroposterior projection MR angiography image obtained 8 months later. On the follow-up study, the narrowing and the distal flow appear to have worsened, and an aneurysmal component is identified in the middle of the M1 segment (*arrow*).

Intervention

The procedure was performed under general anesthesia via a right femoral access (4-French arterial sheath), using a 4-French diagnostic catheter as a guide (DAV, Cook, Bloomington, Indiana). A loading dose of 160 mg of aspirin was administered rectally shortly before the procedure, and a bolus of 1000 IU of heparin was given after arterial access was secured. A 1.9-French microcatheter (Echelon 10, ev3 Neurovascular, Irvine, California) was advanced over a 0.010 guidewire (Transend 10, Boston Scientific Neurovascular) into the aneurysm, which was coiled using six detachable microcoils (one GDC 3D and five GDC 360 soft, Boston Scientific Neurovascular) (**Fig. 15.9**). A total of 27.5 mL (1.9 cc/kg) of contrast agent (Omnipaque 300, Amersham Health, Little Chalfont, Buckinghamshire, UK) was injected, with a combined anteroposterior and lateral fluoroscopy time of 26.6 minutes. Femoral hemostasis was obtained by gentle manual compression after normalization of the partial thromboplastin time (PTT) ratio. Heparin was restarted 3 hours later with a target PTT ratio of 2.0 to 2.5 for 20 hours. The procedure was uneventful, and the patient was discharged 2 days later in her baseline neurologic condition. Daily aspirin was restarted at the preprocedural dosage in regard to the MCA stenosis.

Discussion

Our obligation to provide children with optimal, up-to-date therapy needs to be carefully balanced with our duty to protect them from harm related to inadequate procedures. Being able to recommend a particular therapeutic strategy, whether it be conservative, endovascular, or surgical, requires a good understanding of its risks and benefits. Many of the risks and benefits of strategies for aneurysm treatment in children, however, remain less well characterized than they are for adults. Therefore, it is of fundamental importance for individual clinicians, and for the field as a whole, to innovate prudently, by continuing to support, pursue, and collaborate in well-designed clinical research aimed at better quantifying the respective risks and benefits of endovascular and surgical treatments of pediatric aneurysms. Only high-quality data from pediatric studies will help clinicians choose the intervention with the highest likelihood of success and the lowest likelihood of harm for a particular clinical situation. Where high-quality data in children are lacking or when data conflict regarding the best

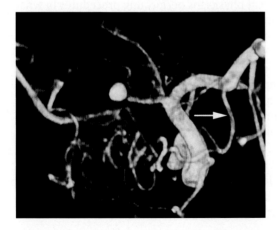

Fig. 15.8 Three-dimensional digital subtraction angiography of a right carotid rotational angiogram (here shown in a right anterior oblique view) reveals a diffusely abnormal M1 segment, with a preocclusive focal stenosis of its midportion and a saccular-looking aneurysm located at the proximal end. These findings are consistent with a right middle cerebral artery dissection. There is a conspicuous collateral network within the sylvian fissure, in front of the aneurysm, principally supplied by a branch of the right anterior cerebral artery (*arrow*).

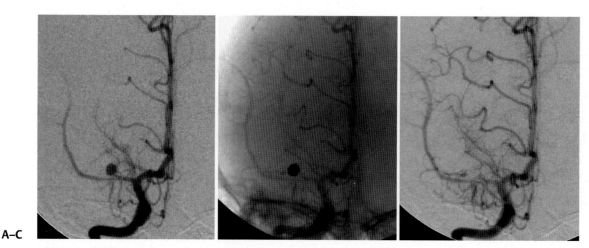

A–C

Fig. 15.9 Endovascular therapy. **(A)** Anteroposterior view of the right internal carotid angiogram prior to treatment. **(B)** Nonsubtracted image shows that the aneurysm has been embolized, with the aneurysmal cavity densely packed with coils. **(C)** Final angiogram documents the absence of flow within the aneurysm, as well as the preserved patency of the M1 segment.

therapeutic strategy, various biases may play a larger role, such as biases related to the invasive versus minimally invasive nature of the treatment, physicians' aspirations to pioneer novel methods, and financial interests in the marketability of new techniques or devices. As an example, let us consider here the case of a 6-month-old child with a giant skull base aneurysm. Will this patient be better treated by a deconstructive method (occlusion of the ICA) or by a constructive method (stent-assisted coiling)? Currently, there are no strong data regarding a direct comparison of the risks and benefits of each method. In general, we know that stent-assisted coiling is associated with potential drawbacks, such as the risks inherent to a relatively complex procedure (arterial dissection or rupture, clot migration); the need for longer fluoroscopy times, resulting in a higher radiation dose (to which pediatric patients are more sensitive); the need for antiplatelet therapy, which reduces but does not remove the risk of delayed thromboembolic events; the burden of unclear long-term efficacy (i.e., recanalization, need for follow-up imaging); and the still unknown long-term effects of an intravascular device placed in a child's vasculature. Nevertheless, stent-assisted coiling is more elegant in that it will preserve the parent artery, and it benefits from a positive "modern" flavor. Parent artery occlusion, by contrast, may seem a crude and old-fashioned method, but it is known to be successful at treating skull base giant aneurysms with minimal periprocedural risks, in particular when adequate collateral circulation is demonstrated by pretreatment angiography and balloon test occlusion, and is associated with excellent long-term results. In the absence of a strong argument in favor of one or the other option (e.g., the absence of collateral pathways precluding parent artery sacrifice), the input from the parents/guardians, after they have been presented with a

clear explanation of what is known about the respective advantages and drawbacks of each available option, may become decisive in the choice of therapy. The need for an honest and informative consent process cannot be emphasized enough, in particular when discussing novel procedures whose exact benefits and risks remain to be established. The assessment and acceptance of new devices or methods must work both ways, welcoming novel procedures with due circumspection, yet offering them first as treatment alternatives, and then as primary options if their role and value are validated by our growing knowledge and experience. In that regard, it is of particular importance that physicians performing procedures in what remains a limited patient population, that is, children with cerebral aneurysms, try sharing their experience, positive or negative, with the rest of the community. Although the publication of case reports and case-based series represents an important step in that direction, only appropriately controlled studies involving multiple centers can allow gathering meaningful data from a statistically adequate sample size in a limited time period and without local biases. Early enthusiasm for endovascular management of aneurysms ("all saccular aneurysms are endovascular"), followed by delayed publication of mitigated results and significant recurrence rates, must be avoided, as it does little, if anything, to advance our field in the right direction.

In summary, constructive and deconstructive endovascular methods represent major components of our armamentarium for the treatment of cerebral aneurysms in children. They must not be understood as competing with microsurgical options, but complementing them. Only a multidisciplinary approach can adequately address the variety and complexity of these lesions through a case-by-case decision process. When a deconstructive method is contemplated, endovascular access is the method of choice. Although endovascular coiling is clearly superior to surgical access in certain situations, the long-term efficacy of surgical clipping sets the standard that endovascular treatment must reach to be considered a primary constructive therapeutic option. The constant developments made in the endovascular field support progress. It remains doubtful, however, that either approach will ever claim superiority for all aneurysms that need be treated.

♦ Lessons Learned

The endovascular approach to pathologies of the nervous system's vascular supply is an enormous success story of innovation and rapid application of basic science in the clinical setting. This is exemplified in the contribution of Pearl et al. Due to the special challenges posed by pediatric patients, the downsides and uncertainties of the various embolization techniques become more apparent than in the adult setting. New understanding of potential side effects of used embolic materials, particularly their unknown long-term problems, are raising concern about their use in the pediatric population. The same is true for implants, the use of which may require long-term antiplatelet medication. The authors thoughtfully balance the promise of the many avenues opened by these innovative treatment techniques with the concern for long-term side effects. They also stress the relative rarity of aneurysms in the pediatric population and their relative inhomogeneity when compared with the adult disease. Consequently, they emphasize the need for interdisciplinary cooperation and careful individualization of a treatment plan for each patient.

The surgical approach is tailored to the stated differences between adult and pediatric disease. The common theme, which very much appeals to the philosophy of the pediatric neurosurgeon, is the concept of early and aggressive treatment, either endovascular or microsurgical. Chandela and Langer remind us that there is a significant genetic component to the pathogenesis of aneurysms, probably more so in the pediatric than the adult population. The concept of hemodynamic stresses applies to aneurysms in children in the same way as it does to those in adults. It is noteworthy that the carotid bifurcation aneurysms are overrepresented in the pediatric population when compared with the "usual" adult series, and that these aneurysms tend to be large. The microsurgical treatment of aneurysms appears to be much more variable and more frequently complex in children than in adults. The authors cite reports of relatively large series of complex aneurysm surgery that included obliteration of the parent vessel, even the carotid, bypass procedures and complex combinations of clip placement, entrapment, and other creative techniques.

Retrospective evidence points toward an advantage of microsurgical treatment over endovascular approaches. Children appear to tolerate both complex procedures and parent vessel obliteration significantly better than adults, either because of the retained flexibility of the neurovascular system or superior neural plasticity, or both. This, combined with the many caveats expressed about the long-term durability of endovascular aneurysm obliteration techniques, is a significant argument toward the continued use of microsurgery, however complex, for children with aneurysms, albeit with highly individualized treatment planning and evidently a large role for interdisciplinary cooperation.

References

1. Blount J, Oakes WJ, Tubbs S, Humphreys R. History of surgery for cerebrovascular disease in children: 1. Intracranial arterial aneurysms. Neurosurg Focus 2006;20(6):E10
2. Eppinger H. Stenosis Aortae Congenital seu Isthmus Persistens. Vrtljschr Prakt Heilk 1871;112:31–67
3. McDonald C, Korb M. Intracranial aneurysms. Arch Neurol Psychiatry 1939;42:298–328
4. Strassman F. Der plotzliche Tod bei Stenose des Isthmus Aortae. Beitr Gerichtl Med 1922;5:91–97
5. Dell S. Asymptomatic cerebral aneurysm: assessment of its risk of rupture. Neurosurgery 1982;10(2):162–166
6. Laughlin S, terBrugge KG, Willinsky RA, Armstrong DC, Montanera W, Humphreys RP. Endovascular management of paediatric intracranial aneurysms. Intervent Neuroradiol 1997;3:205–214
7. Burke MJ. Occult aneurysmal hemorrhage in a child: case report and literature review. Pediatr Neurosurg 2000;33(5):274–277
8. Gerosa M, Licata C, Fiore DL, Iraci G. Intracranial aneurysms of childhood. Childs Brain 1980;6(6):295–302
9. Heiskanen O, Vilkki J. Intracranial arterial aneurysms in children and adolescents. Acta Neurochir (Wien) 1981;59(1–2):55–63
10. Herman JM, Rekate HL, Spetzler RF. Pediatric intracranial aneurysms: simple and complex cases. Pediatr Neurosurg 1991–1992;17(2):66–72, discussion 73
11. Huang J, McGirt MJ, Gailloud P, Tamargo RJ. Intracranial aneurysms in the pediatric population: case series and literature review. Surg Neurol 2005;63(5):424–432, discussion 432–433
12. Husson RN, Saini R, Lewis LL, Butler KM, Patronas N, Pizzo PA. Cerebral artery aneurysms in children infected with human immunodeficiency virus. J Pediatr 1992;121(6):927–930

13. Kanaan I, Lasjaunias P, Coates R. The spectrum of intracranial aneurysms in pediatrics. Minim Invasive Neurosurg 1995;38(1):1–9

14. Meyer FB, Sundt TM Jr, Fode NC, Morgan MK, Forbes GS, Mellinger JF. Cerebral aneurysms in childhood and adolescence. J Neurosurg 1989;70(3):420–425

15. Norris JS, Wallace MC. Pediatric intracranial aneurysms. Neurosurg Clin N Am 1998;9(3):557–563

16. Proust F, Toussaint P, Garniéri J, et al. Pediatric cerebral aneurysms. J Neurosurg 2001;94(5):733–739

17. Sandberg DI, Lamberti-Pasculli M, Drake JM, Humphreys RP, Rutka JT. Spontaneous intraparenchymal hemorrhage in full-term neonates. Neurosurgery 2001;48(5):1042–1048, discussion 1048–1049

18. Patel AN, Richardson AE. Ruptured intracranial aneurysms in the first two decades of life: a study of 58 patients. J Neurosurg 1971; 35(5):571–576

19. Ostergaard JR, Voldby B. Intracranial arterial aneurysms in children and adolescents. J Neurosurg 1983;58(6):832–837

20. Young WF, Pattisapu JV. Ruptured cerebral aneurysm in a 39-day-old infant. Clin Neurol Neurosurg 2000;102(3):140–143

21. LeRoux P, Winn HR, Newell DW, eds. Management of Cerebral Aneurysms. Philadelphia: WB Saunders; 2003

22. Allison JW, Davis PC, Sato Y, et al. Intracranial aneurysms in infants and children. Pediatr Radiol 1998;28(4):223–229

23. Sekhar LN, Heros RC. Origin, growth, and rupture of saccular aneurysms: a review. Neurosurgery 1981;8(2):248–260

24. Stehbens WE. Etiology of intracranial berry aneurysms. J Neurosurg 1989;70(6):823–831

25. Schievink WI. Genetics of intracranial aneurysms. Neurosurgery 1997;40(4):651–662, discussion 662–663

26. Lipper S, Morgan D, Krigman MR, Staab EV. Congenital saccular aneurysm in a 19-day-old neonate: case report and review of the literature. Surg Neurol 1978;10(3):161–165

27. Ostergaard JR. Aetiology of intracranial saccular aneurysms in childhood. Br J Neurosurg 1991;5(6):575–580

28. Ostergaard JR, Reske-Nielsen E, Buhl J. Deficiency of reticular fibers in cerebral arteries: on the etiology of saccular aneurysms in childhood. Br J Neurosurg 1989;3(1):113–115

29. Stehbens WE, Manz HJ, Uszinski R, Schellinger D. Atypical cerebral aneurysm in a young child. Pediatr Neurosurg 1995;23(2):97–100

30. Lee KS, Liu SS, Spetzler RF, Rekate HL. Intracranial mycotic aneurysm in an infant: report of a case. Neurosurgery 1990;26(1):129–133

31. Piatt JH Jr, Clunie DA. Intracranial arterial aneurysm due to birth trauma: case report. J Neurosurg 1992;77(5):799–803

32. Roach ES, Riela AR, eds. Intracranial aneurysms. In: Pediatric Cerebrovascular Disorders. Armonk, NY: 1995

33. Shucart WA, Wolpert SM. Intracranial arterial aneurysm in childhood. Am J Dis Child 1974;127(2):288–293

34. Storrs BB, Humphreys RP, Hendrick EB, Hoffman HJ. Intracranial aneurysms in the pediatric age-group. Childs Brain 1982;9(5):358–361

35. Amacher LA, Drake CG. Cerebral artery aneurysms in infancy, childhood and adolescence. Childs Brain 1975;1(1):72–80

36. Weir BK. Aneurysms Affecting the Nervous System. Baltimore: Williams &Wilkins; 1987

37. Kangasniemi M, Mäkelä T, Koskinen S, Porras M, Poussa K, Hernesniemi J. Detection of intracranial aneurysms with two-dimensional and three-dimensional multislice helical computed tomographic angiography. Neurosurgery 2004;54(2):336–340, discussion 340–341

38. Lena G, Choux M. Giant intracranial aneurysms in children 15 years old or under: case reports and literature review. J Pediatr Neurosci 1985;1:84–93

39. Humphreys RP, Hendrick EB, Hoffman HJ. Cerebrovascular disease in children. Can Med Assoc J 1972;107(8):774–776, passim

40. Ito M, Yoshihara M, Ishii M, Wachi A, Sato K. Cerebral aneurysms in children. Brain Dev 1992;14(4):263–268

41. Choux M, Lena G, Genitori L. Intracranial aneurysms in children. In: Cerebrovascular Diseases in Children. New York: Springer Verlag; 1991

42. Kassell NF, Torner JC, Haley EC Jr, Jane JA, Adams HP, Kongable GL. The International Cooperative Study on the Timing of Aneurysm Surgery: 1. Overall management results. J Neurosurg 1990;73(1): 18–36

43. Hacker RJ. Intracranial aneurysms of childhood: a statistical analysis of 500 cases from the world literature. Neurosurgery 1982; 10:775

44. Chandela S, Langer D, Sen C, Berenstein A, Niimi, Song. Side-to-side PICA-PICA bypass in treatment of a complex posterior fossa aneurysm in a pediatric patient. J Neurosurg 2007

45. Amacher AL, Drake CG, Ferguson GG. Posterior circulation aneurysms in young people. Neurosurgery 1981;8(3):315–320

46. Amacher AL, Drake CG. The results of operating upon cerebral aneurysms and angiomas in children and adolescents: 1. Cerebral aneurysms. Childs Brain 1979;5(3):151–165

47. Wong JH, Mitha AP, Willson M, Hudon ME, Sevick RJ, Frayne R. Assessment of brain aneurysms by using high-resolution magnetic resonance angiography after endovascular coil delivery. J Neurosurg 2007;107(2):283–289

48. Sanai N, Quinones-Hinojosa A, Gupta NM, et al. Pediatric intracranial aneurysms: durability of treatment following microsurgical and endovascular management. J Neurosurg 2006;104(2, Suppl): 82–89

49. Krishna H, Wani AA, Behari S, Banerji D, Chhabra DK, Jain VK. Intracranial aneurysms in patients 18 years of age or under, are they different from aneurysms in adult population? Acta Neurochir (Wien) 2005;147(5):469–476, discussion 476

50. Ferrante L, Fortuna A, Celli P, Santoro A, Fraioli B. Intracranial arterial aneurysms in early childhood. Surg Neurol 1988;29(1):39–56

51. Agid R, Souza MP, Reintamm G, Armstrong D, Dirks P, ter Brugge KG. The role of endovascular treatment for pediatric aneurysms. Childs Nerv Syst 2005;21(12):1030–1036

52. Eddleman C, Nikas D, Shaibani A, Khan P, Dipatri AJ Jr, Tomita T. HydroCoil embolization of a ruptured infectious aneurysm in a pediatric patient: case report and review of the literature. Childs Nerv Syst 2007;23(6):707–712

53. Locksley HB. Natural history of subarachnoid hemorrhage, intracranial aneurysms and arteriovenous malformations: based on 6368 cases in the cooperative study. J Neurosurg 1966;25(2):219–239

54. Patel AN, Richardson AE. Ruptured intracranial aneurysms in the first two decades of life: a study of 58 patients. J Neurosurg 1971;35(5):571–576

55. Proust F, Toussaint P, Garniéri J, et al. Pediatric cerebral aneurysms. J Neurosurg 2001;94(5):733–739

56. Ventureyra EC. Pediatric intracranial aneurysms: a different perspective. J Neurosurg 2006;104(2, Suppl):79–80, discussion 80–81

57. Molyneux A, Kerr R, Stratton I, et al; International Subarachnoid Aneurysm Trial (ISAT) Collaborative Group. International Subarachnoid Aneurysm Trial (ISAT) of neurosurgical clipping versus endovascular coiling in 2143 patients with ruptured intracranial aneurysms: a randomised trial. Lancet 2002;360(9342):1267–1274

58. Molyneux AJ, Kerr RS, Yu LM, et al; International Subarachnoid Aneurysm Trial (ISAT) Collaborative Group. International Subarachnoid Aneurysm Trial (ISAT) of neurosurgical clipping versus endovascular coiling in 2143 patients with ruptured intracranial aneurysms: a randomised comparison of effects on survival, dependency, seizures, rebleeding, subgroups, and aneurysm occlusion. Lancet 2005;366(9488):809–817

59. Britz GW. ISAT trial: coiling or clipping for intracranial aneurysms? Lancet 2005;366(9488):783–785

60. Saatci I, Cekirge HS, Ozturk MH, et al. Treatment of internal carotid artery aneurysms with a covered stent: experience in 24 patients with mid-term follow-up results. AJNR Am J Neuroradiol 2004; 25(10):1742–1749

61. Alexander MJ. Endovascular treatment of cerebral aneurysms in children. In: Alexander MJ, Spetzler RF, eds. Pediatric Neurovascular Disease: Surgical, Endovascular, and Medical Management. New York: Thieme Medical Publishers; 2006:145–151

62. Murayama Y, Nien YL, Duckwiler G, et al. Guglielmi detachable coil embolization of cerebral aneurysms: 11 years' experience. J Neurosurg 2003;98(5):959–966

63. Piotin M, Spelle L, Mounayer C, et al. Intracranial aneurysms: treatment with bare platinum coils—aneurysm packing, complex coils, and angiographic recurrence. Radiology 2007;243(2):500–508

64. Sanai N, Quinones-Hinojosa A, Gupta NM, et al. Pediatric intracranial aneurysms: durability of treatment following microsurgical and endovascular management. J Neurosurg 2006;104(2, Suppl): 82–89

65. Kimchi TJ, Willinsky RA, Spears J, Lee SK, ter Brugge K. Endovascular treatment of intracranial aneurysms with matrix coils: immediate posttreatment results, clinical outcome and follow-up. Neuroradiology 2007;49(3):223–229

66. Cloft HJ. Have you been smoking something that is biologically active? AJNR Am J Neuroradiol 2006;27(2):240–242

67. Kang HS, Han MH, Lee TH, et al. Embolization of intracranial aneurysms with hydrogel-coated coils: result of a Korean multicenter trial. Neurosurgery 2007;61(1):51–58, discussion 58–59

68. Kang HS, Han MH, Kwon BJ, et al. Short-term outcome of intracranial aneurysms treated with polyglycolic acid/lactide copolymer-coated coils compared to historical controls treated with bare platinum coils: a single-center experience. AJNR Am J Neuroradiol 2005;26(8):1921–1928

69. Lubicz B, Leclerc X, Gauvrit JY, Lejeune JP, Pruvo JP. Endovascular treatment of intracranial aneurysms with matrix coils: a preliminary study of immediate post-treatment results. AJNR Am J Neuroradiol 2005;26(2):373–375

70. Fiorella D, Albuquerque FC, McDougall CG. Durability of aneurysm embolization with matrix detachable coils. Neurosurgery 2006;58(1):51–59, discussion 51–59

71. Taschner CA, Leclerc X, Rachdi H, Barros AM, Pruvo JP. Matrix detachable coils for the endovascular treatment of intracranial aneurysms: analysis of early angiographic and clinical outcomes. Stroke 2005;36(10):2176–2180

72. Workman MJ, Cloft HJ, Tong FC, et al. Thrombus formation at the neck of cerebral aneurysms during treatment with Guglielmi detachable coils. AJNR Am J Neuroradiol 2002;23(9):1568–1576

73. Murayama Y, Tateshima S, Gonzalez NR, Vinuela F. Matrix and bioabsorbable polymeric coils accelerate healing of intracranial aneurysms: long-term experimental study. Stroke 2003;34(8): 2031–2037

74. Cloft HJ. HydroCoil for Endovascular Aneurysm Occlusion (HEAL) study: periprocedural results. AJNR Am J Neuroradiol 2006;27(2): 289–292

75. Gaba RC, Ansari SA, Roy SS, Marden FA, Viana MA, Malisch TW. Embolization of intracranial aneurysms with hydrogel-coated coils versus inert platinum coils: effects on packing density, coil length and quantity, procedure performance, cost, length of hospital stay, and durability of therapy. Stroke 2006;37(6):1443–1450

76. Ding YH, Dai D, Lewis DA, Cloft HJ, Kallmes DF. Angiographic and histologic analysis of experimental aneurysms embolized with platinum coils, Matrix, and HydroCoil. AJNR Am J Neuroradiol 2005;26(7):1757–1763

77. Berenstein A, Song JK, Niimi Y, et al. Treatment of cerebral aneurysms with hydrogel-coated platinum coils (HydroCoil): early single-center experience. AJNR Am J Neuroradiol 2006;27(9): 1834–1840

78. Im SH, Han MH, Kwon BJ, Jung C, Kim JE, Han DH. Aseptic meningitis after embolization of cerebral aneurysms using hydrogel-coated coils: report of three cases. AJNR Am J Neuroradiol 2007;28(3):511–512

79. Meyers PM, Lavine SD, Fitzsimmons BF, et al. Chemical meningitis after cerebral aneurysm treatment using two second-generation aneurysm coils: report of two cases. Neurosurgery 2004;55(5):1222

80. Pickett GE, Laitt RD, Herwadkar A, Hughes DG. Visual pathway compromise after hydrocoil treatment of large ophthalmic aneurysms. Neurosurgery 2007;61(4):E873–E874, discussion E874

81. Schmidt GW, Oster SF, Golnik KC, et al. Isolated progressive visual loss after coiling of paraclinoid aneurysms. AJNR Am J Neuroradiol 2007;28(10):1882–1889

82. Cohen JE, Ferrario A, Ceratto R, Miranda C, Lylyk P. Reconstructive endovascular approach for a cavernous aneurysm in infancy. Neurol Res 2003;25(5):492–496

83. Higashida RT, Halbach VV, Dowd CF, Juravsky L, Meagher S. Initial clinical experience with a new self-expanding nitinol stent for the treatment of intracranial cerebral aneurysms: the Cordis Enterprise stent. AJNR Am J Neuroradiol 2005;26(7):1751–1756

84. Biondi A, Janardhan V, Katz JM, Salvaggio K, Riina HA, Gobin YP. Neuroform stent-assisted coil embolization of wide-neck intracranial aneurysms: strategies in stent deployment and midterm follow-up. Neurosurgery 2007;61(3):460–468, discussion 468–469

85. Lubicz B, Leclerc X, Levivier M, et al. Retractable self-expandable stent for endovascular treatment of wide-necked intracranial aneurysms: preliminary experience. Neurosurgery 2006;58(3): 451–457, discussion 451–457

86. Weber W, Bendszus M, Kis B, Boulanger T, Solymosi L, Kühne D. A new self-expanding nitinol stent (Enterprise) for the treatment of wide-necked intracranial aneurysms: initial clinical and angiographic results in 31 aneurysms. Neuroradiology 2007;49(7): 555–561

87. Howington JU, Hanel RA, Harrigan MR, Levy EI, Guterman LR, Hopkins LN. The Neuroform stent, the first microcatheter-delivered stent for use in the intracranial circulation. Neurosurgery 2004;54(1):2–5

88. Benitez RP, Silva MT, Klem J, Veznedaroglu E, Rosenwasser RH. Endovascular occlusion of wide-necked aneurysms with a new intracranial microstent (Neuroform) and detachable coils. Neurosurgery 2004;54(6):1359–1367, discussion 1368

89. Fiorella D, Albuquerque FC, Han P, McDougall CG. Preliminary experience using the Neuroform stent for the treatment of cerebral aneurysms. Neurosurgery 2004;54(1):6–16, discussion 16–17

90. Fiorella D, Albuquerque FC, Woo H, Rasmussen PA, Masaryk TJ, McDougall CG. Neuroform in-stent stenosis: incidence, natural history, and treatment strategies. Neurosurgery 2006;59(1):34–42, discussion 34–42

91. Lee YJ, Kim DJ, Suh SH, Lee SK, Kim J, Kim DI. Stent-assisted coil embolization of intracranial wide-necked aneurysms. Neuroradiology 2005;47(9):680–689

92. Turk AS, Niemann DB, Ahmed A, Aagaard-Kienitz B. Use of self-expanding stents in distal small cerebral vessels. AJNR Am J Neuroradiol 2007;28(3):533–536

93. Finkelstein Y, Nurmohamed L, Avner M, Benson LN, Koren G. Clopidogrel use in children. J Pediatr 2005;147(5):657–661

94. Israels SJ, Michelson AD. Antiplatelet therapy in children. Thromb Res 2006;118(1):75–83

95. Tamargo RJ, Rigamonti D, Murphy K, Gailloud P, Conway JE, Clatterbuck RE. Treatment of intracranial aneurysms: surgical clipping or endovascular coiling? Ann Neurol 2001;49(5):682–684

96. Kanaan I, Lasjaunias P, Coates R. The spectrum of intracranial aneurysms in pediatrics. Minim Invasive Neurosurg 1995;38(1):1–9

97. Pasqualin A, Mazza C, Cavazzani P, Scienza R, DaPian R. Intracranial aneurysms and subarachnoid hemorrhage in children and adolescents. Childs Nerv Syst 1986;2(4):185–190

98. terBrugge KG. Neurointerventional procedures in the pediatric age group. Childs Nerv Syst 1999;15(11–12):751–754

99. Agid R, terBrugge KG. Pediatric aneurysms. J Neurosurg 2007;106(4, Suppl):328, author reply 328–329

100. Piotin M, Mandai S, Murphy KJ, et al. Dense packing of cerebral aneurysms: an in vitro study with detachable platinum coils. AJNR Am J Neuroradiol 2000;21(4):757–760

II   Intraspinal

16 Myelomeningocele

♦ Fetal Repair

Nalin Gupta

Fetal surgery was developed to treat conditions such as congenital diaphragmatic hernia and sacrococcygeal teratoma that were otherwise fatal.[1] An open neural tube defect, however, is compatible with a term gestation, and a child with such a defect in the modern era should expect a long life span, particularly if concurrent medical problems are managed appropriately.[2] As with any surgical intervention, the procedural risks must be balanced against the potential benefit, which in this case is a reduction in the burden of disability for the affected child. A particular ethical consideration specific for this fetal procedure is the risk borne by the mother, and whether she is able to dispassionately balance the risk to herself against the benefit to her unborn child. Currently, the reported benefits of fetal surgery include a reduction in shunt insertion rates and an improvement in the hindbrain abnormality.[3–5] Published reports of results from fetal myelomeningocele procedures are mostly retrospective case series compared with historical controls. To obtain more conclusive data, the potential benefit of fetal surgery for myelomeningocele is being examined in a clinical trial directly comparing patients randomized into pre- and postnatal treatment groups.

Neurologic Deficits and Myelomeningocele

The neurologic deficits associated with a myelomeningocele can be separated into two groups: primary and secondary. Primary neurologic deficits are those caused by the arrested development of the neural tube.[6] Because neural tube closure occurs during the 3rd and 4th week of gestation, the spinal cord is very immature at the stage when a myelomeningocele develops. It is clear that the normal anatomy of the spinal cord is severely disrupted at the level of the placode.[7] The functional neurologic level is either at the same level as the vertebral anomaly or actually higher than the vertebral level, resulting in worse neurologic function in > 80% of patients with spina bifida aperta, but not

with spina bifida occulta.[8] There is little that can be done in the postnatal setting to reverse the primary developmental abnormality of the affected spinal cord. It is unknown whether the unclosed neural tube retains the capacity for further development.

The appearance of a repaired myelomeningocele lesion on magnetic resonance imaging (MRI) invariably shows a dysplastic spinal cord terminating and adherent to the overlying soft tissues at the site of the defect. The presence of the conus at the level of the repair site means that virtually all of these patients have a tethered spinal cord by radiologic criteria. A symptomatic tethered spinal cord can occur in childhood or many decades later. Patients develop secondary neurologic deficits, such as loss of motor function, paresthesias, and worsening bowel and bladder control. Orthopedic problems, such as progressive foot deformities and scoliosis, can also occur. It is not clear why some patients with a myelomeningocele remain free of symptoms related to a tethered spinal cord. One possibility is that these patients are likely to maintain normal viscoelasticity of the filum terminale, preventing the lumbosacral cord from unnecessary stretching.[9]

Rationale for Fetal Repair of Myelomeningocele

The theoretical benefit of an early fetal myelomeningocele repair is that the neural tube is covered and protected many months before the anticipated delivery date. The basis for expecting improved neurologic function is that restoration of the dysplastic neural placode within the spinal canal isolates it from the amniotic fluid and prevents ongoing injury.[10,11] Evidence supporting this hypothesis was obtained from experiments performed on fetal sheep. Mueli et al surgically created a spinal cord lesion in fetal sheep at 75 days of gestation that simulated a spontaneous spina bifida lesion.[12] After delivery at term, these animals were incontinent and had loss of sensation and motor function below the lesion level. The gross and microscopic appearance of the exposed spinal cord resembled a human myelomeningocele lesion. Animals with surgically created spina bifida lesions were then treated using a musculocutaneous flap at 100 days of gestation. These animals were then carried to full-term gestation and had near-normal motor function and normal bowel and bladder control. The results of these experiments suggest that early repair of an exposed spinal cord may preserve neurologic function and allow improvement through plasticity.[13] Although provocative and interesting, these large animal experiments clearly rely on a model system that does not recapitulate all the features of the human disease.

Timing for Fetal Surgery

Fetal surgery for myelomeningoceles would be expected to have the best results if performed as early as possible. However, this is limited by the timing of diagnosis and the technical limitations of the actual surgical procedure. Ultrasonography allows detection of most fetuses with myelomeningoceles by the midportion of the second trimester.[14] From a practical point of view, this means that a diagnosis of a myelomeningocele is usually made between 18 and 22 weeks of gestation. Taking into consideration current obstetrical practice, it is unlikely that the detection of fetal myelomeningoceles will occur any earlier unless new, more sensitive screening tests are discovered.

Preoperative Imaging Studies

Preoperative fetal imaging studies begin with a detailed ultrasound examination. The specific goals of the exam are to identify anomalies in ventricular shape and size, the position of the cerebellar tonsils, the level of the spinal defect, and the presence of lower-extremity deformities. In many cases, the dimensions of the anatomical defect can be accurately measured by ultrasound examination, although there can be difficulty determining the exact dysraphic level.[14] Most patients being considered for fetal surgery will also undergo an MRI study. The preferred technique performed at the University of California, San Francisco is a single-shot, fast spin echo T2-weighted sequence. The parameters of this sequence are repetition time, 4000 msec; echo time, 90 msec; field of view, 24 cm; slice thickness, 3 mm; no skip; bandwidth, 25 kHz; matrix, 192 × 160; and number of excitations, 0.5. These images are acquired in the axial, sagittal, and coronal planes, although adequate image quality is sometimes difficult to obtain because of fetal motion.[15] There is some evidence that MRI may improve the ability to detect coexisting spinal and brain anomalies that may not be apparent on ultrasound studies.[16,17]

Surgical Technique

Fetal surgery cannot be performed without the participation of a well-trained team. Successful completion of a procedure requires specialized maternal and fetal anesthesia, the ability to perform uterine opening (hysterotomy) and closure with control of uterine contractions, and continuous intraoperative fetal monitoring. These techniques are described elsewhere and will not be addressed further in this chapter.[18]

The steps involved in the fetal procedure are similar to the standard postnatal procedure. They include (1) identification of the neural placode, (2) separation of the placode from the surrounding epithelium, (3) closure of the dura and overlying soft tissues, and (4) closure of the skin. There are several differences, however, between a fetal procedure and that done upon a term infant. First, all tissues during dissection and closure must be handled with great care. The neural placode is extremely fragile, and even limited manipulation leads to loss of tissue integrity. Although the nerve roots are able to withstand some handling, excessive tension causes avulsion. The dura is often insubstantial, transparent when mobilized, and has the physical characteristics of arachnoid in older children. The skin is able to handle surgical dissection, but excessive tension leads to tearing.

A second limitation is the inability to place the fetus in a neutral position at all times during the procedure. The location of the hysterotomy is determined in part by the position of the fetus but also by the location of the placenta (**Fig. 16.1**). The orientation of the fetus can be confirmed prior to hysterotomy with intraoperative ultrasound, but it can be difficult to maintain the lumbar spine in a horizontal position, which interferes with the visualization of the lesion. Additional assistants are sometimes required to stabilize the fetus.

The fetal neural placode is more easily distinguished from the surrounding arachnoid and skin than in the term infant. The edges of the placode are contiguous with the arachnoid, which is extremely thin and translucent. If the myelomeningocele sac is intact, the placode will be lifted upward away from the surface of the back. The epithelium of the skin usually does not reach the edge of the placode. The clear identification of the intervening arachnoid usually allows the placode to be divided from its attachments with sharp dissection. Depending on the consistency of the placode, the neural tube can be retubularized; however, if the placode is particularly fragile, this step may not be possible. The dura is loosely attached to the underlying subcutaneous tissues just lateral to the spinal canal. After incising the dura at its lateral junction with the dermis, gentle instillation of saline into the epidural plane lifts the dura away from the underlying tissues, which minimizes the manipulation of the dura. Between 18 and 20 weeks of gestation, the dura can be very thin and difficult to handle. After 22

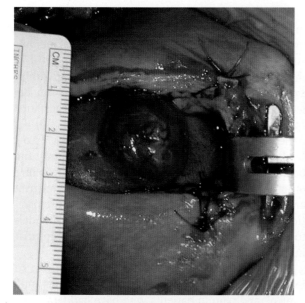

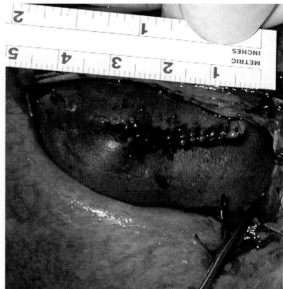

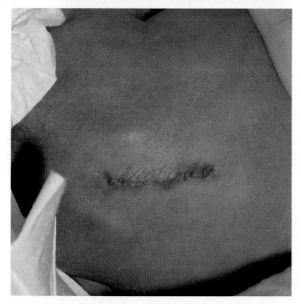

Fig. 16.1 Fetal closure of a myelomeningocele lesion. **(A)** The fetal myelomeningocele is framed in the hysterotomy incision. The fetus is not removed from the uterus, and every effort is made to maintain the amniotic fluid volume. The actual sac consists of thin membranous tissue with a minimum of skin extending upward toward the placode. **(B)** The skin is closed as a single layer, in this case without a patch required. **(C)** After delivery at 36 weeks, the wound appears well closed, although the sutures, which are the monofilament absorbable type, are still visible.

weeks of gestation, the dura becomes more substantial and can be handled more easily.

Once the dura is detached from the dermis and separated from the underlying lumbar fascia, it can be closed using a running suture. If the amount of dura is insufficient, then a patch is used to close the opening. The use of acellular human dermis to repair the dura may contribute to the formation of intracellular dermoid cysts.[19] For this reason, a synthetic collagen matrix (DuraGen, Integra Life Sciences, New Jersey) can be used to create a dural barrier. Following dural closure, the skin is closed as a single layer incorporating the superficial and deeper tissues. In general, dissection of the underlying muscle and fascia is not attempted because excessive fetal blood loss must be avoided and the

duration of the procedure minimized. Elevation of the skin and separation from the underlying subcutaneous tissues are relatively easy, although increased tension on the skin inevitably leads to tearing. Small openings in the skin caused by handling with forceps or tension from suture points generally close rapidly. If the skin can be brought together, the final postnatal appearance is often excellent (**Fig. 16.1**). For situations where insufficient skin is available to close the lesion, skin flaps, relaxing incisions, or synthetic material can be used.

There are substantial complications associated with open hysterotomy. These include placental separation, blood loss, premature labor, and delayed uterine rupture.[20,21] All of these reasons have led to most fetal procedures evolving toward endoscopic techniques. The treatment goals for myelomeningocele can be achieved by using endoscopic or open procedures, but the quality of the repair is substantially better with an open procedure.[22,23] Because endoscopic procedures are associated with fewer complications, new techniques may allow this approach to be reevaluated in the future.

Results

Data from centers performing fetal surgery for myelomeningocele have indicated that the benefits of surgery are a reduction in the rate of cerebrospinal fluid (CSF) shunt insertion and improvement in the appearance of the Chiari II malformation (**Fig. 16.2**) on imaging studies.[3,24] It is unknown whether the structural improvement in the hindbrain abnormality results in an improvement of clinical signs and symptoms caused by the Chiari II malformation. The shunt rate in a cohort of 116 children treated with fetal surgery and followed in the postnatal period for at least 12 months was 54%.[25] The strongest predictor for postnatal shunt placement was the upper level of the spinal lesion, with those above L3 showing the highest rates of shunt insertion. This trend is similar to a historical series where lesion level affected shunt rates.[8] The overall percentage of patients requiring shunt placement, based on retrospective series, is usually in the range of 80 to 95%. By this measure, the reduction in shunt insertion rates reported in the fetal surgery group is encouraging. However, it is possible that selection bias alone may account for this benefit.

Experimental evidence suggested that early closure of myelomeningoceles should improve neurologic function by preventing secondary injury to the exposed nervous tissue.[10,12] Early clinical results from fetal repair of human myelomeningoceles have been disappointing. Tubbs et al examined a cohort of patients ($n = 37$) who had undergone fetal repair between 20 and 28 weeks of gestation and compared their neurologic function to a cohort ($n = 40$) of patients who underwent postnatal procedures.[26] No statistical difference was observed in lower-extremity function between the two groups. Although this study, along with others, has limitations inherent with any retrospective analysis, the lack of clear improvement in neurologic function with fetal surgery suggests that the animal models used to study this disorder do not adequately recapitulate the human disease.

The incidence of delayed signs and symptoms such as lower extremity weakness, worsening of bladder and bowel control, and pain in patients who have had fetal surgery is unknown. Based on anecdotal cases, reexploration in patients who have had previous fetal repair appears to be more difficult because tissue planes in the area of the placode are poorly defined. Postnatal imaging studies of the distal spinal cord in patients who have had fetal repair, however, do not show an obvious anatomical difference compared with patients who have had postnatal repair. Urodynamics performed on a small group of children who had undergone fetal surgery showed clear abnormalities such as vesicoureteral reflux and a significant postvoid residual urine volume. These results were indistinguishable

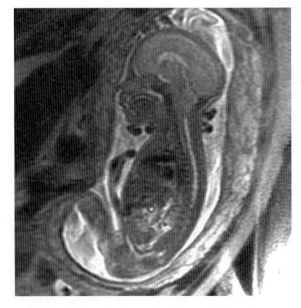
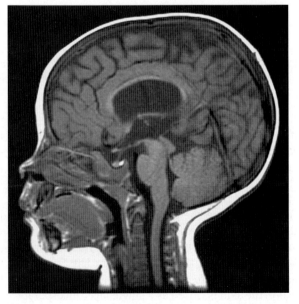

A

B

Fig. 16.2 Effect of fetal closure on hindbrain appearance. **(A)** Fetal magnetic resonance imaging (MRI) sagittal image showing a tight posterior fossa with tonsillar descent into the upper cervical spine.

(B) MRI (T1-weighted sagittal sequence) of the same patient after delivery showing the near normal appearance of the cerebellum with normal-appearing brainstem and the presence of a cisterna magna.

from those of patients who had undergone postnatal repair.[27] This is not unexpected, as urological function should be strongly related to sacral spinal cord function.

Conclusion

Fetal surgery for myelomeningocele can be performed safely with acceptable maternal and fetal risks. Whether these risks are balanced by a benefit to the child over many years of follow-up is unknown. To measure the presumed reduction in shunt insertion rates and to assess maternal and fetal risks, a randomized, prospective clinical trial sponsored by the National Institutes of Health is under way. The Management of Myelomeningoceles Study compares patients who are randomly assigned to either postnatal or fetal surgery. In addition to shunt insertion rates, other measures, such as the Bayley Scale of Infant Development and neurologic functional level, will be used to assess the effect of fetal surgery. Wider adoption of fetal surgery for myelomeningocele should await definitive evidence of clinical benefit.

♦ Postnatal Repair

Ulrich W. Thomale

The arguments for postnatal myelomeningocele or intrauterine myelomeningocele repair are based on different aspects. In terms of the prenatal diagnosis of a neural tube defect and the decision to continue the pregnancy to full term, the treatment should be associated with low risk for the mother and with preparing good conditions of development for the child. Also, a safe technique of plastic reconstruction of the neural tube defect should be achieved. The technique should be well evolved with clear exposure and good control of anatomical structures. Another aim is to deal accurately with the expected complications in the neurofunctional development of the fetus as well as to acquire sufficient data of experience of the incidence and impact of these complications for long-term outcome. These factors will be further elucidated in this discussion.

Pregnancy and Delivery

In many centers, cesarean section has become the recommended method of delivery for infants with prenatally diagnosed myelomeningocele defects.[28,29] Although none of the controlled trials have proven the significant benefit of cesarean section regarding lower morbidity or better neurofunctional outcome,[30,31] postmortem and clinical studies have postulated mechanical damage to the neural tube defect caused by repeated uterine contractions as well as by vaginal breech delivery.[32] Another advantage of cesarean section is the rather controlled situation of delivery, which can be scheduled precisely in terms of good availability of experienced staff for immediate postnatal treatment. In particular, the neurosurgical availability within 24 hours for postnatal myelomeningocele repair can be scheduled accordingly. Furthermore, the entire procedure can be discussed in detail with the parents in an interdisciplinary appointment weeks before the scheduled date of birth.

The morbidity and mortality rates for cesarean section in combination with postnatal myelomeningocele repair are known to be fairly low, not only because of the rather high degree of routine experience, but also because of the minimal amount of invasiveness during the term of pregnancy. In a series of 202 children, no delivery-related morbidity was reported over a 20-year period.[33]

In contrast to that, the technique of intrauterine repair reported both mother- and fetus-associated morbidity as well as mortality. Despite the fact that all mothers underwent at least two operative procedures during pregnancy, Bruner et al had to admit that 2 of 29 mothers in their study experienced wound dehiscence, and 1 of them had a complicated bowel obstruction.[34] There is no evidence so far that future pregnancies are affected by such intrauterine procedures. In a study by Sutton et al on fetus mortality, 1 of 10 was delivered prematurely after intrauterine repair and died thereafter.[35] Combining the series by Bruner and Sutton and colleagues, 8 of 38 fetuses delivered before the 30th week of gestation, 3 had further complications due to prematurity, and 1 suffered CSF fistula necessitating further surgery. A more recent study showed an overall fetus mortality rate of 6%.[36] Although a learning curve must be considered for new interventions techniques, these complications need to be weighed against the benefits of the intrauterine procedure.

Surgical Repair

The major goals of postnatal surgical repair are to prevent central nervous system infection, to reconstruct anatomical layers within the defect region, and to preserve remaining neurologic function. Therefore, surgery needs to be well planned before the date of birth. It is known that the risk of infection in a nonoperated child with myelomeningocele increases with the time after delivery, which can provoke further functional morbidity.[33,37] Surgery should be scheduled 24 to 48 hours after cesarean section. Cardiopulmonary conditions can be stabilized during the early hours, and safe

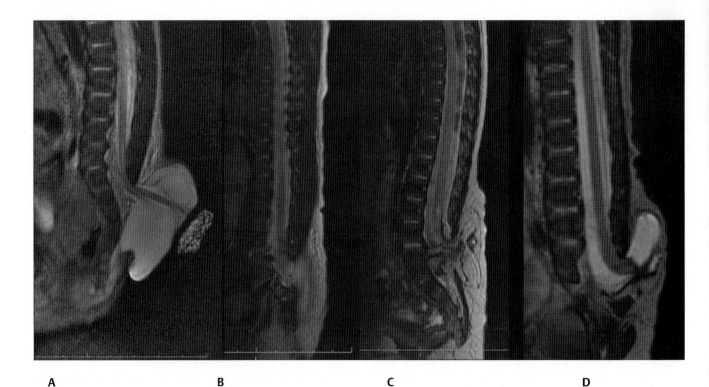

A   B   C   D

Fig. 16.3 MRIs depicting various conditions of the dysraphic malformation involving the lumbosacral region as the most common localization. **(A)** Sacral myelomeningocele with low myelon attachment developing a superficial placode. **(B)** Lateralized sac of the myelomeningocele. **(C)** Lipomeningomyelocele with split cord malformation and a lumbar diastema. **(D)** Sacral skin-covered myelomeningocele.

conditions for surgery can be prepared. We prefer to perform cranial as well as spinal MRI prior to surgery to visualize the defect and to define all associated anomalies (**Fig. 16.3**).[38] This allows the surgeon to prepare for all kinds of atypical anatomical conditions by visualizing the entire extent of spinal deformity as well as by locating the neural structures within the defect (**Fig. 16.4**). This may facilitate more accurate planning of the surgical repair. Moreover, a fatal developmental abnormality involving the brain can be identified, which can influence decisions regarding therapeutical measures in those cases at an early stage. During the preoperative period, a strict protocol must be established to prevent desiccation and mechanical manipulation of the placode. Sterile saline-soaked gauze for coverage, as well as adequate handling of the neonate by avoiding supine positioning and direct pressure or manipulation to the defect, is essential. We prefer perioperative antibiotic coverage starting after delivery. During the surgical procedure itself, in general no major blood loss is expected. Thus, anemic conditions are rare; however, hypothermia and hypoglycemia must be avoided before and during surgery.[39] The surgical technique itself is performed on a routine basis under strict microscopical conditions.[40] In the entire circumference, the anatomical layers of the arachnoid, dura, skin, and placode are divided meticulously. We start the procedure with an intraspinal approach in the adjacent

intact anatomical area cranially or caudally to the lesion. If necessary, a small laminotomy is performed to identify the intact dura layer. The dura is opened, and the subdural space is dissected bilaterally, if possible leaving the arachnoid layer intact. In a similar fashion, the epidural space is prepared bilaterally. Next, the layers of the skin and dura are sharply dissected at the structure's normal appearance at the most adjacent level toward the surface by leaving the medial parts of the neural placode untouched. The layers are ligated, respectively, along the bilateral incision for better identification at later steps. If the entire circumference is dissected, the preparation of the medial placode is performed. Epithelialized remnants from the placode are resected. Special care must be taken not to injure the possible U-shaped course of the nerve roots, which may be originating radially from the placode.

This standardized technique of microsurgical preparation warrants a high degree of visual control to enable as much preservation of neurologic function as possible. The fact that anatomical conditions are well developed, and thus have become less fragile, enables a safer separation of the respective layers in a microsurgical fashion. Untethering of the terminal filum, if identifiable, is performed to ensure free intraspinal motion of the neural structures. Following complete separation and reduction from the epithelial edges, the placode itself is laterally rolled up, and a tube is

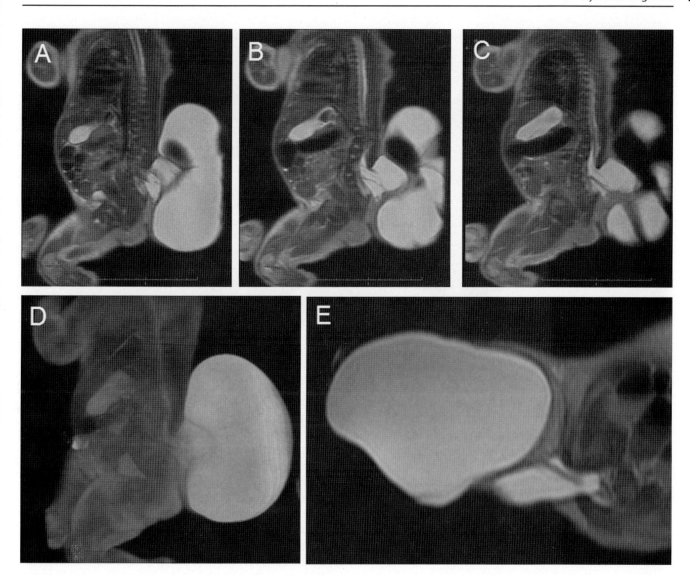

Fig. 16.4 Large myelomeningocele with lateralized placode evolving as an internal cystic membrane and partially attached to the adjacent skin as visualized in the thin-sliced sagittal reconstructed T2 images (A-C) as well as in the axial reconstruction (E). Additional kyphotic spinal malformation at the thoracolumbar region. A three-dimensional reconstructed dataset with translucent surface rendering may help for better presurgical planning (D).

formed and fixated with microsutures at the dorsal margins. A plastic reconstruction of the dura is performed in a watertight fashion to prevent any CSF leakage. Additionally, the overlying soft tissue must be readapted as far as possible. The skin incision is straightened and mobilized laterally to allow a linear skin closure. Reconstructive skin flaps are rarely necessary, even in larger myelomeningocele defects, if the mobilization of the skin is performed down to the ventrolateral regions bilaterally to the surgical site (**Fig. 16.5**).[41] This entire technique of open postnatal myelomeningocele repair is well established and can be performed in a routine fashion, with a reasonable rate of complications.[33]

The intrauterine closure of the fetal myelomeningocele is still an experimental treatment. Major disadvantages are the limited exposure of the defect and the fragility of the anatomical structures, both of which may lead to a higher risk of further neurologic dysfunction. Reported complications are postnatal CSF leakage and early tethering of the spinal cord.[36] The potential benefits of early fetal repair must be weighed against the drawbacks. Spontaneous elevation of the spinal cord and spontaneous replacement of the cerebellar structures from the spinal canal back into the posterior fossa, as well as the more normal development of a regular cisterna magna and the size of the posterior fossa during the remaining pregnancy, have been reported for intrauterine repair.[35] Moreover, the number of shunt-dependent infants was reported to be reduced in this cohort.[34,36] All of these factors are giving hope for a promising technique that may lead to a better quality of life for a highly disabled population of patients. However, as long as

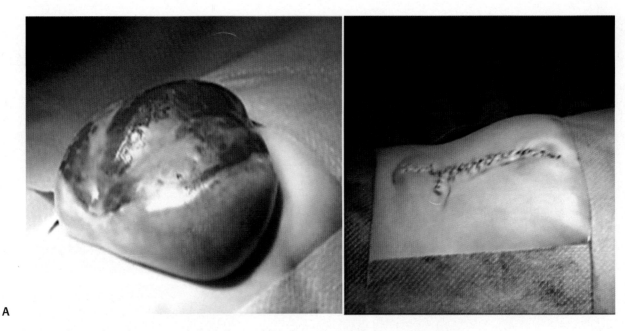

Fig. 16.5 Lumbosacral myelomeningocele **(A)** before and **(B)** after postnatal plastic reconstruction.

the complications are still reported in rather significant numbers, the overall benefits remain to be proven. The higher amount of prematurity causes its own mortality and morbidity additional to that of spina bifida. A potentially higher rate of early tethered cord syndrome, as well as potentially higher neurologic morbidity, due to less accurate closure and reconstructions of the respective layers in more challenging conditions may decrease the potential benefits of the procedure. Thus, longer follow-up data of patients need to be acquired before finalizing these arguments.[42]

Outcome Measures

Hydrocephalus is a major factor in spina bifida. Clear indications for shunt placement are still under debate. Nevertheless, the necessity for treatment depends on the severity and progression of the hydrocephalus. The literature reports 80 to 85% of patients with hydrocephalus are shunt dependent after myelomeningocele repair.[33,43] In the long run, only ~5% of these patients are able to become shunt independent later.[44] Complicated courses of treatment with several revisions of the CSF shunt have been shown to correlate with a decrease in intelligence quotient measures in these patients. Moreover, complications in hydrocephalus treatment affect the rates of mortality and morbidity.[45] Technically, the initial implantation of CSF shunts in infants has potential complications, such as overdrainage, underdrainage, and infection. Up to 64% of patients experience shunt failure within the first year. In 20% of cases, multiple shunt revisions are necessary.[46] Looking at the recent progress in shunt technology with adjustable valves and antibiotic-impregnated catheters,

a decrease in the rate of such complications may be proven in the near future.[47-50] Even a reduced rate of shunting to 51% could be accomplished after open myelomeningocele repair with stricter shunt indication protocols.[51] However, shunt complications will remain relevant in the treatment of newborns with spina bifida as well as in their long-term follow-up. Hence, any way to prevent hydrocephalus is more than welcome. Using intrauterine myelomeningocele repair, we are looking at a shunt rate that seems to be significantly decreased compared with conditions after conventional postnatal surgery.[34,36] These data were not acquired in a controlled prospective fashion and remain questionable so far. Better trials are needed to quantify the worth of the new treatment.[42]

Displacement of the cerebellar tonsils in patients with spina bifida described as Chiari II malformation occurs in almost all patients with myelomeningocele. Hydrocephalus often contributes to the clinical manifestations of Chiari II malformation; additionally, ventricular CSF diversion reduces the extent of tonsillar displacement and may completely reverse this malformation.[52,53] Anatomical relations of Chiari II malformation not only consist of tonsillar displacement but also involve a medullary kinking at the upper cervical level and brainstem malformations. Although only 20 to 30% of cases of Chiari II malformation become clinically relevant, it remains a significant contributing factor for secondary dependent disability and mortality.[52,54] In general, the severity of Chiari-associated symptoms occurring at a younger age correlates with a worse outcome, thus requiring more intensive treatment of these patients. Surgical treatment in symptomatic cases consists of shunt insertion or revision and craniocervical decompression. In addition, tethered cord syndrome may be associated with Chiari II malformation and requires untethering for potential elevation of cerebellar and medullary structures. Early treatment in cases with mild to moderate progressing symptoms ameliorates the outcome.[53] Moreover, better knowledge of effective surgical treatment options, including advanced techniques of shunting, microsurgical options, and less invasiveness for craniocervical decompression, was related to decreased surgery-associated secondary morbidity.[33] In comparing postnatal and intrauterine myelomeningocele repair with respect to Chiari II malformation, we are looking at only one fifth to one third of patients becoming neurologically affected and requiring surgical treatment. One may argue that only this proportion of patients will benefit directly from early elevation of intraspinal and posterior fossa neural structures. Again, this must be weighed against the potentially increased risks of intrauterine repair.

Syringomyelia is often a secondary result of either Chiari II malformation or the existence of general CSF dynamic disturbances.[55,56] Most often the visualization of syringomyelia does not directly correlate with clinical symptoms. Treating the primary cause of syringomyelia by either shunt revision or osteodural decompression often results in a decrease of its extent on MRI or in the clinical symptoms themselves. Malformative cysts, without any signs of progression, almost never require any treatment. Only very few intramedullary cysts have an independent dynamic course of development, and only these need specific treatment options.[33] Although the potential treatment modalities are often frustrating, we prefer cystoarachnoid shunting using a Teflon wick.

A further significant complication in the long-term follow-up of patients with myelomeningocele is secondary tethered cord syndrome. Scar tissue evolving from the site of myelomeningocele repair causes connectivity of neural structures toward the dural surface. The elongation of the tethered spinal cord during body growth and daily activity is believed to cause mechanical stress, structural damage, and disturbances in microcirculation.[57] Fixation of the spinal cord and the low-lying position of the conus are observed in almost every patient. However, only 20 to 30% of patients become clinically symptomatic.[58,59] Surgical treatment consists of microsurgical detethering. Indication for surgery is based mainly on clinical progression, but also on ultrasonographic pulsatility studies of the myelon and electrophysiologic monitoring of somatosensory evoked potentials.[60] Because almost all patients suffer scar adhesion of the myelon, the potentially better surgical techniques must be weighed against the proportion of patients who develop clinical symptoms of tethered cord syndrome. The number of patients and the time when surgical repair is needed may serve as outcome measures. Comparing postnatal and intrauterine repair in regards to the occurrence of tethered cord syndrome will require long follow-up periods for valid evaluation. In one study, early untethering was reported to become necessary in patients after intrauterine myelomeningocele repair.[34] This result may become one of the crucial factors in comparing the techniques. Less exposure and higher fragility of tissue layers during intrauterine repair may lead to decreased quality in plastic reconstruction and higher rates of early spinal cord tethering. However, better technical evolution of fetal myelomeningocele repair may lessen these drawbacks. Regarding postnatal repair, recent progress was made to prevent tethered cord syndrome using the tubing technique to reconstruct the neural placode. Furthermore, the application of hyaluronic acid at the end of the initial surgery may result in less scar tissue development.[33] Nevertheless, tethered cord syndrome remains a significant factor and is not expected to become positively affected by the intrauterine technique.

Conclusion

Postnatal myelomeningocele repair remains the gold standard for the treatment of patients with spinal neural tube defects. Major advantages are the development of standardized procedures and the well-developed expertise of many surgeons for adequate microsurgical open repair. This technique is currently available in most countries.

However, because complications associated with postnatal surgery are still significant, it behooves researchers to examine intrauterine myelomeningocele repair. Strict evaluation will be necessary to define the additional risks and potential benefits of this technique.

♦ Lessons Learned

There has been considerable controversy about the management of myelomeningoceles. Early arguments concerned the need to treat, but that has been resolved.

The issue of how aggressive pediatric neurosurgeons should be in the prophylactic treatment of the various manifestations of spinal dysraphism is an almost eternal discussion. That an open myelomeningocele must be closed shortly after birth is undisputed. But whether or not there is benefit in the enormously complex undertaking of prenatal intrauterine repair of myelomeningocele is much less clear, both from an ethical standpoint and from a presentation of preliminary outcome data from case series. Gupta's contribution gives us a clear understanding of the issues involved, issues that carry a lot of ethical baggage, in addition to the purely medical and technical considerations involved. The chapter clearly states the medical questions. It appears that the framework of obtaining a near-normal anatomy early to prevent subsequent injury to the exposed placode is not only logical but also based on sound experimental evidence gathered in experiments with sheep. However, the results of the human trials have been much less convincing, in that the postnatal neurologic and urological findings differ little if at all from the data gathered from untreated children born with myelomeningoceles. Nonetheless, there appears to be some benefit, as the rates of shunt insertion and the severity of hindbrain abnormalities appear to be lowered.

From an ethical perspective, even when leaving the question of societal values and religious prerogatives untouched, the question of maternal morbidity is huge. Are the risks of blood loss, uterine rupture, and early delivery indeed justified? One can argue that this is not for doctors to decide but for the affected individuals. But we feel that we do have a responsibility of having and expressing a professional and personal opinion as to what can be sensibly recommended to a pregnant woman in this ominous predicament. Patients will invariably look to us for guidance, recommendation, and reassurance.

The issue is in utero closure or postnatal surgery for the myelomeningocele. Both camps offer reasonable arguments and methods for the closure. What we know from the ongoing in utero study is that the functional outcome of lower extremity function is unchanged, but the need for shunt placement is less when these children are treated early. We also learn that the surgery, though with risks, can be performed at specialized centers in a safe fashion for both the infant and the mother. Emerging techniques may include endoscopic closure. Regarding postnatal closure, the techniques are refined and easily performed regardless of the size of the placode. The issue concerning shunt placement will remain surgeon dependent. The modality of the delivery type is also dependent upon the center.

References

1. Harrison MR. Surgically correctable fetal disease. Am J Surg 2000;180(5):335–342

2. Mitchell LE, Adzick NS, Melchionne J, Pasquariello PS, Sutton LN, Whitehead AS. Spina bifida. Lancet 2004;364(9448):1885–1895

3. Bruner JP, Tulipan N, Paschall RL, et al. Fetal surgery for myelomeningocele and the incidence of shunt-dependent hydrocephalus. JAMA 1999;282(19):1819–1825

4. Johnson MP, Sutton LN, Rintoul N, et al. Fetal myelomeningocele repair: short-term clinical outcomes. Am J Obstet Gynecol 2003;189(2):482–487

5. Tulipan N, Hernanz-Schulman M, Lowe LH, Bruner JP. Intrauterine myelomeningocele repair reverses preexisting hindbrain herniation. Pediatr Neurosurg 1999;31(3):137–142

6. Copp AJ, Greene ND, Murdoch JN. The genetic basis of mammalian neurulation. Nat Rev Genet 2003;4(10):784–793

7. Hutchins GM, Meuli M, Meuli-Simmen C, Jordan MA, Heffez DS, Blakemore KJ. Acquired spinal cord injury in human fetuses with myelomeningocele. Pediatr Pathol Lab Med 1996;16(5):701–712

8. Rintoul NE, Sutton LN, Hubbard AM, et al. A new look at myelomeningoceles: functional level, vertebral level, shunting, and the implications for fetal intervention. Pediatrics 2002;109(3):409–413

9. Yamada S, Knerium DS, Mandybur GM, Schultz RL, Yamada BS. Pathophysiology of tethered cord syndrome and other complex factors. Neurol Res 2004;26(7):722–726

10. Heffez DS, Aryanpur J, Hutchins GM, Freeman JM. The paralysis associated with myelomeningocele: clinical and experimental data implicating a preventable spinal cord injury. Neurosurgery 1990;26(6):987–992

11. Heffez DS, Aryanpur J, Rotellini NA, Hutchins GM, Freeman JM. Intrauterine repair of experimental surgically created dysraphism. Neurosurgery 1993;32(6):1005–1010

12. Meuli M, Meuli-Simmen C, Hutchins GM, et al. In utero surgery rescues neurological function at birth in sheep with spina bifida. Nat Med 1995;1(4):342–347

13. Walsh DS, Adzick NS, Sutton LN, Johnson MP. The rationale for in utero repair of myelomeningocele. Fetal Diagn Ther 2001;16(5):312–322

14. Patel TR, Bannister CM, Thorne J. A study of prenatal ultrasound and postnatal magnetic imaging in the diagnosis of central nervous system abnormalities. Eur J Pediatr Surg 2003;13(Suppl 1):S18–S22

15. Coakley FV, Glenn OA, Qayyum A, Barkovich AJ, Goldstein R, Filly RA. Fetal MRI: a developing technique for the developing patient. AJR Am J Roentgenol 2004;182(1):243–252

16. Glenn OA, Goldstein RB, Li KC, et al. Fetal magnetic resonance imaging in the evaluation of fetuses referred for sonographically suspected abnormalities of the corpus callosum. J Ultrasound Med 2005;24(6):791–804

17. von Koch CS, Glenn OA, Goldstein RB, Barkovich AJ. Fetal magnetic resonance imaging enhances detection of spinal cord anomalies in patients with sonographically detected bony anomalies of the spine. J Ultrasound Med 2005;24(6):781–789

18. Harrison MR, Evans MI, Adzick NS, eds. The Unborn Patient: The Art and Science of Prenatal Diagnosis. 3rd ed. Philadelphia: WB Saunders; 2000

19. Mazzola CA, Albright AL, Sutton LN, Tuite GF, Hamilton RL, Pollack IF. Dermoid inclusion cysts and early spinal cord tethering after fetal surgery for myelomeningocele. N Engl J Med 2002;347(4):256–259

20. Wilson RD, Johnson MP, Crombleholme TM, et al. Chorioamniotic membrane separation following open fetal surgery: pregnancy outcome. Fetal Diagn Ther 2003;18(5):314–320

21. Wilson RD, Johnson MP, Flake AW, et al. Reproductive outcomes after pregnancy complicated by maternal-fetal surgery. Am J Obstet Gynecol 2004;191(4):1430–1436

22. Bruner JP, Tulipan NB, Richards WO, Walsh WF, Boehm FH, Vrabcak EK. In utero repair of myelomeningocele: a comparison of endoscopy and hysterotomy. Fetal Diagn Ther 2000;15(2):83–88

23. Farmer DL, von Koch CS, Peacock WJ, et al. In utero repair of myelomeningocele: experimental pathophysiology, initial clinical experience, and outcomes. Arch Surg 2003;138(8):872–878

24. Tulipan N, Hernanz-Schulman M, Bruner JP. Reduced hindbrain herniation after intrauterine myelomeningocele repair: a report of four cases. Pediatr Neurosurg 1998;29(5):274–278

25. Bruner JP, Tulipan N, Reed G, et al. Intrauterine repair of spina bifida: preoperative predictors of shunt-dependent hydrocephalus. Am J Obstet Gynecol 2004;190(5):1305–1312

26. Tubbs RS, Chambers MR, Smyth MD, et al. Late gestational intrauterine myelomeningocele repair does not improve lower extremity function. Pediatr Neurosurg 2003;38(3):128–132

27. Holmes NM, Nguyen HT, Harrison MR, Farmer DL, Baskin LS. Fetal intervention for myelomeningocele: effect on postnatal bladder function. J Urol 2001;166(6):2383–2386

28. Bensen JT, Dillard RG, Burton BK. Open spina bifida: does cesarean section delivery improve prognosis? Obstet Gynecol 1988;71(4):532–534

29. Cochrane D, Aronyk K, Sawatzky B, Wilson D, Steinbok P. The effects of labor and delivery on spinal cord function and ambulation in patients with meningomyelocele. Childs Nerv Syst 1991;7(6):312–315

30. Hill AE, Beattie F. Does caesarean section delivery improve neurological outcome in open spina bifida? Eur J Pediatr Surg 1994;4(Suppl 1):32–34

31. Hadi HA, Loy RA, Long EM Jr, Martin SA, Devoe LD. Outcome of fetal meningomyelocele after vaginal delivery. J Reprod Med 1987;32(8):597–600

32. Rális ZA. Traumatizing effect of breech delivery on infants with spina bifida. J Pediatr 1975;87(4):613–616

33. Talamonti G, D'Aliberti G, Collice M. Myelomeningocele: long-term neurosurgical treatment and follow-up in 202 patients. J Neurosurg 2007;107(5, Suppl):368–386

34. Bruner JP, Tulipan N, Paschall RL, et al. Fetal surgery for myelomeningocele and the incidence of shunt-dependent hydrocephalus. JAMA 1999;282(19):1819–1825

35. Sutton LN, Adzick NS, Bilaniuk LT, Johnson MP, Crombleholme TM, Flake AW. Improvement in hindbrain herniation demonstrated by serial fetal magnetic resonance imaging following fetal surgery for myelomeningocele. JAMA 1999;282(19):1826–1831

36. Johnson MP, Sutton LN, Rintoul N, et al. Fetal myelomeningocele repair: short-term clinical outcomes. Am J Obstet Gynecol 2003;189(2):482–487

37. Dias MS. Neurosurgical management of myelomeningocele (spina bifida). Pediatr Rev 2005;26(2):50–60, discussion 50–60

38. Cabraja M, Thomale UW, Vajkoczy P. [Spinal disorders and associated CNS anomalies: tethered cord and Arnold-Chiari malformation.] Orthopade 2008;37(4):347–355 Review. German.

39. Conran AM, Kahana M. Anesthetic considerations in neonatal neurosurgical patients. Neurosurg Clin N Am 1998;9(1):181–185

40. Gaskill SJ. Primary closure of open myelomeningocele. Neurosurg Focus 2004;16(2):E3

41. Luce EA. Discussion of "a new technique for closure of large meningomyelocele defects." Ann Plast Surg 2007;59(5):544–545

42. Fichter MA, Dornseifer U, Henke J, et al. Fetal spina bifida repair—current trends and prospects of intrauterine neurosurgery. Fetal Diagn Ther 2008;23(4):271–286

43. Bowman RM, McLone DG, Grant JA, Tomita T, Ito JA. Spina bifida outcome: a 25-year prospective. Pediatr Neurosurg 2001;34(3):114–120

44. Iannelli A, Rea G, Di Rocco C. CSF shunt removal in children with hydrocephalus. Acta Neurochir (Wien) 2005;147(5):503–507, discussion 507

45. Nejat F, Kazmi SS, Habibi Z, Tajik P, Shahrivar Z. Intelligence quotient in children with meningomyeloceles: a case-control study. J Neurosurg 2007;106(2, Suppl):106–110

46. Tuli S, Drake J, Lamberti-Pasculli M. Long-term outcome of hydrocephalus management in myelomeningoceles. Childs Nerv Syst 2003;19(5–6):286–291

47. Marlin AE. Management of hydrocephalus in the patient with myelomeningocele: an argument against third ventriculostomy. Neurosurg Focus 2004;16(2):E4

48. Parker SL, Attenello FJ, Sciubba DM, et al. Comparison of shunt infection incidence in high-risk subgroups receiving antibiotic-impregnated versus standard shunts. Childs Nerv Syst 2009;25(1):77–83, discussion 85

49. Rohde V, Haberl EJ, Ludwig H, Thomale UW. First experiences with an adjustable gravitational valve in childhood hydrocephalus. J Neurosurg Pediatr 2009;3(2):90–93

50. Weinzierl MR, Rohde V, Gilsbach JM, Korinth M. Management of hydrocephalus in infants by using shunts with adjustable valves. J Neurosurg Pediatr 2008;2(1):14–18

51. Chakraborty A, Crimmins D, Hayward R, Thompson D. Toward reducing shunt placement rates in patients with myelomeningocele. J Neurosurg Pediatr 2008;1(5):361–365

52. McLone DG, Dias MS. The Chiari II malformation: cause and impact. Childs Nerv Syst 2003;19(7–8):540–550

53. Stevenson KL. Chiari type II malformation: past, present, and future. Neurosurg Focus 2004;16(2):E5

54. Vandertop WP, Asai A, Hoffman HJ, et al. Surgical decompression for symptomatic Chiari II malformation in neonates with myelomeningocele. J Neurosurg 1992;77(4):541–544

55. McLone DG. Results of treatment of children born with a myelomeningocele. Clin Neurosurg 1983;30:407–412

56. Oldfield EH. Cerebellar tonsils and syringomyelia. J Neurosurg 2002;97(5):1009–1010, discussion 1010

57. Yamada S, Won DJ, Pezeshkpour G, et al. Pathophysiology of tethered cord syndrome and similar complex disorders. Neurosurg Focus 2007;23(2):1–10

58. Bowman RM, Mohan A, Ito J, Seibly JM, McLone DG. Tethered cord release: a long-term study in 114 patients. J Neurosurg Pediatr 2009;3(3):181–187

59. Hudgins RJ, Gilreath CL. Tethered spinal cord following repair of myelomeningocele. Neurosurg Focus 2004;16(2):E7

60. Haberl H, Tallen G, Michael T, Hoffmann KT, Benndorf G, Brock M. Surgical aspects and outcome of delayed tethered cord release. Zentralbl Neurochir 2004;65(4):161–167

17 Lipomyelomeningocele/Tethered Cord

♦ Prophylactic Untethering

Jeffrey A. Pugh, R. Shane Tubbs, and W. Jerry Oakes

Spinal cord tethering and the tethered cord syndrome are seen with relative frequency in pediatric neurosurgery. Seen primarily in cases of myelomeningocele, occult spinal dysraphisms, and thickened or fatty fila terminale, as well as secondarily following closure of spinal dysraphisms, traction on the spinal cord results in several neurologic, urologic, and orthopedic sequelae. Limited data exist on the incidence and natural history of tethered spinal cord; however, there is evidence to suggest that patients whose spinal cord is tethered will demonstrate progressive injury in the form of pain, sensory loss, weakness, bladder dysfunction, and orthopedic deformity. Furthermore, the clinical picture may not improve completely following release of the tethered spinal cord. The challenge facing pediatric neurosurgeons is determining if the progressive neurologic deficit can be avoided with prophylactic surgical intervention, and if so, at what cost? Should we wait until the child develops symptoms, which may be irreversible, or act prophylactically and accept the risks of potential neurologic injury at the time of surgery? The balance lies in understanding the true surgical risks to the patient and the expected efficacy of surgical intervention. In coming to this understanding, we must consider each of the clinical conditions causing spinal cord tethering separately and acknowledge that patient age and surgeon experience play an important role in the overall outcome.

Clinical Presentation

The conclusion that tethered spinal cord leads to progressive neurologic injury and subsequent neurologic, urologic, and orthopedic disability comes from observations of clinical series that older patients generally present with more serious symptomatology. Neonates and infants often present with cutaneous stigmata of occult spinal dysraphism and tethered spinal cord and normal neurologic function.[1–7] Older children and adults are more likely to present with neurologic or urologic dysfunction, orthopedic deformity, and pain.[7–10] Few studies have followed the natural history of asymptomatic tethered spinal cord; however, with time, it is clear that neurologic and urologic deficits develop and may not be reversible with surgery.[7,8,11] Hoffman et al reported on 97 patients with lipomyelomeningoceles.[7] They found that of those presenting in the first 6 months of life, 35 of 56 (62%) had a completely normal neurologic exam. In contrast, only 12 of 41 patients (29%) over the age of 6 months were normal. Early treatment was associated with maintained or, in some cases, improved neurologic function, whereas delayed surgical untethering resulted in poorer neurologic outcome.[7] Thus, although prophylactic surgery has the risk of inducing neurologic injury, early surgery before symptoms develop offers the best opportunity for normal neurologic function. Similarly, Kanev and Bierbrauer showed that asymptomatic patients having lipomyelomeningocele repair and release of spinal cord tethering retained intact bladder function.[8] That said, detethering operations, particularly of lipomyelomeningoceles, can be challenging, and procedures performed by the technically excellent general neurosurgeon in this difficult patient population are associated with potentially undesirable outcomes.

Myelomeningocele

Myelomeningocele represents the most extreme form of tethered spinal cord. In infancy, the primary goal of closing this type of lesion is to reduce the risk of infection. Closing the placode and reconstructing the dural tube in such fashion as to reduce the risk of retethering is important in the long-term management of patients with spina bifida. Signs and symptoms of delayed retethering include progressive scoliosis, worsening gait in ambulators, back pain, and progressive hand weakness and clumsiness. Retethering should be thought of as a matter of when, not if, following myelomeningocele repair. As such, in following these patients, our clinical suspicion for tethered spinal cord should remain high. We recognize that traction on the distal spinal cord is injurious to neurons and can lead to progressive neurologic deterioration and that such injury is often permanent. Experimental research in animals has demonstrated that traction applied to the spinal cord reduces local blood flow and that both continuous and intermittent traction results in spinal cord ischemia.[12–15] Thus, when early clinical deterioration is recognized, we should actively sort out and resolve spinal cord retethering expeditiously so as to maintain neurologic function in these delicate patients. Importantly, as the majority of these patients have associated hydrocephalus, it is imperative to first ensure adequate shunt function when they present with any clinical deterioration. The clinical impact of spinal cord tethering can be so great that in patients who are nonambulatory and have no voluntary bladder and bowel control, a spinal cord transection immediately above the tethering element is warranted.[16,17]

Occult Spinal Dysraphisms

Lipomas of the conus medullaris and the filum terminale have traditionally been reported as a group as spinal or lumbosacral lipomas. Although their clinical presentation can often overlap, their surgical management and outcome are disparate. Several articles have demonstrated that lipomas of the filum terminale and caudal spinal cord are amenable to surgery with little risk of neurologic injury, whereas dorsal and transitional lipomyelomeningoceles are more difficult owing to the presence of functioning nerve roots passing through the lipoma.[18–21] Thus, it is important to discuss each of these lesions in turn to better understand the risks of surgery.

Lipomyelomeningocele

Lipomas of the conus medullaris with associated spina bifida have been categorized by Chapman into two distinct variants, dorsal and caudal, and a transitional form that has components of both (**Fig. 17.1**).[20] The importance of differentiating lipomyelomeningoceles relates to the relationship of functioning neural tissue within the lipoma. Dorsal lipomyelomeningoceles often have a substantial subcutaneous lipoma continuous with the intradural lipoma through a wide dural defect tethering the spinal cord dorsally. The sensory rootlets emerge from the caudal spinal cord immediately ventral to the fusion line of the lipoma, with the spinal cord and the motor rootlets further ventral. Thus, there are no functional neural elements within the lipoma, which can be resected free from the spinal cord at its interface. Care must be taken when incising the dura lateral to the lipoma to ensure that sensory rootlets are not

injured. In contrast, caudal lipomyelomeningoceles may be entirely intradural or extend subcutaneously through an occult spinal dysraphism. The terminal spinal cord enlarges into the lipoma, and the most caudal nerve roots often run within the more fibrous portion of the lipoma anteriorly and anterolaterally. In some cases, these nerve roots are rudimentary, and the nerves serving the bowel, bladder, and lower extremities are free from the lipoma. Intraoperative nerve root stimulation can be valuable in differentiating functional sacral roots from rudimentary roots within the fibrofatty mass, but it is important to stress that aggressive surgical resection of this lipoma carries a higher risk of neurologic injury, particularly to bowel and bladder function. The most difficult lipomyelomeningocele to manage is the transitional type. The line of fusion between the lipoma and spinal cord is dorsal to the sensory rootlets superiorly, but as the mass continues caudally, this line of fusion is displaced ventrally such that nerve roots are found to emerge from the anterolateral aspect of the lipoma. In most cases, these are sensory rootlets; however, there is often greater variability in the relationship between the lipoma and the spinal cord and neural elements in this type of lipomyelomeningocele. The primary goal of surgery is to relieve the spinal cord from mechanical constraint and not necessarily to remove the lipomatous mass in its entirety (**Fig. 17.2**). Aggressive surgical resection carries increased risk of injury to neural structures, whereas limited resections have an increased risk of retethering. Byrne et al retrospectively reported on the outcomes of children with spinal lipomas and found that those who had a definitive untethering procedure had better long-term neurologic outcome than those who underwent a cosmetic resection of their lipoma, who in all cases, went on to have a symptomatic tethered cord and late postoperative deterioration.[22] Additionally, they reported that in those patients presenting with neurologic deficits, 39% improved, and 3% deteriorated following surgery. No asymptomatic patient deteriorated postoperatively, and 93% remained symptom free at 4-year follow-up.[22] Surgical experience is of great value in understanding the relationship of the lipoma with the spinal cord to provide the greatest resection safely on the first attempt. Subsequent operations for retethering are always made more difficult due to the presence of scar and the disruption of tissue planes. This is especially true when the neural elements are rotated in the axial plane.

Lipoma of the Filum Terminale: "Fatty Filum"

Spinal cord tethering by a tight or fatty filum is more straightforward than in the presence of a spinal dysraphism. The principle of surgery is the same: release the mechanical constraint and prevent retethering. Upon opening the dura, nerve roots will often be dorsally displaced

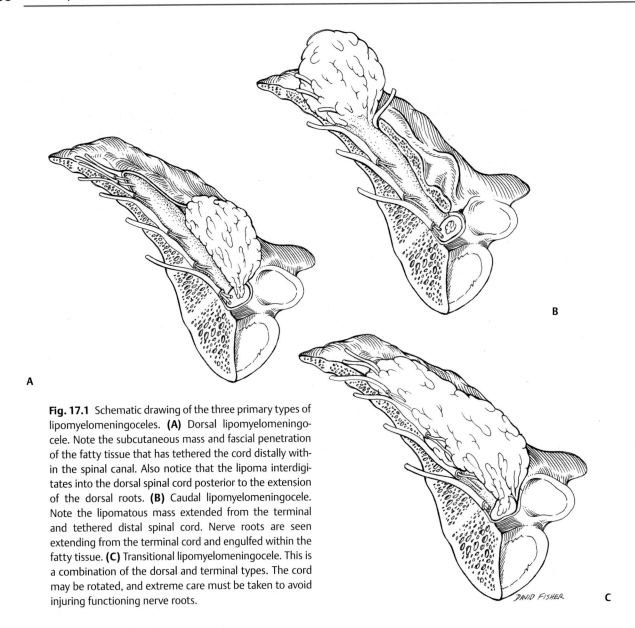

Fig. 17.1 Schematic drawing of the three primary types of lipomyelomeningoceles. **(A)** Dorsal lipomyelomeningocele. Note the subcutaneous mass and fascial penetration of the fatty tissue that has tethered the cord distally within the spinal canal. Also notice that the lipoma interdigitates into the dorsal spinal cord posterior to the extension of the dorsal roots. **(B)** Caudal lipomyelomeningocele. Note the lipomatous mass extended from the terminal and tethered distal spinal cord. Nerve roots are seen extending from the terminal cord and engulfed within the fatty tissue. **(C)** Transitional lipomyelomeningocele. This is a combination of the dorsal and terminal types. The cord may be rotated, and extreme care must be taken to avoid injuring functioning nerve roots.

and need to be protected from injury. Some authors advocate sectioning the filum immediately as it arises from the conus medullaris, whereas others prefer to open the dural inferiorly over the cauda equina and identify the nerve roots as they exit laterally through the intervertebral foramen and to follow the filum as it continues inferiorly and exits the dura dorsally. The decision as to which technique to employ is surgeon dependent based on personal preference and experience as long as the filum can be definitively identified and sectioned without injury to neural elements and in such a fashion as to avoid retethering. In experienced hands; a reasonable adjunct to filum section is to advance a flexible endoscope both dorsally and ventrally to ensure the absence of a tandem tethering element, such as thickened arachnoid adhesions. A more controversial issue is the management of patients presenting with symptoms related to a tight filum terminale whose imaging demonstrates a normal-lying conus medullaris. Bao et al demonstrated that these patients benefit from early release of their filum terminale and that surgical and pathologic identification of fibrofatty tissue within the filum may not appear on magnetic resonance imaging (MRI).[23] Unfortunately, the criteria for sectioning the filum with normal imaging have not been clinically established, and the pool of candidate children with bed wetting issues is large. Great care must be taken to limit this procedure to those with intractable medical problems.

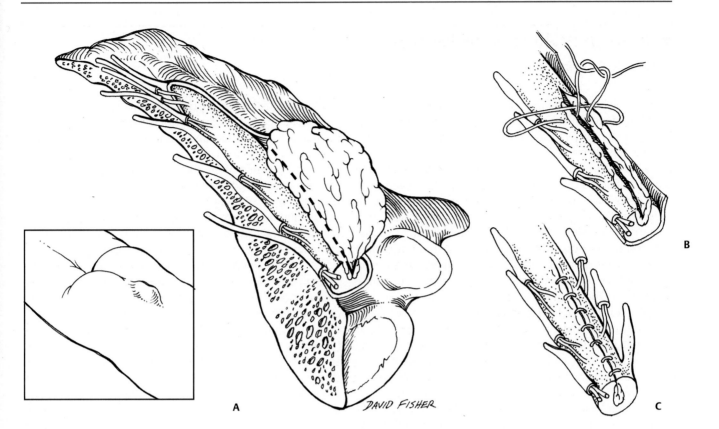

DAVID FISHER

Fig. 17.2 (A) Artist's rendition of the plane (*dotted line*) used for debulking the lipomyelomeningocele. This is an example of a dorsal lipomyelomeningocele. Note that immediately deep to the thoracodorsal fascial defect, there is continuity of the more superficial fat and spinal cord. **(B,C)** Following debulking, the pial edges of the cord defect are opposed with sutures.

Conclusion

In assessing the value of any surgical procedure, the risks and efficacy of the operation must be better than the natural history. This is particularly true for prophylactic operations in which the surgical risks are borne by an asymptomatic patient. Pierre-Kahn and colleagues demonstrated that the surgical risks associated with spinal cord untethering are much better than the natural history. More than half of patients with lumbosacral lipomas (lipomas of the filum terminale or conus medullaris) will show neurologic deterioration with time, whereas surgical release carries low operative risks, and very few patients deteriorate postoperatively.[24–26] That said, outcomes following surgery are largely dependent on surgical pathology. Patients with lipomas of the filum terminale have better outcomes than those with lipomas of the conus medullaris or lipomyelomeningocele. This is true in cases of both symptomatic and asymptomatic fatty filum. These patients have lower rates of postoperative deterioration and improved resolution of symptoms. In contrast, patients with lipomas of the conus medullaris have increased risk of delayed deterioration due to retethering, as well as poorer resolution of symptoms and neurologic recovery following surgical untethering. Additionally, patients' greatest chance for success rests with the first surgeon to release the spinal cord from mechanical tethering, as outcomes following principle untethering are much better than following secondary retethering.[27,28]

The management of patients with spinal cord tethering remains difficult and somewhat controversial.[29] The natural history seems to be one of slow neurologic deterioration, progressive urologic dysfunction and orthopedic deformity, and the development of back pain and radiculopathy. These clinical features are occasionally found in the setting of normal imaging, adding to the complexity of management. In cases of tethered spinal cord secondary to tight or lipomatous filum terminale, the surgical risk-to-benefit ratio is clearly in favor of surgery in both symptomatic and asymptomatic cases. Spinal cord tethering secondary to lipomyelomeningocele or retethering following a spina bifida repair is surgically more complex and is best managed by those experienced with the disorder. That said, asymptomatic patients likely will benefit most from surgical untethering because continuous traction on the spinal cord clearly leads to neurologic injury, and once neurologic deficits exist, they may not be reversible with surgery.

♦ Is Surgery Always Necessary?

Dominic N. P. Thompson

For children born with lumbosacral lipoma, progressive neurologic dysfunction due to spinal cord tethering is inevitable. Timely surgery before the onset of symptoms, however, may prevent this deterioration. Such is the philosophy that has prevailed in the pediatric neurosurgical community for more than a half decade.[30] Indeed, numerous case series and technical notes have been published that show that mechanical untethering of the spinal cord is technically possible, that operative morbidity is low, and that good outcomes can be achieved in most cases. However, the majority of published series are retrospective, single institution/single surgeon series and have commonly grouped together rather disparate populations. For example, in some series, filar lipomas and complex transitional lipomyelomeningoceles have been considered together under the all-embracing title of spinal lipomas, and in others, both symptomatic and asymptomatic patients have been analyzed together. Most surgeons would agree that the surgery to untether a transitional-type lipoma is a major undertaking, and out of experienced hands, morbidity (neurologic, urologic, and wound related) can be significant. By contrast, division of a lipomatous filum terminale is usually a simple procedure with few complications but enduring efficacy.[31–33] Over the past 10 years the dogma that all patients with lipomatous dysraphic malformations should be untethered has been challenged. It has become apparent that the natural history of these conditions may not be as pessimistic as traditionally thought.[34] There are several questions that lie at the heart of this neurosurgical controversy: Is it appropriate to consider all lipomas together and apply the same treatment criteria to each? What is their true natural history if left untreated? and How safe and effective is prophylactic spinal cord untethering for this condition?

What follows is an attempt to examine some of these questions and suggest that a more critical evaluation of the role of early neurosurgery is now appropriate and that, at least for some patients, a conservative approach with close neurologic and urologic surveillance might result in a better long-term outcome.

Classification and Embryogenesis

The classification of lumbosacral lipomas suggested by Chapman[35] is perhaps the most widely known. It is anatomically based, describing the position of the neural placode (the point of attachment of the lipoma to the spinal cord) in relation to the conus and posterior nerve roots. Dorsal lipomas are situated on the dorsal aspect of the lower spinal cord but above the conus, caudal types are attached to the termination of the spinal cord, and transitional types are intermediate between these. Transitional types are complex malformations characteristically involving the conus. They have an intimate association with the elements of the cauda equina; the neural placode is frequently rotated to one side, where nerve roots are commonly horizontally disposed due to the low position of the spinal cord and shortened relative to the opposite side. Additionally, such lipomas are frequently large, obliterating the cerebrospinal fluid (CSF) spaces and associated with significant deficiencies of the terminal dural sac. Each of these features contributes to the complicated surgical anatomy of these lesions.

The embryological basis of lumbosacral lipomas remains unknown. In contrast to the open dysraphic states, there is no animal model in which this entity can be studied. Naidich and associates proposed that these lesions resulted from premature dysjunction.[36] Early separation of the neuroectoderm (before complete tubularization of the neural plate) from the surrounding cutaneous ectoderm exposes the incompletely closed neural plate to the underlying mesoderm, which subsequently differentiates into fat, thus resulting in a lipoma adherent to the neural placode. Although this hypothesis fits well with the surgical anatomy of these lesions, there is an inherent embryological inconsistency. The majority of lumbosacral lipomas have some attachment either at or below the conus. This part of the spinal cord, however, does not undergo primary neurulation or disjunction; instead, it is formed as a result of secondary neurulation, an incompletely understood process (in the human at least) by which mesenchymal cells in the tail bud coalesce around a lumen, thus forming the secondary neural tube, which subsequently becomes incorporated into the rest of the spinal cord.[37–39] This process, which will result in formation of the conus, cauda equina, and filum terminale, is also referred to as retrogressive differentiation. Thus, although the premature disjunction hypothesis remains compatible with the site and anatomy of dorsal-type lipomyelomeningoceles, it is less easy to reconcile with the more common and usually more complex transitional- and caudal-type lipomas. The common occurrence of other tissue types within these latter types of lipoma and the well-recognized coexistence of hindgut and urogenital anomaly[40–43] further support the notion that these are complex regional anatomical malformations involving all germ layers. It is therefore to be expected that, at least in some cases, there is a primary dysplasia of the underlying neurologic tissue that might not be anticipated to be reversed by surgical intervention.

Mechanisms of Deterioration

That lumbosacral lipomas can cause neurologic deficits is beyond doubt; however, it is perhaps worth examining the potential mechanisms by which such deficits may be produced.

- ◆ *Spinal cord tethering:* Mechanical stretching of a low-lying spinal cord and nerve roots in response to movement or growth is the most commonly cited mechanism to explain the neurologic deterioration observed in dysraphic patients, a process thought to be mediated by vascular insufficiency leading to impaired oxygen delivery to the neural tissue.[44] Indeed, it is on the assumption that this is the principal cause of neurologic deterioration that surgical release of the terminal spinal cord, separating it from the fat and surrounding dura (spinal cord untethering), is predicated.
- ◆ *Mass effect:* The intradural component of the lipoma will not infrequently distort or compress the terminal spinal cord (**Fig. 17.3**). That direct pressure from an intraspinal lipoma could lead to neurologic deterioration was suggested almost 50 years ago.[45] Lipomas may reach substantial size and indeed can grow, resulting in mechanical compression of the spinal cord and nerve roots.[46]
- ◆ *Dysplasia:* The parenchyma of the terminal spinal cord and nerve roots are likely be to at least some extent developmentally abnormal. On MRI and at the time of surgery, short nerve roots, rotation of the placode, and a widely open placode (**Fig. 17.4**) suggest a significant primary developmental anomaly.

In clinical practice, it can be extremely difficult to establish the extent to which each of these processes may be contributing to a deficit, or indeed what potential each has to cause a future problem in an asymptomatic patient. Although surgery to reduce the mass effect exerted by a lipoma or to release a stretched spinal cord may lead to demonstrable improvement, the same cannot be anticipated where there is significant underlying neuronal dysplasia.

Clinical Presentation

A cutaneous marker, most usually a subcutaneous mass, is present in ~90% of cases.[33,47–59] From a functional point of view, however, approximately one third of patients have no apparent neurologic, urologic, or orthopedic manifestations of "spinal cord tethering" and so are deemed asymptomatic.[31,32] For the remainder of patients, these have, at the time of presentation, some indication that distal spinal cord function is abnormal and are thus considered symptomatic. Although in most of the larger series the distinction between asymptomatic and symptomatic is made, this is not universally so. This is important, as these may not be comparable groups of patients, and it cannot be assumed that the natural history and thus indication for treatment are the same for each.

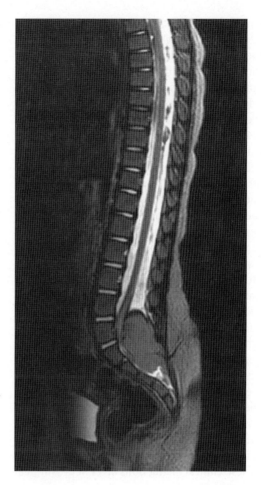

Fig. 17.3 A large transitional lipoma exerting mass effect on the low terminal spinal cord.

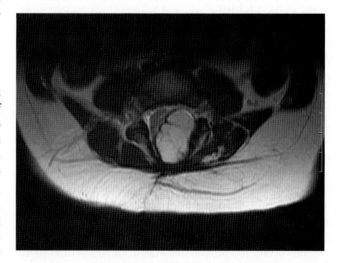

Fig. 17.4 Axial T2-weighted magnetic resonance image demonstrating a complex sacral lipomyelocele. The placode is effaced and rotated by the adherent lipoma.

Distinguishing between the asymptomatic and the symptomatic patient is not as straightforward as might initially appear to be the case, and such a simple classification likely disguises important clinical differences. For example, confirming asymptomatic status in infancy, particularly in respect of bladder function, is extremely difficult. If an infant without "bladder symptoms" at 1 year of age fails to achieve continence by 4 years of age, was the child truly asymptomatic and has deteriorated, or is this "deterioration" simply the reflection of a congenital deficit revealed by the passage of time? It is often not possible to answer this question with certainty, particularly if one relies on clinical symptoms alone. It is hoped that with specialist and ongoing urologic assessment from the outset, one can increase the sensitivity of detecting (or refuting the presence of) a deficit and impart some element of objectivity into the process of surveillance. For the symptomatic patients, too, this designation may obscure clinically distinct groups. First, there are those symptomatic patients who present with symptoms that have been evident since birth, neither worsening nor improving; such symptoms might include a foot deformity, muscle mass/leg length asymmetry, or continuous urinary dribbling. These patients might be referred to as "symptomatic static." Second, there are those whose symptoms are new, such as the development of lower limb pain, gait deterioration, or loss of an acquired skill (e.g., episodic incontinence in a previously continent child). This latter group can be referred to as "symptomatic progressive."

How might these clinical distinctions be of neurosurgical relevance? For "symptomatic progressive" patients, there is good evidence that effective, timely untethering of the spinal cord can provide not only improvement but also resolution of symptoms.[31–33,47] It is important that this group of patients continue to be followed, as late deterioration is well recognized.[50,51] By contrast, asymptomatic patients, particularly those who have attained bladder and bowel continence, have demonstrated neurologic functionality, whatever the appearance on MRI of the terminal spinal cord. Whether in such a scenario the low-lying spinal cord and attached lipoma represent a threat to that neurologic or urologic function cannot be known unless a sufficient number of such asymptomatic patients have been followed without intervention so as to know the natural history. Symptomatic "static" patients also represent a potential area of contention. Such patients have never demonstrated neurologic functionality; indeed, for these children, symptoms are likely a reflection of underlying neurodysplasia. If such symptoms had developed in utero as a result of mechanical tethering, then it would be expected that the symptoms would continue to progress in infancy and would thus be considered progressive. Again, for this symptomatic "static" group, there is insufficient evidence to support intervention for all, as in most series, congenital symptoms are not improved by surgery.[33]

It is, however, the asymptomatic patients with true lumbosacral lipomas (in contrast to simple filar lipomas) that have been at the heart of the current controversy, and it is the issue of offering prophylactic spinal cord untethering to this group that needs to be explored further.

Prophylactic Untethering

It is to be reiterated that the overwhelming majority of contemporary pediatric neurosurgeons recognize that spinal cord untethering for patients with new or progressive symptoms or signs will lead to stabilization or improvement in most cases. Thus, the role of surgery for this subset of patients has been established.

For asymptomatic children, the general body of surgical opinion is to advocate spinal cord untethering to prevent subsequent deterioration, that is, perform a prophylactic procedure. The prophylactic treatment of many medical ailments is well established. Not only does this have clear benefits for the individual, but there may be obvious socioeconomic advantages in that prevention may be more resource efficient than treatment. However, to justify a prophylactic surgical intervention, certain basic criteria need to be satisfied. First, the natural history of the condition must be understood; second, the prophylactic intervention must be safe; and third, that intervention must be effective in beneficially altering the course of the disease. These criteria can be examined for the case of spinal lipoma.

Natural History

". . . [B]y the time [lipoma patients] reach the age of 4 years, none are neurologically intact, and many have a significant deficit."[52] Such has been the pervading view of the natural history of lumbosacral lipomas since. It remains a widely held view that for the child presenting with spinal lipoma, the outlook is one of slow but inevitable deterioration in neurologic and or urologic function. Surprisingly, however, the evidence base for this assumption is extremely limited.

Some authors have observed that the number of asymptomatic patients diminishes in the older age groups. This has been interpreted as evidence that, over time, asymptomatic patients have become symptomatic, indicating a natural tendency to deterioration.[52] This argument is clearly invalid. An asymptomatic older patient may never seek medical attention. Thus, without knowing the true prevalence of spinal lipoma (symptomatic and asymptomatic) at each age group, such an inference regarding natural history cannot be drawn. It is because spinal lipoma may be clinically occult that prevalence rates for this condition do not exist. Reviewing published series of autopsy studies, Pierre-Khan et al estimated the incidence of lipomatous malformations of the spinal cord to be ~0.03%.[33] It is therefore to be expected that any hospital-based published data will be disproportionately skewed toward symptomatic patients.

The surgical literature frequently points out that the outcome for those patients treated before the onset of symptoms is superior to that when surgery is undertaken in the presence of a neurologic deficit.[32,53] Again, this is cited as evidence of a poor long-term prognosis and thus justification for prophylactic intervention. As pointed out by Dorward et al, this assumes that the (young) asymptomatic patients and (older) symptomatic patients are both examples of the same disease considered at different points in time.[54] Although this may be the case, it certainly cannot be assumed to be so. It is possible that these represent different pathophysiologic entities. Asymptomatic patients, by definition, have demonstrated neurologic functionality; symptomatic patients, by contrast, exhibit a deficit that may or may not be amenable to correction by surgery.

Given these criticisms, it is clearly only possible to comment on the natural history of this condition if sufficient children are followed neurologically and urologically beyond a time by which symptoms would have been anticipated to have been manifest. There is a paucity of data on the natural history of this condition.[55] Some centers have begun to collect such data, pursuing a policy of close neurologic and urologic surveillance for those patients deemed to be asymptomatic at the time of presentation. Kulkarni et al reported a series of 53 asymptomatic patients with spinal lipomas followed over a mean period of 4.4 years.[34] During the course of follow-up, only 25% of the cohort exhibited a neurologic deterioration. The authors calculated that at 9 years the actuarial risk of deterioration for an unoperated patient was 33%, compared with 46% for an earlier series of asymptomatic surgically treated patients. That patient cohort has now been followed for 10 years, and the rate of deterioration has remained at 33%. In a similar series from my own institution, 51 children were followed over a mean period of 5.8 years, during which time 27.5% showed deterioration. The estimated rate of deterioration by 12 years was calculated to be 42%.[56] The similarity between the results of these two studies, separate populations in two different countries, supports the notion that these figures are a reasonable reflection of the natural history of this condition.

Clearly, for those asymptomatic patients who develop symptoms or demonstrate loss of a previously acquired function, it would seem reasonable to suppose that mechanical factors (as opposed to intrinsic myelodysplasia) have been responsible for this deterioration. These patients should, in theory at least, have the potential to recover function with appropriately timed intervention. Can this be demonstrated? In the London series, stabilization or improvement in symptoms was seen in all cases following surgery for a demonstrated deterioration, although none where there had been a urologic deterioration returned to normal function as defined by clinical and urologic testing.

By contrast, in the Paris series, 55% of patients who had deteriorated and then received surgery returned to normal function. Thus, adopting a policy of early conservative management and intervening only in the presence of symptomatic deterioration, 88% of the Paris series and 72% of the London series remained clinically asymptomatic at the end of follow-up. The survival curves compare favorably with previously published cohorts of prophylactic surgery. These findings imply that the poor prognosis traditionally attributed to children who are symptomatic at the time of presentation may not be as severe as for the child who becomes symptomatic (and thus receives surgery) during a policy of close clinical surveillance.

Safe Intervention

Untethering of the spinal cord in cases of filar lipoma is in most instances a well-tolerated procedure with low morbidity (0.4%). By contrast, untethering surgery for complex lipoma is technically demanding, and even in experienced hands morbidity can be significant. For large transitional-type lipomas, even after meticulous microsurgical untethering and lipoma resection, the terminal cord is often bulky and difficult to replace in the thecal compartment in a way that is likely to ensure durable mobility of the terminal spinal cord. Furthermore, the neural placode is frequently rotated toward the side where the nerve roots are shorter; these may persist as a tethering element in themselves. These impressions are reinforced by the results of postoperative MRI, which are frequently disappointing, and correlate poorly with clinical outcome.[50,57,58] Complications of neurosurgical interventions, particularly those that result in a new or worsened deficit, are a feared but ever-present risk for the pediatric neurosurgeon. Surgical complications, however, need to be evaluated with particular scrutiny if they occur in the course of undertaking prophylactic treatment. CSF leakage, pseudomeningocele formation, and infection, as well as neurologic impairment resulting in pain, worsening sphincter function, or motor deterioration, are well recognized complications of lipoma surgery. Wound-related complications, mostly CSF leakage, occurred in 11% of the Chicago series[32] and 20% of the Paris series,[33] two of the largest published series and thus representative of a large surgical experience. In other series the incidence of such complications is even greater.[49] Although not usually responsible for any demonstrable long-term adverse consequence, these complications result in prolonged hospital stay, the need for additional surgical procedures, and in some instances meningitis. The risk of neurologic deterioration following surgery for lipoma of the conus is extremely variable. No asymptomatic patients experienced a neurologic deterioration in La Marca et al's series,[32] whereas 4% of the asymptomatic group sustained a new deficit in the study by Pierre-Khan et al; in this latter series, this worsened to 6.4% by the end of the first postoperative year.[33] The most common aggravation is related to sphincter function.

Effective Intervention

The final criterion to be fulfilled to justify a prophylactic intervention is that the results of that intervention should be better compared with natural history. Although the early results of spinal cord untethering for asymptomatic lipoma appear encouraging, in that the majority of patients are not worsened by surgery and so remain asymptomatic, these initial good results deteriorate over time. Therefore, the question arises: Does "technically successful" surgery actually protect against late deterioration? In the series by Xenos et al, 26% of asymptomatic patients showed late deterioration despite surgery.[31] This concern is reflected in other large series. For example, in a study by La Marca et al, at a mean follow-up of 6.2 years, 12.7% of asymptomatic patients deteriorated and required further surgery.[32] In Pierre-Khan et al's series, of those who had undergone prophylactic surgery, 46.9% had symptoms after a mean follow-up of 8.7 years.[33] Similarly, Colak et al calculated the actuarial risk of deterioration to be 40% at 8 years.[50] It thus appears that the rate of symptomatic retethering increases with time. Some have suggested that the time to deterioration following untethering surgery is shorter for those with preoperative symptoms compared with those without,[32] thus supporting the argument for prophylactic untethering. Cochrane and colleagues failed to find any difference in the time to deterioration according to status at the time of surgery and concluded that untethering did not prevent longer-term functional deterioration.[60]

Not All Lipomas Are Equal

It is now accepted that filar lipomas should be considered separately from conus lipomas, as these represent a more simple anatomy that can be safely operated upon, and results are generally excellent.[32,33,61] In several studies examining the role of untethering surgery in dysraphism, filar and conus lipomas have been considered together, risking an overly optimistic interpretation of long-term outcomes.[62] Most surgeons acknowledge the anatomical complexity and surgical challenge posed by the transitional-type lipoma.[63] Within this group, the presence of congenitally short nerve roots, a rotated placode, and bulky lipomatous tissue enveloping the terminal spinal cord represents a scenario in which true untethering is perhaps impossible. However, there have been few studies examining the prognostic significance of the subtype of conus lipomas; these tend to be considered together in most large series. Where a distinction has been made, it appears that the prognosis, particularly in respect to retethering, is worse for the transitional-type compared with the dorsal-type of

lipoma.[50,60,64] In a study performed by this author, all the initially asymptomatic patients who deteriorated had transitional-type lipomas; perhaps noteworthy is that 13 out of 14 deteriorating patients were female.[56]

A Tailored Management Algorithm for Spinal Lipoma

The neurosurgical management of these complex dysraphic anomalies is likely to remain controversial, as there is insufficient evidence at present regarding asymptomatic lipomas to judge whether prophylactic spinal cord untethering should be the treatment of choice. What evidence there is casts some doubt on the traditionally held belief that all children with spinal lipoma will eventually deteriorate and that early surgery confers an advantage over a policy of close multidisciplinary surveillance. Recent publications indicate that perhaps pediatric neurosurgeons are beginning to more critically evaluate the role of prophylactic spinal cord untethering in favor of close surveillance, particularly for complex lipomas.[63,65] Perhaps the burden of proof now lies with those advocating the more aggressive surgical approach. For pediatric neurosurgeons recommending prophylactic untethering, it is for them to appraise their own results and measure these against the emerging knowledge of natural history. This is unlikely to result in a global recommended standard of care, as for those whose results are as good as or better than natural history, their approach is vindicated. However, where results are inferior to natural history, then a more selective approach to management might be pertinent. An algorithm is suggested that recognizes not only the benefits of untethering surgery in selected cases, but also the potentially benign natural history for many of these patients (**Fig. 17.5**). Fundamental to such a policy of management is the need for close regular surveillance, both neurologic and urologic, particularly until such time as urinary continence has been established and the need for patients and their families to be aware of warning symptoms that might herald the onset of tethering.

Conclusion

To consider all lipomas of the lumbosacral region as a single disease entity overlooks the embryological, anatomical, and clinical heterogeneity of this extremely complex group of malformations. For the previously normal child who develops a deficit or who exhibits loss of a previously acquired neurologic function, then, to invoke a mechanical explanation and offer untethering surgery is entirely appropriate and should be considered an evidence-based treatment. For the asymptomatic child with such a malformation, the evidence upon which to base prophylactic untethering of the spinal cord is tenuous. Recent natural history studies suggest that it is no longer appropriate to advise surgery on the

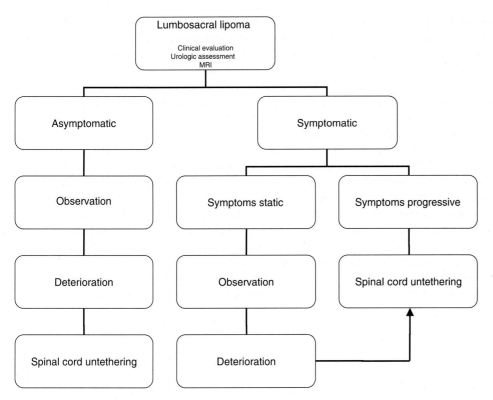

Fig. 17.5 Suggested algorithm that recognizes not only the benefits of untethering surgery in selected cases but also the potentially benign natural history for many patients. Observation comprises neurologic and urologic review, at least 6 monthly until 3 years of age or until the child achieves normal continence and at least annually thereafter. MRI, magnetic resonance imaging.

basis that deterioration is inevitable; furthermore, the intervention is not without risk, and, in most hands, the outcome of surgery may be little better than with conservative treatment. A conservative approach to the asymptomatic patient is therefore advocated, recognizing the need for close neurologic and urologic surveillance and the need for intervention in the event of any evidence of deterioration. Such a policy will spare some patients unnecessary interventions and result in outcomes better than those reported in most series of prophylactic intervention.

♦ Lessons Learned

Whether or not asymptomatic patients with tethered cord syndrome should be offered a prophylactic untethering operation has emerged as a controversial issue only over the last 10 years or so. Prior to that, the intervention-based retrospective case series were the only source of evidence beyond the individual surgeon's experience, and these favored the prophylactic intervention.

However, in recent years, careful analysis of a growing body of data and the study of unoperated patients have created a rift between the "traditional" interventionists, more often represented in North America, and the "conservative" noninterventionists, also sometimes referred to as the "Paris school." The latter group has compiled evidence that there is reason to doubt the concept of prophylactic surgery for asymptomatic children with spinal dysraphism and tethered cord syndrome.

As is beautifully exemplified in the present contributions by Thompson and Pugh and colleagues, the devil lies in the details. Indeed, the question of who is to be considered "asymptomatic" is one that is more difficult to answer than one would expect. We learn that the different forms of spinal dysraphism have been described and understood in terms of morphologic appearance, in terms of conceptual understanding of the form of developmental damage, and in terms of the pathophysiologic understanding of what contributes to symptoms. The latter point is particularly important because symptoms may be caused by a fixed, noncorrectable dysplasia and a secondary, potentially progressive damage caused either by compression from a large lipoma or by the well-known oxidative damage due to chronic stretching of the cord. These three mechanisms may well overlap in degrees that cannot be determined. Consequently, a deficit due to dysplasia cannot be improved by any surgery, but the other two mechanisms may well be influenced positively, either by improving symptoms or by preventing deterioration.

Both contributions to this chapter note the technical difficulty of approaching certain types of conus lipomas where the nerve roots are located within the lipoma. This situation increases the surgical risk, and the inherently short nerve roots naturally limit the extent of untethering that can be accomplished. It should be understood that secondary surgery is clearly more difficult than first operations; thus, all efforts should be made to succeed in the first surgery. This, of course, will be more likely when an experienced pediatric neurosurgeon performs this type of delicate operation rather than a general neurosurgeon or a pediatric surgeon.

Neither contribution spends much time on the question of preventing second surgeries, which may well be necessary in a third of operated children. There is probably a unique variety of surgical techniques, all based more or less on individual experience and "school," on the use of certain types of implants as dural grafts, with the object to reduce postoperative scarring and thus reduce the risk of retethering.

In the editors' view, no optimal surgical technique addressing this problem exists. We use an "inlay" technique to cover the conus and cauda with a synthetic dural graft, over which the dura is closed with or without a fascial patch and tangential sutures, preventing the suture line from making contact with the pia. This works well, but whether or not it prevents retethering more than other techniques remains to be proven.

Prophylactic untethering will occupy room in discussion boards in pediatric neurosurgery for some time.

References

1. Albright AL, Gartner JC, Wiener ES. Lumbar cutaneous hemangiomas as indicators of tethered spinal cords. Pediatrics 1989;83(6):977–980
2. Appignani BA, Jaramillo D, Barnes PD, Poussaint TY. Dysraphic myelodysplasias associated with urogenital and anorectal anomalies: prevalence and types seen with MR imaging. AJR Am J Roentgenol 1994;163(5):1199–1203
3. Davidoff AM, Thompson CV, Grimm JM, Shorter NA, Filston HC, Oakes WJ. Occult spinal dysraphism in patients with anal agenesis. J Pediatr Surg 1991;26(8):1001–1005
4. Lode HM, Deeg KH, Krauss J. Spinal sonography in infants with cutaneous birth markers in the lumbo-sacral region: an important sign of occult spinal dysraphism and tethered cord. Ultraschall Med 2007; 29(5):281–288
5. Long FR, Hunter JV, Mahboubi S, Kalmus A, Templeton JM Jr. Tethered cord and associated vertebral anomalies in children and infants with imperforate anus: evaluation with MR imaging and plain radiography. Radiology 1996;200(2):377–382
6. Tatli MM, Kumral A, Duman N, Ozkan S, Ozkan H. An unusual cutaneous lesion as the presenting sign of spinal dysraphism in a preterm infant. Pediatr Dermatol 2004;21(6):664–666
7. Hoffman HJ, Taecholarn C, Hendrick EB, Humphreys RP. Management of lipomyelomeningoceles: experience at the Hospital for Sick Children, Toronto. J Neurosurg 1985;62(1):1–8
8. Kanev PM, Bierbrauer KS. Reflections on the natural history of lipomyelomeningocele. Pediatr Neurosurg 1995;22(3):137–140
9. Keating MA, Rink RC, Bauer SB, et al. Neurourological implications of the changing approach in management of occult spinal lesions. J Urol 1988;140(5 Pt 2):1299–1301
10. Koyanagi I, Iwasaki Y, Hida K, Abe H, Isu T, Akino M. Surgical treatment supposed natural history of the tethered cord with occult spinal dysraphism. Childs Nerv Syst 1997;13(5):268–274
11. Guthkelch AN. Diastematomyelia with median septum. Brain 1974; 97(4):729–742
12. Tani S, Yamada S, Knighton RS. Extensibility of the lumbar and sacral cord: pathophysiology of the tethered spinal cord in cats. J Neurosurg 1987;66(1):116–123
13. Yamada S, Iacono RP, Andrade T, Mandybur G, Yamada BS. Pathophysiology of tethered cord syndrome. Neurosurg Clin N Am 1995;6(2):311–323
14. Yamada S, Won DJ, Yamada SM. Pathophysiology of tethered cord syndrome: correlation with symptomatology. Neurosurg Focus 2004;16(2):E6
15. Yamada S, Zinke DE, Sanders D. Pathophysiology of "tethered cord syndrome." J Neurosurg 1981;54(4):494–503
16. Blount JP, Tubbs RS, Okor M, et al. Supraplacode spinal cord transection in paraplegic patients with myelodysplasia and repetitive symptomatic tethered spinal cord. J Neurosurg 2005;103(1, Suppl):36–39
17. Ragnarsson TS, Durward QJ, Nordgren RE. Spinal cord tethering after traumatic paraplegia with late neurological deterioration. J Neurosurg 1986;64(3):397–401
18. Arai H, Sato K, Okuda O, et al. Surgical experience of 120 patients with lumbosacral lipomas. Acta Neurochir (Wien) 2001;143(9): 857–864
19. Blount JP, Elton S. Spinal lipomas. Neurosurg Focus 2001;10(1):e3
20. Chapman PH. Congenital intraspinal lipomas: anatomic considerations and surgical treatment. Childs Brain 1982;9(1):37–47
21. Xenos C, Sgouros S, Walsh R, Hockley A. Spinal lipomas in children. Pediatr Neurosurg 2000;32(6):295–307
22. Byrne RW, Hayes EA, George TM, McLone DG. Operative resection of 100 spinal lipomas in infants less than 1 year of age. Pediatr Neurosurg 1995;23(4):182–186, discussion 186–187
23. Bao N, Chen ZH, Gu S, Chen QM, Jin HM, Shi CR. Tight filum terminale syndrome in children: analysis based on positioning of the conus and absence or presence of lumbosacral lipoma. Childs Nerv Syst 2007;23(10):1129–1134
24. Hirsch JF, Pierre-Kahn A. Lumbosacral lipomas with spina bifida. Childs Nerv Syst 1988;4(6):354–360
25. Pierre-Kahn A, Lacombe J, Pichon J, et al. Intraspinal lipomas with spina bifida: prognosis and treatment in 73 cases. J Neurosurg 1986;65(6):756–761
26. Pierre-Kahn A, Zerah M, Renier D, et al. Congenital lumbosacral lipomas. Childs Nerv Syst 1997;13(6):298–334, discussion 335

27. Lee GY, Paradiso G, Tator CH, Gentili F, Massicotte EM, Fehlings MG. Surgical management of tethered cord syndrome in adults: indications, techniques, and long-term outcomes in 60 patients. J Neurosurg Spine 2006;4(2):123–131

28. Fone PD, Vapnek JM, Litwiller SE, et al. Urodynamic findings in the tethered spinal cord syndrome: does surgical release improve bladder function? J Urol 1997;157(2):604–609

29. Steinbok P, Garton HJ, Gupta N. Occult tethered cord syndrome: a survey of practice patterns. J Neurosurg 2006;104(5, Suppl)309–313

30. Bassett RC. The neurologic deficit associated with lipomas of the cauda equina. Ann Surg 1950;131(1):109–116

31. Xenos C, Sgouros S, Walsh R, Hockley A. Spinal lipomas in children. Pediatr Neurosurg 2000;32(6):295–307

32. La Marca F, Grant JA, Tomita T, McLone DG. Spinal lipomas in children: outcome of 270 procedures. Pediatr Neurosurg 1997;26(1):8–16

33. Pierre-Kahn A, Zerah M, Renier D, et al. Congenital lumbosacral lipomas. Childs Nerv Syst 1997;13(6):298–334, discussion 335

34. Kulkarni AV, Pierre-Kahn A, Zerah M. Conservative management of asymptomatic spinal lipomas of the conus. Neurosurgery 2004;54(4):868–873, discussion 873–875

35. Chapman PH. Congenital intraspinal lipomas: anatomic considerations and surgical treatment. Childs Brain 1982;9(1):37–47

36. Naidich TP, McLone DG, Mutluer S. A new understanding of dorsal dysraphism with lipoma (lipomyeloschisis): radiologic evaluation and surgical correction. AJR Am J Roentgenol 1983;140(6):1065–1078

37. Copp AJ, Brook FA. Does lumbosacral spina bifida arise by failure of neural folding or by defective canalisation? J Med Genet 1989;26(3):160–166

38. Müller F, O'Rahilly R. The primitive streak, the caudal eminence and related structures in staged human embryos. Cells Tissues Organs 2004;177(1):2–20

39. Saitsu H, Yamada S, Uwabe C, Ishibashi M, Shiota K. Development of the posterior neural tube in human embryos. Anat Embryol (Berl) 2004;209(2):107–117

40. De Gennaro M, Rivosecchi M, Lucchetti MC, Silveri M, Fariello G, Schingo P. The incidence of occult spinal dysraphism and the onset of neurovesical dysfunction in children with anorectal anomalies. Eur J Pediatr Surg 1994;4(Suppl 1):12–14

41. Karrer FM, Flannery AM, Nelson MD Jr, McLone DG, Raffensperger JG. Anorectal malformations: evaluation of associated spinal dysraphic syndromes. J Pediatr Surg 1988;23(1 Pt 2):45–48

42. Qi BQ, Beasley SW, Arsic D. Abnormalities of the vertebral column and ribs associated with anorectal malformations. Pediatr Surg Int 2004;20(7):529–533

43. Warf BC, Scott RM, Barnes PD, Hendren WH III. Tethered spinal cord in patients with anorectal and urogenital malformations. Pediatr Neurosurg 1993;19(1):25–30

44. Tani S, Yamada S, Knighton RS. Extensibility of the lumbar and sacral cord: pathophysiology of the tethered spinal cord in cats. J Neurosurg 1987;66(1):116–123

45. James CC, Lassman LP. Spinal dysraphism: spinal cord lesions associated with spina bifida occulta. Physiotherapy 1962;48:154–157

46. Hirsch JF, Pierre-Kahn A. Lumbosacral lipomas with spina bifida. Childs Nerv Syst 1988;4(6):354–360

47. Byrne RW, Hayes EA, George TM, McLone DG. Operative resection of 100 spinal lipomas in infants less than 1 year of age. Pediatr Neurosurg 1995;23(4):182–186, discussion 186–187

48. Kanev PM, Lemire RJ, Loeser JD, Berger MS. Management and long-term follow-up review of children with lipomyelomeningocele, 1952–1987. J Neurosurg 1990;73(1):48–52

49. McLone DG, Thompson DNP. Lipomas of the spine. In: McLone DG, ed. Pediatric Neurosurgery: Surgery of the Developing Nervous System. Philadelphia: WB Saunders; 2001:289–301

50. Colak A, Pollack IF, Albright AL. Recurrent tethering: a common long-term problem after lipomyelomeningocele repair. Pediatr Neurosurg 1998;29(4):184–190

51. Van Calenbergh F, Vanvolsem S, Verpoorten C, Lagae L, Casaer P, Plets C. Results after surgery for lumbosacral lipoma: the significance of early and late worsening. Childs Nerv Syst 1999;15(9):439–442, discussion 443

52. Hoffman HJ, Taecholarn C, Hendrick EB, Humphreys RP. Management of lipomyelomeningoceles: experience at the Hospital for Sick Children, Toronto. J Neurosurg 1985;62(1):1–8

53. Oi S, Nomura S, Nagasaka M, et al. Embryopathogenetic surgicoanatomical classification of dysraphism and surgical outcome of spinal lipoma: a nationwide multicenter cooperative study in Japan. J Neurosurg Pediatr 2009;3(5):412–419

54. Dorward NL, Scatliff JH, Hayward RD. Congenital lumbosacral lipomas: pitfalls in analysing the results of prophylactic surgery. Childs Nerv Syst 2002;18(6–7):326–332

55. Jamil M, Bannister CM. A report of children with spinal dysraphism managed conservatively. Eur J Pediatr Surg 1992;2(Suppl 1):26–28

56. Wykes V, Thompson D. Asymptomatic lumbosacral lipomas: to operate or not? Childs Nerv Syst 2008;24:1231

57. O'Neill P, Stack JP. Magnetic resonance imaging in the pre-operative assessment of closed spinal dysraphism in children. Pediatr Neurosurg 1990-1991;16(4–5):240–246

58. Vernet O, O'Gorman AM, Farmer JP, McPhillips M, Montes JL. Use of the prone position in the MRI evaluation of spinal cord retethering. Pediatr Neurosurg 1996;25(6):286–294

59. Zide BM, Epstein FJ, Wisoff J. Optimal wound closure after tethered cord correction: technical note. J Neurosurg 1991;74(4):673–676

60. Cochrane DD, Finley C, Kestle J, Steinbok P. The patterns of late deterioration in patients with transitional lipomyelomeningocele. Eur J Pediatr Surg 2000;10(Suppl 1):13–17

61. Bulsara KR, Zomorodi AR, Villavicencio AT, Fuchs H, George TM. Clinical outcome differences for lipomyelomeningoceles, intraspinal lipomas, and lipomas of the filum terminale. Neurosurg Rev 2001;24(4):192–194

62. Kasliwal MK, Mahapatra AK. Surgery for spinal cord lipomas. Indian J Pediatr 2007;74(4):357–362

63. Drake JM. Occult tethered cord syndrome: not an indication for surgery. J Neurosurg 2006;104(5, Suppl):305–308

64. Arai H, Sato K, Okuda O, et al. Surgical experience of 120 patients with lumbosacral lipomas. Acta Neurochir (Wien) 2001;143(9):857–864

65. Cochrane DD. Occult spinal dysraphism. In: Albright AL, Pollack IF, Adelson PD, eds. Principles and Practice of Pediatric Neurosurgery. New York: Thieme; 2008:367–393

18 Intramedullary Spinal Cord Tumors

♦ **Biopsy and Adjuvant Therapy**

Donald J. Blaskiewicz and Mark R. Proctor

The optimal treatment of intramedullary spinal cord tumors (IMSCTs) has long been controversial; however, the evolving opinion of contemporary surgeons has been in favor of an aggressive surgical resection with or without postoperative adjuvant therapy.[1–3]

Technological advances in neuroimaging, microsurgical technique, neurophysiologic monitoring, and operative equipment have permitted neurosurgeons to undertake a more aggressive surgical approach, often achieving gross total resection (GTR) or subtotal resection (STR) based on intraoperative inspection of the tumor surgical site and postoperative magnetic resonance imaging (MRI).[4–27] Despite these advances, the risk of morbidity associated with aggressive surgical resection remains substantial, and the true benefit of aggressive surgical therapy has not been validated in terms of survival curves and functional outcomes scales when compared with less aggressive measures, such as biopsy for tissue diagnosis, along with adjuvant radiotherapy and/or chemotherapy.[8,28]

Furthermore, the current body of literature supporting aggressive resection is based on retrospective series, case reports, and expert opinions. Class I data comparing aggressive surgical resection with tissue biopsy and adjuvant therapy are unavailable.

In this chapter we have been asked to support the use of a minimally aggressive surgical approach in the management of IMSCT. Data will be presented to support the point of view that biopsy followed as necessary by adjuvant therapy is a safe and effective way to manage these lesions and may be preferable to aggressive surgical excision.

Epidemiology

Intramedullary spinal cord tumors are rarely encountered neoplasms, particularly in the pediatric population, where the incidence is 4 to 10 per 10 million.[29,30] Among neoplasms of the central nervous system (CNS), IMSCTs account for 6 to 8% of all tumors.[6,29,31] In the pediatric population, astrocytomas are more prevalent, being 3 times more common than ependymomas, whereas the opposite holds true in the adult population.[9,32,33] Among pediatric astrocytomas, 25% are of malignant histology, being either anaplastic astrocytomas or glioblastoma multiforme.[1,34]

Clinical Presentation

At the time of presentation, the most common findings are motor regression, pain, and gait abnormality. A smaller percentage may present with scoliosis or orthopedic abnormalities. In general, patients with more malignant lesions have a shorter prodrome of complaints before the correct diagnosis of spinal cord tumor is established.

Outcomes Analysis

To date, the body of literature supporting the aggressive surgical management of IMSCT is based on class IV evidence, comprised of uncontrolled studies, case series, case reports, and expert opinions.[1,2,6–8,10,11,13,14,35–39]

The largest pediatric series to date on IMSCT is that by Constantini et al, which comprises the surgical series of Dr. Fred Epstein.[1] In this series, the authors retrospectively reviewed 164 children and young adults who underwent surgery for IMSCT. GTR was achieved in 76.8% and STR in 20.1%, with 79% of the lesions being histologically low grade. Over time there was an increasing bias toward use of neurophysiologic monitoring and laminoplasty. Pre- and postoperative functional evaluations were assessed with the Modified McCormick Scale (**Table 18.1**).[1] Twenty-three percent of patients worsened at least one functional grade after surgery, 60% were unchanged, and 17% improved. Patients with poor preoperative functioning had a greater risk of surgical morbidity, and in general, high-grade lesions were more disabled at presentation. Histologic analysis

Table 18.1 Modified McCormick Scale for Functional Evaluation of Patients with Intramedullary Spinal Cord Tumors

Grade	Explanation
I	Neurologically intact; ambulates normally; may have minimal dyesthesia
II	Mild motor or sensory deficit; patient maintains functional independence
III	Moderate deficit; limitation of function; independent with external aid
IV	Severe motor or sensory deficit; limitation of function with a dependent patient
V	Paraplegia or quadriplegia, even if there is flickering movement

revealed low-grade tumors in 124, intermediate-grade in 19, and high-grade in 12 patients. Twenty-six percent of the group went on to have adjuvant therapy, including radiation and chemotherapy. Progression-free survival was estimated using the Kaplan-Meier technique. This revealed that GTR and STR were equally efficacious for low-grade tumors, and there was no survival benefit to GTR. Patients who underwent biopsy alone did fare worse, but these appear to have been almost exclusively high-grade lesions that behaved poorly regardless of attempted surgical approach. In fact, tumor histology was the only reliable predictor of patient survival. In summary, this study showed us that radical surgery can be performed in the majority of patients, but it did not prove that survival was superior to biopsy alone for low-grade lesions; furthermore, the patients were more likely to worsen than to improve their functional status with aggressive surgery.[1]

Dr. Epstein had a unique practice with an unusually high volume of patients with IMSCTs, and the data derived from his study are important to our understanding of these children. His work accurately describes the clinical course of pediatric patients undergoing aggressive resection of IMSCTs; however, a prospective, randomized control study or prospective matched group cohort study comparing aggressive surgical therapy with biopsy and adjuvant therapy has not been performed.

Radiotherapy

Many institutions reserve external beam radiotherapy for patients in whom GTR was not possible, in patients who have disease recurrence, or for high-grade lesions. Many authors have advocated aggressive surgery alone over subtotal resection or biopsy followed by radiation so as to avoid late complications of radiation. The current body of literature, however, does not necessarily support this rationale. In addition, in looking at the late effects of radiation, one must then equally consider the late effects of surgery on the pediatric spine to have an accurate comparison.

The largest, most comprehensive review of IMSCT in children treated at a single institution with surgery followed by external beam radiation was performed by O'Sullivan et al reviewing the data from the Hospital for Sick Children in Toronto.[34] Included in this study were 11 ependymomas and 15 astrocytomas, of which 12 were low grade, 3 high grade, and 5 other tumor types. Biopsy alone was performed in 35%, STR in 45%, and GTR in 19%. All patients received local high-dose radiation. The relapse rate based on the extent of resection was 37%, 14%, and 33%, for biopsy, STR, and GTR, respectively; thus, the extent of resection seemed to have no effect on the likelihood of recurrence. Local control of the tumor was achieved in 26 cases (84%), despite either grossly incomplete resection or biopsy alone in 25 of these cases (81%). Two patients did suffer from second malignancies that were felt to be radiation induced. Based on their results, the authors concluded that radiation treatment without resection may achieve long-term control in children with astrocytoma or ependymoma of the spinal cord, and in fact the results of progression-free survival were similar to the large surgical series of Constantini et al.[1] It was more difficult to determine any differences in functional outcome between the two studies.[1,34] Of note, 68% of the patients did go on to suffer from progressive spinal deformity, therefore indicating that biopsy and adjuvant therapy may not be protective against deformity.[34] Other authors have shown that in low- and intermediate-grade astrocytomas, postoperative radiation therapy has improved overall survival or progression-free survival.[40–46]

Chemotherapy

The role of chemotherapy in the management of IMSCTs has not been clearly defined. Its use has been reserved primarily as an adjuvant modality in cases of unresectable or recurrent lesions. There has been documentation in the literature of successful and inspiring treatment of intramedullary astrocytomas with chemotherapeutic agents; however, these have been isolated to case reports.[47–53]

Postsurgical Spinal Deformity

The incidence of progressive spinal deformity following either laminectomy or laminoplasty for any indication has been previously reviewed.[54] Risk factors associated with increased incidence of deformity include the extent of facet resection, the number of lamina removed, the spinal segment involved, the presence of preoperative deformity, the growth potential of the spine (more common in pediatric patients), and IMSCTs.[55–67]

The developing spine is especially susceptible to postlaminectomy deformity for several reasons. There is increased ligamentous laxity when compared with that of more mature skeletal systems. Furthermore, in the pediatric cervical spine, the orientation of the facet complex is more in the horizontal plane as compared with the vertical plane arrangement in the adult spine and therefore protects less against anterior subluxation.[65,68] Finally, surgical disruption of the growth dynamics of the pediatric spine tends to propagate further deformities.[55,56,64–66]

IMSCTs, in and of themselves, are known to be associated with sagittal plane deformity.[60,64,65] It has been postulated that involvement of the ventral horns may cause neuromuscular insufficiency, thus weakening the muscular support of the spine and leading to progressive spinal column deformity.[69,70] At the time of initial presentation, 15 to 40% of patients presenting with IMSCTs have an existing deformity, which is a known risk factor for progressive deformity following surgical resection of IMSCT.[61,64] Furthermore, when compared with those undergoing cervical decompression for degenerative conditions of the spine, patients with IMSCTs are twice as likely to develop deformity, with postoperative deformity being reported in 16 to 100% of patients in various studies.[56,57,71,72]

Yao et al described the risk factors for progressive spinal deformity in children undergoing surgical resection of IMSCT: age younger than 13 years, the presence of preoperative deformity, and involvement of the thoracic or thoracolumbar segments increased the odds ratio of a subsequent spinal deformity requiring surgery for stabilization by 4.4, 3.2, and 2.6, respectively.[65] Although the extent of resection as an independent risk factor did not have a statistically significant predictive value on progression of deformity, children undergoing GTR (resection > 95%) or STR (80–95% resection) had an odds ratio of 2.31 and 0.565, respectively, of developing postoperative deformity that required further surgery for stabilization, whereas those undergoing biopsy alone had an odds ratio of 0.001.[65]

Efforts to reduce postoperative deformity by performing laminoplasty have shown marginal clinical reduction in the progression of sagittal imbalance.[54] Some authors advocate preemptive fusion at the time of the initial resection in patients who present with a preoperative kyphotic deformity.[68]

Conclusion

Aggressive resection of IMSCTs carries a substantial risk of surgical morbidity, including neurologic decline and subsequent spinal column deformity requiring further surgical intervention for stabilization. In cases of ependymomas or low-grade astrocytomas, aggressive surgery may confer long-term survival benefits that outweigh the surgical risks, although this has not been established in any prospective study, and current data would indicate that the survival is similar to children undergoing biopsy and adjuvant radiotherapy. For patients with intermediate or high-grade lesions, surgical intervention does not appear to improve the overall survival, while subjecting these patients to high rates of surgical morbidity.

We respect the authors who have meticulously compiled and analyzed their experiences with IMSCTs. In light of the rarity of IMSCTs, however, it will require a multicenter, randomized, prospective study to formally address this controversial topic, especially for patients with low-grade lesions. Future studies should have specific emphasis on comparing survival, functional outcomes, and progression of spinal deformity. Currently, the literature does not define the optimal treatment algorithm for managing these complex patients, and the data supporting a conservative approach of initial biopsy followed by adjuvant therapy compare favorably to aggressive surgical approaches.

◆ The Case for Surgery

Karl F. Kothbauer

Tumors arising from within the spinal cord are a small subgroup of CNS tumors occurring in childhood. Nonetheless, they are regarded as particularly problematic because of the densely packed fiber tracts and neural networks within the cord substance and the subsequent threat of severe spinal cord dysfunction. There is an ongoing debate on how these tumors should be treated.

Due to the small numbers of patients treated by each individual pediatric neurosurgeon or even at leading pediatric institutions, no evidence robust enough to withstand a Cochrane review exists to support any management strategy for patients suffering from these tumors. Thus, we have to make do with the existing series-based evidence, with the evidence about surgical technology and that derived from treatment modalities applied in other areas of the nervous

system reapplied to the spinal cord. Consequently, the treatment choices will be made mostly based on experience.

Surgery for spinal cord tumors has a surprisingly long history, given the presumed difficulty of safely operating on the spinal cord. The first successful resection of an intramedullary spinal cord tumor was accomplished by Anton von Eiselsberg in Vienna in the fall of 1907.[73] A two-stage surgical resection strategy (based on two cases) was developed shortly after that by Charles Elsberg in New York and published in 1911.[74]

These bold pioneers had nothing of what is commonplace today: no useful imaging, no surgical technology, no microsurgery, no monitoring, no neuroanesthesia. In subsequent decades, humanity was preoccupied with wars and economic disaster. There were no resources to further develop such seemingly "outlandish" surgeries. The neurologic risk of resecting intramedullary neoplasms was considered unacceptably high, and a conservative treatment concept was followed with a small role for surgery: an often timid biopsy, at best, combined with dural decompression to relieve the compartment-like compression of the swollen cord within the dural sac. Radiation therapy regardless of the histologic diagnosis was the factual treatment.[75]

Only in better times, and just prior to the advent of microsurgery, were new attempts made to remove tumors from the spinal cord.[76,77] Microneurosurgery reopened the door to a serious effort to establish surgical resection of intramedullary tumors as a management strategy superior to the biopsy–radiation concept. In the 1980s, after the microscope had established itself as an indispensable tool in neurosurgery, MRI dramatically improved the preoperative anatomical assessment of the spinal cord. Preoperative planning and postoperative follow-up became a reality. Thus, the conservative treatment strategy for intramedullary tumors gradually developed, and still continues to evolve, to a more active treatment concept with a larger role for aggressive surgical resection. This is aided by increased knowledge about the natural history of the disease and the response to surgery. Because most intramedullary tumors are low-grade neoplasms, complete and even near-complete resection appears to result in long-term progression-free survival with acceptable neurologic morbidity.[78–85] After the imaging revolution of the 1980s, the 1990s brought the development and application of intraoperative neurophysiologic monitoring. Understanding the functional integrity of the cord, particularly of the motor system, during surgery and in the process of neurologic recovery thereafter improved the surgeons' ability to resect tumors with low neurologic morbidity.[86–89]

Nevertheless, differences of opinion still exist about the proper referral of the relatively few children suffering from intramedullary tumors and their optimal individualized treatment. Despite the advances in surgical treatment, the old concept of "biopsy and radiation" is not extinct.[90,91] Lack of controlled evidence for a benefit of surgery has been suggested as an argument for a conservative treatment.

New drugs used for chemotherapeutic management of CNS tumors have not been widely used to treat intramedullary tumors. Only higher-grade glial tumors have been treated with a combination approach that includes chemotherapy.[92] For low-grade tumors, little, if any, experience exists as to the impact of medical treatment of these neoplasms.[93] Given recent advances in the chemotherapeutic treatment of malignant gliomas of the brain,[94] it is reasonable to use the same regimen for glioblastomas of the spinal cord, and there may be further chemotherapy for spinal cord neoplasms in the future.

Epidemiology and Pathology

Intrinsic tumors of the spinal cord are rare. They comprise ~20 to 35% of all intradural neoplasms, with a higher percentage (55% of all intradural neoplasms) in children.[95] The most common intramedullary tumors in children are astrocytomas. Intramedullary ependymomas are the most frequent type in the adult age group but are rare exceptions in children.[85] Other tumors, such as hemangioblastomas[96] and cavernomas,[97] occur.

The great majority of spinal cord tumors in children are benign, being either pilocytic or, less frequently, fibrillary astrocytomas. Like astrocytomas in the brain, the latter are poorly demarcated from normal tissue. Pilocytic tumors frequently have large areas of good demarcation, as well as cystic components, and smaller areas of diffuse growth next to the normal cord tissue.

Gangliogliomas are also low grade and occur primarily in children and young adults. Most frequently, intramedullary gangliogliomas grow slowly and thus have an indolent course and may present only when exceedingly large.[98]

Ependymomas are the most common intramedullary neoplasm in adults,[99,100] whereas in children they account for only 12% of all intramedullary tumors.[101] Typically, they have a central location in the spinal cord. Most often they are well circumscribed and clearly delineated from the surrounding spinal cord tissue. Practically all ependymomas are histologically benign.

Myxopapillary ependymomas are a subgroup of ependymomas with characteristic microcystic histologic features.[102] They are usually located in the conus–cauda region.[103] They may grossly enlarge the filum and displace the nerve roots laterally and anteriorly. Despite their benign histology, a small percentage of them tend to subarachnoid dissemination.[104]

Hemangioblastomas account for only 3 to 7% of intramedullary spinal cord tumors.[96,105] They occur mostly sporadically, but up to 25% of patients have von Hippel-Lindau disease.[106]

Surgery

Arguments for an attempt at surgical resection for any newly diagnosed intramedullary tumor in a child or an adult are threefold: first, to ascertain the histologic diagnosis; second, as the by far most effective oncologic treatment; and third, to prevent long-term motor dysfunction.

Standard microsurgical techniques with suction and bipolar coagulation should be used together with a limited set of specialized instruments that aid in minimizing surgical trauma to normal spinal cord tissue. Depending on the specific nature of the tumor, the surgical technique must be adjusted. For instance, the removal of a hemangioblastoma significantly differs from the resection of an astrocytoma.

Ultrasonic Aspirator

The introduction of the now ubiquitously used Cavitron ultrasonic aspirator (CUSA)[107] system (Integra Life Sciences, Plainsboro, New Jersey) was a significant advancement in the resection of spinal cord tumors.[108] Experience with intraoperative monitoring has shown that, not infrequently, partial injury to the motor pathways occurred exactly at the time that the CUSA was used. Therefore, its utilization has been modified: it is considered safe to remove an already partially detached tumor mass but less safe to internally decompress tumor bulk still in situ.

Laser

The microsurgical laser is an excellent surgical tool for spinal cord surgery.[109] The Nd:YAG (neodymium:yttrium-aluminum-garnet) Contact Laser System (PhotoMedex, Inc., Montgomeryville, Pennsylvania) is used by this author. It is particularly useful in myelotomies and for demarcating the glia–tumor interface. Using laser and suction allows the tumor to be removed in a piecemeal fashion. Also, laser does not cause an electric artifact, unlike bipolar cautery. Thus, intraoperative monitoring is not hampered by amplifier blockade. If the texture of the tumor is particularly firm, as in rare types of intramedullary tumors, it can only be removed with reasonable safety with laser because such a lesion cannot be manipulated with bipolar cautery and scissors, and it is too firm for the CUSA.

Surgical Technique

Surgery is always performed with the patient in the prone position.[77,110,111] A rigid head holder, either Sugita or Mayfield, is used for cervical and cervicothoracic tumors to secure the head and the spinous processes in the neutral position.

An osteoplastic laminotomy[112] is performed with a high-power drill using the craniotome attachment. The bone removal must expose the solid tumor but not necessarily the rostral or caudal cysts unless their wall enhances and they are considered intratumoral cysts. Paratumoral cysts usually disappear after the neoplasm is resected, as the walls of these "capping" cysts are usually composed of non-neoplastic glial tissue.

Intraoperative ultrasound usually shows the full extent of the tumor and thus confirms that the bone opening is sufficient.[113]

The dura is usually opened in the midline. The spinal cord is often expanded, rotated, and distorted. The asymmetric expansion and rotation of the spinal cord may make identification of the midline raphe difficult. However, it is important to localize this landmark because it is the standard approach into the cord. An alternative for asymmetrical tumors is to enter the cord through the dorsal root entry zone. This may be useful if an asymmetric deficit is present, and it is essential to preserve the "good" arm.

This author uses the microsurgical laser to perform the myelotomy. A cord–tumor interface can be separated with dissectors and a specially designed plated bayoneted

forceps[114] or the microsurgical laser.[109] It is useful to start at one pole of the tumor and identify the cleavage plane, then separate the tumor from there in the craniocaudal direction. It is absolutely essential not to injure the anterior spinal artery. Astrocytomas or gangliogliomas typically have a heterogeneous composition and texture. They are usually removed in an inside-out fashion until the cord–tumor interface is recognized. There is almost never a true plane between the tumor and the normal spinal cord, at least not throughout the tumor length, as in ependymomas. Injury to the cord at this area may cause neurologic dysfunction.[115] The CUSA, microsurgical laser, and suction–bipolar dissection are used where appropriate and with the caveats described earlier.

Following tumor removal, hemostasis is obtained with saline irrigation and, if necessary, by local application of microfibrillar collagen (Avitene, C. R. Bard, Inc., Murray Hill, New Jersey). Bipolar coagulation may be necessary for bleeding vessels that cannot be otherwise controlled. However, retrograde thrombosis into the anterior spinal artery or local thermal injury has resulted in significant injury, and using intraoperative monitoring at the time of injury has unequivocally been linked to the time of coagulation of bleeding vessels, particularly those close to the anterior midline of the cord. The dura is closed primarily in a watertight fashion usually with a running locked nonabsorbable suture. If an osteoplastic laminotomy was performed, all segments of bone are replaced and secured with a size 1 or 0 nonabsorbable suture on each lamina bilaterally[112] or with miniplates, such as those used for cranioplasty. The spinal muscle fascia must be closed in a watertight fashion without lateral tension to prevent cerebrospinal fluid leakage. The skin is closed with running locked sutures.

Intraoperative Neurophysiologic Monitoring

Spinal orthopedic surgeons first used evoked potentials for intraoperative assessment of spinal cord functional integrity.[116,117] The use of somatosensory evoked potentials with primitive and unreliable[118,119] technology has evolved into the combined use of D-wave monitoring[86,120–124] and monitoring of muscle motor evoked potentials,[125–129] which provide practically real-time feedback about the current state of the functional integrity of the motor pathways with high reliability[88] and proven impact on neurologic outcome.[130]

Surgical Complications

The feared complication of intramedullary tumor surgery is paralysis. Its true incidence, however, is surprisingly small.[85,99,130,131] In general, the occurrence of postoperative motor deficits of any magnitude is related to the state of preoperative neurologic function. Patients who have no or minimal preoperative motor deficits have a small risk for motor deterioration. Patients who already have a significant motor deficit before surgery are more likely to deteriorate postoperatively.[86]

The resection radicality in intramedullary glioma surgery is almost always < 100%. Only ependymomas,[77,99,100] hemangioblastomas,[96] and cavernomas[97] can be resected in an anatomically complete fashion. Complete removal, particularly of the last bits and pieces of tumor tissue in astrocytoma resection, carries a high risk of major neurologic dysfunction. GTR is feasible in ~70 to 80% of cases and a subtotal (80–97%) in the remainder.

Short-term motor dysfunction is significant: one third of patients experience a transient motor deficit, which resolves within hours to days[88] or months.[131] The long-term motor outcome is much better and directly related to the preoperative neurologic function.[86] Therefore, it is advisable that patients with intramedullary tumors undergo surgery before the development of significant neurologic deficits.

Impaired joint position sense may be a component of serious postsurgical functional disability and is more commonly seen after ependymoma than astrocytoma removal. Patients with impaired proprioception require physical therapy to train to compensate for this deficit. In addition, patients may experience a variety of pain syndromes, autonomic symptoms, and decreased endurance. It is a common complaint that all symptoms tend to get worse during the cold season and better during the summer.

Scoliosis and kyphosis can occur after surgery.[132–135] This is of particular importance for children, where about one third of patients with a significant deformity eventually require a stabilizing spinal operation. Osteoplastic laminotomy is believed to reduce the incidence of spinal deformity in children.[112]

Neurologic Outcome

There is no doubt that resection of an intramedullary tumor is a very serious undertaking in terms of neurologic morbidity. Both in children and adults a significant degree of long-term sensory dysfunction and dysesthetic pain may be present.[131] However, the rate of significant motor disturbance up to paraplegia is low,[85,88,130,131] and, most importantly, both clinical[86,136] and experimental evidence[137] favors early rather than late surgery because motor outcome tends to be superior as long as motor function is good. There is unequivocal surgical experience that once a patient is nonambulatory, no surgery can reverse this disability.

Oncologic Outcome

Obviously, in tumors such as hemangioblastomas and cavernomas, the surgical resection provides cure of the disease, and neurologic morbidity is a function of presurgical damage to the cord by the tumor and of surgical damage to the cord.

In glial tumors, as stated earlier, even with GTRs, some residual microscopic fragments always remain in the resection bed no matter how "good" a surgery may have been. This residual tissue may remain dormant or involute over time. The available evidence strongly suggests that a resection that exceeds 80 to 90% removal is as good as 98 to 100% removal in terms of long-term progression-free survival.[85] This allows the conclusion that it may not be necessary to attempt a "total" removal to achieve the optimally possible outcome. This helps in determining to stop the resection before it gets very close to the normal spinal cord tissue, which would carry a high risk of surgical injury and subsequent neurologic dysfunction.

Not surprisingly, long-term survival is better for low-grade neoplasms when compared with the high-grade group[1]. Five- and 10-year survival rates were 88 and 82%, respectively, for low-grade neoplasms. The cause of death in these patients was progression of disease. Patients with high-grade neoplasms have an 18% 5-year survival rate despite surgery and adjuvant therapy.

Adjuvant Therapy

Some experts still recommend radiotherapy even for benign intramedullary spinal cord tumors.[90,138,139]

Radiation therapy has an undisputed role for patients with malignant tumors, those who have tumor recurrence, and those with substantial residual tumor for whom further surgery is considered too risky.

Intramedullary ependymomas should be resected, and radiotherapy is an option only in exceptional circumstances.

The future role of chemotherapy is uncertain at this time for intramedullary tumors. There are few reports and experiences with chemotherapy in low-grade tumors.[93] There is certainly a role for chemotherapy in high-grade tumor management,[92] but it does not appear to provide a big survival benefit. The new treatment protocol with temozolomide established for cerebral glioblastomas[94] is a reasonable choice for spinal cord glioblastomas as well. So far, no experience with this approach has been reported.

The deleterious effect of radiation with myelopathy induced by doses > 30 Gy[140] is known, and no study has demonstrated a beneficial effect of radiation therapy on survival or neurologic function for low-grade spinal cord tumors. A spinal deformity may also be a result of radiation therapy used to treat epidural tumors.[141,142] Mayfield et al reported that 32 of 57 children with neuroblastomas treated with radiation therapy and chemotherapy developed significant spinal deformities. A higher rate of deformity was associated with younger age at time of radiation, doses > 20 Gy, and asymmetrical radiation fields.[143] This serves also as evidence that radiation treatment is not a "noninvasive" therapeutic alternative to surgery.

Conclusion

Intramedullary spinal cord tumors are a serious illness. The great majority are benign, completely resectable lesions or low-grade glial tumors. Both types can be surgically removed with relatively low morbidity and good oncologic outcome. Significant resection of glial tumors achieves long-term progression-free survival in the majority of patients, and advanced microsurgical technique, coupled with the use of intraoperative neurophysiologic monitoring, minimizes neurologic morbidity. The optimal treatment for malignant tumors remains resection followed by radiation therapy, with a likely benefit from combination with temozolomide chemotherapy.

No study exists to compare the oncologic and neurologic outcomes of management with aggressive surgery and management with primary radiation treatment. The experience and evidence appear to favor the surgical approach.

♦ Lessons Learned

Intramedullary spinal cord tumors represent a small proportion of all CNS tumors in children. These two surgeons highlight the different surgical management for these tumors. Tumors that are symptomatic and have demonstrated growth warrant a surgical procedure in an attempt to remove the tumor with the aid of neurophysiologic monitoring or biopsy followed by adjuvant radiotherapy. There have been no prospective randomized clinical studies that have determined the best treatment course for these tumors. The data available are thus the aggressive surgery modality as advocated by Fred Epstein and the earlier literature advocating biopsy and radiation therapy. Each of these approaches has disadvantages, such as scoliosis, risk of permanent paralysis, radiation necrosis, and radiation injury to the surrounding structures. The best approach depends on the surgeon's skill and experience with neurophysiologically guided surgery. The surgeon must weigh the risks and benefits of each treatment.

References

1. Constantini S, Miller DC, Allen JC, Rorke LB, Freed D, Epstein FJ. Radical excision of intramedullary spinal cord tumors: surgical morbidity and long-term follow-up evaluation in 164 children and young adults. J Neurosurg 2000; 93(2, Suppl):183–193
2. Fischer G, Mansuy L. Total removal of intramedullary ependymomas: follow-up study of 16 cases. Surg Neurol 1980;14(4): 243–249
3. Jallo GI, Danish S, Velasquez L, Epstein F. Intramedullary low-grade astrocytomas: long-term outcome following radical surgery. J Neurooncol 2001;53(1):61–66
4. Ahyai A, Woerner U, Markakis E. Surgical treatment of intramedullary tumors (spinal cord and medulla oblongata): analysis of 16 cases. Neurosurg Rev 1990;13(1):45–52
5. Brotchi J, Dewitte O, Levivier M, et al. A survey of 65 tumors within the spinal cord: surgical results and the importance of preoperative magnetic resonance imaging. Neurosurgery 1991;29(5):651–656, discussion 656–657
6. Constantini S, Epstain F. Intraspinal tumors in children and infants. In: Youmans JR, Becker DP, Dunsker SB, et al, eds. Neurological Surgery. 4th ed. Philadelphia: Saunders; 1996:3123–3133
7. Constantini S, Houten J, Miller DC, et al. Intramedullary spinal cord tumors in children under the age of 3 years. J Neurosurg 1996; 85(6):1036–1043
8. Cooper PR. Outcome after operative treatment of intramedullary spinal cord tumors in adults: intermediate and long-term results in 51 patients. Neurosurgery 1989;25(6):855–859
9. Cooper PR, Epstein F. Radical resection of intramedullary spinal cord tumors in adults: recent experience in 29 patients. J Neurosurg 1985; 63(4):492–499
10. Cristante L, Herrmann HD. Surgical management of intramedullary spinal cord tumors: functional outcome and sources of morbidity. Neurosurgery 1994;35(1):69–74, discussion 74–76
11. Epstein FJ, Farmer JP, Freed D. Adult intramedullary spinal cord ependymomas: the result of surgery in 38 patients. J Neurosurg 1993;79(2):204–209
12. Epstein FJ, Farmer JP, Schneider SJ. Intraoperative ultrasonography: an important surgical adjunct for intramedullary tumors. J Neurosurg 1991;74(5):729–733
13. Fornari M, Pluchino F, Solero CL, et al. Microsurgical treatment of intramedullary spinal cord tumours. Acta Neurochir Suppl (Wien) 1988;43:3–8
14. Garrido E, Stein BM. Microsurgical removal of intramedullary spinal cord tumors. Surg Neurol 1977;7(4):215–219
15. Hoshimaru M, Koyama T, Hashimoto N, Kikuchi H. Results of microsurgical treatment for intramedullary spinal cord ependymomas: analysis of 36 cases. Neurosurgery 1999;44(2):264–269
16. Knake JE, Gabrielsen TO, Chandler WF, Latack JT, Gebarski SS, Yang PJ. Real-time sonography during spinal surgery. Radiology 1984; 151(2):461–465
17. Koyanagi I, Iwasaki Y, Isu T, Abe H, Akino M, Kuroda S. Spinal cord evoked potential monitoring after spinal cord stimulation during surgery of spinal cord tumors. Neurosurgery 1993;33(3):451–459, discussion 459–460
18. Li MH, Holtås S. MR imaging of spinal intramedullary tumors. Acta Radiol 1991;32(6):505–513
19. Maiuri F, Iaconetta G, Gallicchio B, Stella L. Intraoperative sonography for spinal tumors: correlations with MR findings and surgery. J Neurosurg Sci 2000;44(3):115–122

20. McLone DG, Naidich TP. Laser resection of fifty spinal lipomas. Neurosurgery 1986;18(5):611–615

21. Miyazawa N, Hida K, Iwasaki Y, Koyanagi I, Abe H. MRI at 1.5 T of intramedullary ependymoma and classification of pattern of contrast enhancement. Neuroradiology 2000;42(11):828–832

22. Quinones-Hinojosa A, Gulati M, Lyon R, Gupta N, Yingling C. Spinal cord mapping as an adjunct for resection of intramedullary tumors: surgical technique with case illustrations. Neurosurgery 2002;51(5):1199–1206, discussion 1206–1207

23. Quiñones-Hinojosa A, Lyon R, Zada G, et al. Changes in transcranial motor evoked potentials during intramedullary spinal cord tumor resection correlate with postoperative motor function. Neurosurgery 2005;56(5):982–993, discussion 982–993

24. Rothwell CI, Jaspan T, Worthington BS, Holland IM. Gadolinium-enhanced magnetic resonance imaging of spinal tumours. Br J Radiol 1989;62(744):1067–1074

25. Sala F, Palandri G, Basso E, et al. Motor evoked potential monitoring improves outcome after surgery for intramedullary spinal cord tumors: a historical control study. Neurosurgery 2006;58(6):1129–1143, discussion 1129–1143

26. Sze G. Magnetic resonance imaging in the evaluation of spinal tumors. Cancer 1991; 67(4, Suppl)1229–1241

27. Sze G, Bravo S, Krol G. Spinal lesions: quantitative and qualitative temporal evolution of gadopentetate dimeglumine enhancement in MR imaging. Radiology 1989;170(3 Pt 1):849–856

28. Sandalcioglu IE, Gasser T, Asgari S, et al. Functional outcome after surgical treatment of intramedullary spinal cord tumors: experience with 78 patients. Spinal Cord 2005;43(1):34–41

29. Bowers DC, Weprin BE. Intramedullary spinal cord tumors. Curr Treat Options Neurol 2003;5(3):207–212

30. Clarke E, Marrett L, Kreiger N: Twenty years of cancer incidence, 1964–83. Ontario Cancer Registry 1987

31. Barker DJ, Weller RO, Garfield JS. Epidemiology of primary tumours of the brain and spinal cord: a regional survey in southern England. J Neurol Neurosurg Psychiatry 1976;39(3):290–296

32. Rawlings CE III, Giangaspero F, Burger PC, Bullard DE. Ependymomas: a clinicopathologic study. Surg Neurol 1988;29(4):271–281

33. Whitaker SJ, Bessell EM, Ashley SE, Bloom HJ, Bell BA, Brada M. Postoperative radiotherapy in the management of spinal cord ependymoma. J Neurosurg 1991;74(5):720–728

34. O'Sullivan C, Jenkin RD, Doherty MA, Hoffman HJ, Greenberg ML. Spinal cord tumors in children: long-term results of combined surgical and radiation treatment. J Neurosurg 1994;81(4):507–512

35. Epstein FJ, Farmer JP, Freed D. Adult intramedullary astrocytomas of the spinal cord. J Neurosurg 1992;77(3):355–359

36. Gori G, Nucci U. [Considerations on 60 intramedullary tumors with long-term follow-up.] G Psichiatr Neuropatol 1965;93(4):1113–1128

37. Greenwood J Jr. Intramedullary tumors of spinal cord: a follow-up study after total surgical removal. J Neurosurg 1963;20:665–668

38. Shrivastava RK, Epstein FJ, Perin NI, Post KD, Jallo GI. Intramedullary spinal cord tumors in patients older than 50 years of age: management and outcome analysis. J Neurosurg Spine 2005;2(3):249–255

39. Xu QW, Bao WM, Mao RL, Yang GY. Aggressive surgery for intramedullary tumor of cervical spinal cord. Surg Neurol 1996;46(4):322–328

40. Abdel-Wahab M, Etuk B, Palermo J, et al. Spinal cord gliomas: a multi-institutional retrospective analysis. Int J Radiat Oncol Biol Phys 2006;64(4):1060–1071

41. Hulshof MC, Menten J, Dito JJ, Dreissen JJ, van den Bergh R, González González D. Treatment results in primary intraspinal gliomas. Radiother Oncol 1993;29(3):294–300

42. Jyothirmayi R, Madhavan J, Nair MK, Rajan B. Conservative surgery and radiotherapy in the treatment of spinal cord astrocytoma. J Neurooncol 1997;33(3):205–211

43. Katoh N, Shirato H, Aoyama H, et al. Hypofractionated radiotherapy boost for dose escalation as a treatment option for high-grade spinal cord astrocytic tumor. J Neurooncol 2006;78(1):63–69

44. Nishio S, Morioka T, Fujii K, Inamura T, Fukui M. Spinal cord gliomas: management and outcome with reference to adjuvant therapy. J Clin Neurosci 2000;7(1):20–23

45. Rodrigues GB, Waldron JN, Wong CS, Laperriere NJ. A retrospective analysis of 52 cases of spinal cord glioma managed with radiation therapy. Int J Radiat Oncol Biol Phys 2000;48(3):837–842

46. Shirato H, Kamada T, Hida K, et al. The role of radiotherapy in the management of spinal cord glioma. Int J Radiat Oncol Biol Phys 1995;33(2):323–328

47. Balmaceda C. Chemotherapy for intramedullary spinal cord tumors. J Neurooncol 2000;47(3):293–307

48. Bouffet E, Amat D, Devaux Y, Desuzinges C. Chemotherapy for spinal cord astrocytoma. Med Pediatr Oncol 1997;29(6):560–562

49. Henson JW, Thornton AF, Louis DN. Spinal cord astrocytoma: response to PCV chemotherapy. Neurology 2000;54(2):518–520

50. Lowis SP, Pizer BL, Coakham H, Nelson RJ, Bouffet E. Chemotherapy for spinal cord astrocytoma: can natural history be modified? Childs Nerv Syst 1998;14(7):317–321

51. Mora J, Cruz O, Gala S, Navarro R. Successful treatment of childhood intramedullary spinal cord astrocytomas with irinotecan and cisplatin. Neuro-oncol 2007;9(1):39–46

52. Townsend N, Handler M, Fleitz J, Foreman N. Intramedullary spinal cord astrocytomas in children. Pediatr Blood Cancer 2004;43(6):629–632

53. Weiss E, Klingebiel T, Kortmann RD, Hess CF, Bamberg M. Intraspinal high-grade astrocytoma in a child—rationale for chemotherapy and more intensive radiotherapy? Childs Nerv Syst 1997;13(2): 108–112

54. Ratliff JK, Cooper PR. Cervical laminoplasty: a critical review. J Neurosurg 2003; 98(3, Suppl):230–238

55. Bell DF, Walker JL, O'Connor G, Tibshirani R. Spinal deformity after multiple-level cervical laminectomy in children. Spine (Phila Pa 1976) 1994;19(4):406–411

56. de Jonge T, Slullitel H, Dubousset J, Miladi L, Wicart P, Illés T. Late-onset spinal deformities in children treated by laminectomy and radiation therapy for malignant tumours. Eur Spine J 2005; 14(8):765–771

57. Fraser RD, Paterson DC, Simpson DA. Orthopaedic aspects of spinal tumors in children. J Bone Joint Surg Br 1977;59(2):143–151

58. Haft H, Ransohoff J, Carter S. Spinal cord tumors in children. Pediatrics 1959;23(6):1152–1159

59. Katsumi Y, Honma T, Nakamura T. Analysis of cervical instability resulting from laminectomies for removal of spinal cord tumor. Spine (Phila 1976) 1989;14(11):1171–1176

60. Lonstein JE. Post-laminectomy kyphosis. Clin Orthop Relat Res 1977;128:93–100

61. Matson DD, Tachdjian MO. Intraspinal tumors in infants and children: review of 115 cases. Postgrad Med 1963;34:279–285

62. Mikawa Y, Shikata J, Yamamuro T. Spinal deformity and instability after multilevel cervical laminectomy. Spine (Phila 1976) 1987;12(1):6–11

63. Raynor RB, Pugh J, Shapiro I. Cervical facetectomy and its effect on spine strength. J Neurosurg 1985;63(2):278–282

64. Tachdjian MO, Matson DD. Orthopaedic aspects of intraspinal tumors in infants and children. J Bone Joint Surg Am 1965;47:223–248

65. Yao KC, McGirt MJ, Chaichana KL, Constantini S, Jallo GI. Risk factors for progressive spinal deformity following resection of intramedullary spinal cord tumors in children: an analysis of 161 consecutive cases. J Neurosurg 2007;107(6, Suppl):463–468

66. Yasuoka S, Peterson HA, MacCarty CS. Incidence of spinal column deformity after multilevel laminectomy in children and adults. J Neurosurg 1982;57(4):441–445

67. Zdeblick TA, Abitbol JJ, Kunz DN, McCabe RP, Garfin S. Cervical stability after sequential capsule resection. Spine (Phila 1976) 1993; 18(14):2005–2008

68. Fassett DR, Clark R, Brockmeyer DL, Schmidt MH. Cervical spine deformity associated with resection of spinal cord tumors. Neurosurg Focus 2006;20(2):E2

69. Epstein JA. The surgical management of cervical spinal stenosis, spondylosis, and myeloradiculopathy by means of the posterior approach. Spine (Phila 1976) 1988;13(7):864–869

70. Sim FH, Svien HJ, Bickel WH, Janes JM. Swan-neck deformity following extensive cervical laminectomy: a review of twenty-one cases. J Bone Joint Surg Am 1974;56(3):564–580

71. Papagelopoulos PJ, Peterson HA, Ebersold MJ, Emmanuel PR, Choudhury SN, Quast LM. Spinal column deformity and instability after lumbar or thoracolumbar laminectomy for intraspinal tumors in children and young adults. Spine (Phila 1976) 1997; 22(4): 442–451

72. Yeh JS, Sgouros S, Walsh AR, Hockley AD. Spinal sagittal malalignment following surgery for primary intramedullary tumours in children. Pediatr Neurosurg 2001;35(6):318–324

73. Av E, Ranzi E. Über die chirurgische Behandlung der Hirn- und Rückenmarkstumoren. Arch Klin Chir 1913;102:309–468

74. Elsberg CA, Beer E. The operability of intramedullary tumors of the spinal cord: a report of two operations with remarks upon the extrusion of intraspinal tumors. Am J Med Sci 1911;142:636–647

75. Wood EH, Berne AS, Taveras JM. The value of radiation therapy in the management of intrinsic tumors of the spinal cord. Radiology 1954;63(1):11–24

76. Greenwood J Jr. Intramedullary tumor of the spinal cord: a follow-up study after total surgical removal. J Neurosurg 1963;20: 665–668

77. Greenwood J Jr. Surgical removal of intramedullary tumors. J Neurosurg 1967;26(2):276–282

78. Malis LI. Intramedullary spinal cord tumors. Clin Neurosurg 1978;25:512–539

79. Stein BM. Surgery of intramedullary spinal cord tumors. Clin Neurosurg 1979;26:529–542

80. Fischer G, Mansuy L. Total removal of intramedullary ependymomas: follow-up study of 16 cases. Surg Neurol 1980;14(4):243–249

81. Guidetti B, Mercuri S, Vagnozzi R. Long-term results of the surgical treatment of 129 intramedullary spinal gliomas. J Neurosurg 1981;54(3):323–330

82. Epstein FJ, Epstein N. Surgical treatment of spinal cord astrocytomas of childhood. A series of 19 patients. J Neurosurg 1982; 57(5): 685–689

83. Brotchi J, Dewitte O, Levivier M, et al. A survey of 65 tumors within the spinal cord: surgical results and the importance of preoperative magnetic resonance imaging. Neurosurgery 1991;29(5): 651–656, discussion 656–657

84. Constantini S, Houten J, Miller DC, et al. Intramedullary spinal cord tumors in children under the age of 3 years. J Neurosurg 1996; 85(6):1036–1043

85. Constantini S, Miller DC, Allen JC, Rorke LB, Freed D, Epstein FJ. Radical excision of intramedullary spinal cord tumors: surgical morbidity and long-term follow-up evaluation in 164 children and young adults. J Neurosurg 2000;93(2, Suppl):183–193

86. Morota N, Deletis V, Constantini S, Kofler M, Cohen H, Epstein FJ. The role of motor evoked potentials during surgery for intramedullary spinal cord tumors. Neurosurgery 1997;41(6):1327–1336

87. Kothbauer KF, Deletis V, Epstein FJ. Intraoperative spinal cord monitoring for intramedullary surgery: an essential adjunct. Pediatr Neurosurg 1997;26(5):247–254

88. Kothbauer KF, Deletis V, Epstein FJ. Motor-evoked potential monitoring for intramedullary spinal cord tumor surgery: correlation of clinical and neurophysiological data in a series of 100 consecutive procedures. Neurosurg Focus 1998;4(5):e1

89. Kothbauer KF. Motor evoked potential monitoring for intramedullary spinal cord tumor surgery. In: Deletis V, Shils J, eds. Neurophysiology in Neurosurgery. Vol 1. Amsterdam: Academic Press, Elsevier Science; 2002:73–92

90. O'Sullivan C, Jenkin RD, Doherty MA, Hoffman HJ, Greenberg ML. Spinal cord tumors in children: long-term results of combined surgical and radiation treatment. J Neurosurg 1994;81(4):507–512

91. Houten JK, Weiner HL. Pediatric intramedullary spinal cord tumors: special considerations. J Neurooncol 2000;47(3):225–230

92. Allen JC, Aviner S, Yates AJ, et al; Children's Cancer Group. Treatment of high-grade spinal cord astrocytoma of childhood with "8-in-1" chemotherapy and radiotherapy: a pilot study of CCG-945. J Neurosurg 1998;88(2):215–220

93. Chamoun RB, Alaraj AM, Al Kutoubi AO, Abboud MR, Haddad GF. Role of temozolomide in spinal cord low grade astrocytomas: results in two paediatric patients. Acta Neurochir (Wien) 2006;148(2):175–179, discussion 180

94. Stupp R, Mason WP, van den Bent MJ, et al; European Organisation for Research and Treatment of Cancer Brain Tumor and Radiotherapy Groups; National Cancer Institute of Canada Clinical Trials Group. Radiotherapy plus concomitant and adjuvant temozolomide for glioblastoma. N Engl J Med 2005;352(10):987–996

95. Yamamoto Y, Raffel C. Spinal extradural neoplasms and intradural extramedullary neoplasms. In: Albright AL, Pollack IF, Adelson PD, eds. Principles and Practice of Pediatric Neurosurgery. New York: Thieme Medical Publishers; 1999:685–696

96. Roonprapunt C, Silvera VM, Setton A, Freed D, Epstein FJ, Jallo GI. Surgical management of isolated hemangioblastomas of the spinal cord. Neurosurgery 2001;49(2):321–327, discussion 327–328

97. Deutsch H, Jallo GI, Faktorovich A, Epstein F. Spinal intramedullary cavernoma: clinical presentation and surgical outcome. J Neurosurg 2000;93(1, Suppl):65–70

98. Lang FF, Epstein FJ, Ransohoff J, et al. Central nervous system gangliogliomas: 2. Clinical outcome. J Neurosurg 1993;79(6):867–873

99. McCormick PC, Torres R, Post KD, Stein BM. Intramedullary ependymoma of the spinal cord. J Neurosurg 1990;72(4):523–532

100. Epstein FJ, Farmer J-P, Freed D. Adult intramedullary spinal cord ependymomas: the result of surgery in 38 patients. J Neurosurg 1993;79(2):204–209

101. DeSousa AL, Kalsbeck JE, Mealey J Jr, Campbell RL, Hockey A. Intraspinal tumors in children: a review of 81 cases. J Neurosurg 1979;51(4):437–445

102. Bagley CA, Kothbauer KF, Wilson S, Bookland MJ, Epstein FJ, Jallo GI. Resection of myxopapillary ependymomas in children. J Neurosurg 2007;106(4, Suppl):261–267

103. Schweitzer JS, Batzdorf U. Ependymoma of the cauda equina region: diagnosis, treatment, and outcome in 15 patients. Neurosurgery 1992;30(2):202–207

104. Rezai AR, Woo HH, Lee M, Cohen H, Zagzag D, Epstein FJ. Disseminated ependymomas of the central nervous system. J Neurosurg 1996;85(4):618–624

105. Lonser RR, Weil RJ, Wanebo JE, DeVroom HL, Oldfield EH, Oldfield MD. Surgical management of spinal cord hemangioblastomas in patients with von Hippel-Lindau disease. J Neurosurg 2003;98(1): 106–116

106. Wanebo JE, Lonser RR, Glenn GM, Oldfield EH. The natural history of hemangioblastomas of the central nervous system in patients with von Hippel-Lindau disease. J Neurosurg 2003;98(1):82–94

107. Flamm ES, Ransohoff JP, Wuchinich D, Broadwin A. Preliminary experience with ultrasonic aspiration in neurosurgery. Neurosurgery 1978;2(3):240–245

108. Epstein FJ, Farmer J-P. Trends in surgery: laser surgery, use of the cavitron, and debulking surgery. Neurol Clin 1991;9(2):307–315

109. Jallo GI, Kothbauer KF, Epstein FJ. Contact laser microsurgery. Childs Nerv Syst 2002;18(6-7):333–336

110. Jallo GI, Kothbauer KF, Epstein FJ. Intrinsic spinal cord tumor resection. Neurosurgery 2001;49(5):1124–1128

111. Brotchi J. Intrinsic spinal cord tumor resection. Neurosurgery 2002;50(5):1059–1063

112. Raimondi AJ, Gutierrez FA, Di Rocco C. Laminotomy and total reconstruction of the posterior spinal arch for spinal canal surgery in childhood. J Neurosurg 1976;45(5):555–560

113. Dohrmann GJ, Rubin JM. Intraoperative ultrasound imaging of the spinal cord: syringomyelia, cysts, and tumors—a preliminary report. Surg Neurol 1982;18(6):395–399

114. Epstein FJ, Ozek M. The plated bayonet: a new instrument to facilitate surgery for intra-axial neoplasms of the spinal cord and brain stem. Technical note. J Neurosurg 1993;78(3):505–507

115. Epstein FJ, Farmer J-P, Freed D. Adult intramedullary astrocytomas of the spinal cord. J Neurosurg 1992;77(3):355–359

116. Kothbauer KF. Intraoperative neurophysiological monitoring for spinal cord surgery. Touch Briefings 2008;3:56–58

117. Nash CL Jr, Lorig RA, Schatzinger LA, Brown RH. Spinal cord monitoring during operative treatment of the spine. Clin Orthop Relat Res 1977;126(126):100–105

118. Ginsburg HH, Shetter AG, Raudzens PA. Postoperative paraplegia with preserved intraoperative somatosensory evoked potentials: case report. J Neurosurg 1985;63(2):296–300

119. Jones SJ, Buonamassa S, Crockard HA. Two cases of quadriparesis following anterior cervical discectomy, with normal perioperative somatosensory evoked potentials. J Neurol Neurosurg Psychiatry 2003;74(2):273–276

120. Patton HD, Amassian VE. Single and multiple-unit analysis of cortical stage of pyramidal tract activation. J Neurophysiol 1954; 17(4):345–363

121. Boyd SG, Rothwell JC, Cowan JMA, et al. A method of monitoring function in corticospinal pathways during scoliosis surgery with a note on motor conduction velocities. J Neurol Neurosurg Psychiatry 1986;49(3):251–257

122. Katayama Y, Tsubokawa T, Maejima S, Hirayama T, Yamamoto T. Corticospinal direct response in humans: identification of the

123. Katayama Y, Tsubokawa T, Yamamoto T, Hirayama T, Maejima S. Separation of upper and lower extremity components of the corticospinal mep (D-wave) recorded at the cervical level. In: Jones SJ, Boyd S, Hetreed M, Smith NJ, eds. Handbook of Spinal Cord Monitoring. Dordrecht, the Netherlands: Kluwer Academic Publishers; 1994:312–320

124. Burke D, Hicks RG, Stephen JPH. Corticospinal volleys evoked by anodal and cathodal stimulation of the human motor cortex. J Physiol 1990;425:283–299

125. Taniguchi M, Cedzich C, Schramm J. Modification of cortical stimulation for motor evoked potentials under general anesthesia: technical description. Neurosurgery 1993;32(2):219–226

126. Jones SJ, Harrison R, Koh KF, Mendoza N, Crockard HA. Motor evoked potential monitoring during spinal surgery: responses of distal limb muscles to transcranial cortical stimulation with pulse trains. Electroencephalogr Clin Neurophysiol 1996;100(5):375–383

127. Pechstein U, Cedzich C, Nadstawek J, Schramm J. Transcranial high-frequency repetitive electrical stimulation for recording myogenic motor evoked potentials with the patient under general anesthesia. Neurosurgery 1996;39(2):335–343, discussion 343–344

128. Katayama Y, Tsubokawa T, Yamamoto T, Hirayama T, Maejima S. Changes in the corticospinal MEP (D wave) during microsurgical removal of intramedullary spinal cord tumours: experience in 16 cases. In: Jones SJ, Boyd S, Hetreed M, Smith NJ; eds. Handbook of Spinal Cord Monitoring. Dordrecht, the Netherlands: Kluwer Academic Publishers; 1994:321–326

129. Calancie B, Harris W, Broton JG, Alexeeva N, Green BA. "Threshold-level" multipulse transcranial electrical stimulation of motor cortex for intraoperative monitoring of spinal motor tracts: description of method and comparison to somatosensory evoked potential monitoring. J Neurosurg 1998;88(3):457–470

130. Sala F, Palandri G, Basso E, et al. Motor evoked potential monitoring improves outcome after surgery for intramedullary spinal cord tumors: a historical control study. Neurosurgery 2006;58(6): 1129–1143, discussion 1129–1143

131. McGirt MJ, Chaichana KL, Atiba A, Attenello F, Yao KC, Jallo GI. Resection of intramedullary spinal cord tumors in children: assessment of long-term motor and sensory deficits. J Neurosurg Pediatr 2008;1(1):63–67

132. Reimer R, Onofrio BM. Astrocytomas of the spinal cord in children and adolescents. J Neurosurg 1985;63(5):669–675

133. Winter RB, Hall JE. Kyphosis in childhood and adolescence. Spine (Phila 1976) 1978;3(4):285–308

134. Yasuoka S, Peterson HA, MacCarty CS. Incidence of spinal column deformity after multilevel laminectomy in children and adults. J Neurosurg 1982;57(4):441–445

135. McGirt MJ, Chaichana KL, Attenello F, et al. Spinal deformity after resection of cervical intramedullary spinal cord tumors in children. Childs Nerv Syst 2008;24(6):735–739

136. Woodworth GF, Chaichana KL, McGirt MJ, et al. Predictors of ambulatory function after surgical resection of intramedullary spinal cord tumors. Neurosurgery 2007;61(1):99–105, discussion 105–106

137. Pennant WA, Sciubba DM, Noggle JC, Tyler BM, Tamargo RJ, Jallo GI. Microsurgical removal of intramedullary spinal cord gliomas in a rat spinal cord decreases onset to paresis, an animal model for

intramedullary tumor treatment. Childs Nerv Syst 2008;24(8): 901–907

138. Minehan KJ, Shaw EG, Scheithauer BW, Davis DL, Onofrio BM. Spinal cord astrocytoma: pathological and treatment considerations. J Neurosurg 1995;83(4):590–595

139. Houten JK, Cooper PR. Spinal cord astrocytomas: presentation, management and outcome. J Neurooncol 2000;47(3):219–224

140. Sundaresan N, Gutierrez FA, Larsen MB. Radiation myelopathy in children. Ann Neurol 1978;4(1):47–50

141. Katzman H, Waugh T, Berdon W. Skeletal changes following irradiation of childhood tumors. J Bone Joint Surg Am 1969;51(5):825–842

142. Riseborough EJ, Grabias SL, Burton RI, Jaffe N. Skeletal alterations following irradiation for Wilms' tumor: with particular reference to scoliosis and kyphosis. J Bone Joint Surg Am 1976;58(4): 526–536

143. Mayfield JK, Riseborough EJ, Jaffe N, Nehme ME. Spinal deformity in children treated for neuroblastoma. J Bone Joint Surg Am 1981; 63(2):183–193

19 Spasticity

♦ Intrathecal Baclofen

A. Leland Albright

The pairing of lumbodorsal rhizotomy (LDR) and intrathecal baclofen (ITB) in this book might suggest that the two treatment modalities were competing for the same group of children. In reality, they are complementary; there are almost no children for whom LDR and ITB are equally appropriate. LDR is an excellent treatment for children with spastic diplegia or with spastic quadriparesis but little spasticity in the arms. It can be used effectively into the midteens and occasionally thereafter if patients have adequate underlying strength, and their associated contractures are mild.

ITB is indicated in very different circumstances. Although there are few controversies about patient selection for ITB, controversies exist about surgical techniques and about ITB outcomes—such as the relationship between ITB and seizures or the relationship between ITB and the development of scoliosis—and will be discussed here.

Indications for Intrathecal Baclofen in Spasticity

Spastic Diplegia

ITB is infrequently indicated for children with spastic diplegia, but it is indicated for them in three circumstances.

1. It is appropriate for ambulatory children with relatively weak lower extremity muscles but moderate or severe spasticity (3 to 4 on the 5-point Ashworth scale) that is impeding gait and causing progressive contractures, since LDR in these children may result in such hypotonia that they are unable to walk because of their underlying weakness.
2. ITB is appropriate for older individuals (older than 16 years, particularly those in their 20s and 30s) with spastic diplegia whose gait is deteriorating as a result of stiffness or pain because they have a harder time learning better gait patterns after LDR than do young children. ITB is helpful in these patients because their

spasticity can be gradually decreased, with baclofen doses increasing as muscles stretch and strengthen with physical therapy.
3. Spastic diplegia in children with hereditary spastic paraparesis (HSP) can be effectively treated with ITB.[1] In children with HSP, spasticity is typically reduced, although gait is not always better because of their associated proximal leg weakness. In my experience, an LDR in one child with HSP improved spasticity for 6 weeks, at which point it returned to the prerhizotomy level.

Spastic Quadriparesis

Spastic quadriparesis is the classic indication for ITB. It is related to cerebral palsy in the majority of cases but may be secondary to severe head injuries. Regardless of etiology, ITB appears to improve spastic quadriparesis.[2,3] Although LDR has been shown to decrease spasticity in the upper extremities, that decrease is mild and considerably less than can be obtained with ITB.[4] Most children who receive ITB for spastic quadriparesis have mean scores of 3 on the 5-point Ashworth scale in both the upper and lower extremities and have been ineffectively treated by oral medications and botulinum toxin injections.

Spastic Hemiparesis

Some clinicians predicted that the use of ITB in spastic hemiparesis would be contraindicated because of concern that the normal side would become hypotonic. In my experience, including with one of the first children to receive a pump in 1988, that is not so: spasticity in the affected side is reduced, and tone in the normal side seems to be unaffected. In patients with spastic hemiparesis, spasticity is usually decreased in the upper extremity, often resulting in improved positioning and functioning of the affected arm and hand.

Mixed Spasticity and Dystonia

Children with mixed spasticity and dystonia in the lower extremities should not be treated with LDR if there is a significant component of dystonia, as it is unaffected by dorsal rhizotomies (although it may be improved by ventral rhizotomies). Conversely, ITB has been shown to improve both spasticity and dystonia, whether in the lower extremities or in both the upper and lower extremities.[5]

Patient Selection

ITB is usually offered to children who have failed oral medications (e.g., baclofen, tizanidine, and dantrolene), although sometimes children present with such severe generalized spasticity that trials of oral medications seem futile, and a decision is made to proceed directly to ITB. There is no controversy about the fact that the response to oral baclofen correlates poorly with the response to ITB, as so little oral baclofen enters the cerebrospinal fluid (CSF).

Before recommending ITB, it is essential to define the treatment goals and to have the parents concur with those goals. Common goals include (1) increasing comfort, (2) increasing ease of care, (3) improving function, and (4) decreasing the development of musculoskeletal contractures. It has been said that "illusion is the parent of disillusion," and if treatment expectations are inappropriate, disappointment is almost invariable.

The reliability of the caregiver to return at appropriate intervals for pump refills should be considered before recommending a pump. We occasionally decide not to put a pump into a child who would probably benefit from it because the parents or caregivers seem to be unreliable. In such cases, we sometimes order a physical therapy regimen twice a week for 6 to 8 weeks, partly to improve the child's condition prior to surgery, but more so to evaluate the consistency with which the child is brought to therapy.

Screening Trials

There is considerable controversy about the necessity of screening trials before a pump is inserted. When the use of ITB began some 20 years ago, bolus injections were always given, primarily to determine if intrathecal baclofen significantly decreased lower extremity spasticity. Since then, thousands of screening injections have been given, and we have learned that spasticity virtually always responds, whether of spinal or cerebral origin. Children who are thought not to respond usually have dystonia or athetosis rather than spasticity, although occasionally a dose higher than the usual 50 μg is needed to cause a 1-point decrease in mean Ashworth score in the lower extremity.

Bolus screening trials are currently advocated in several circumstances: (1) centers that are just starting ITB therapy

that have minimal experience with the changes caused by ITB, (2) individual cases where parents insist on demonstrating that a bolus dose decreases tone before submitting their child to a pump, and (3) cases in which a screening dose is mandated by insurance companies. I used screening doses in the first 200 or so spasticity cases but have not used them in patients with spasticity in probably 10 years.

If a screening bolus—usually 50 μg—is given, the sole purpose of doing the trial is to confirm that spasticity in the lower extremities is decreased. The purpose is not to determine if function, particularly ambulation, is improved. Some investigators have inserted a lumbar catheter and used a continuous baclofen infusion in an attempt to determine if ambulation is improved. That technique provides more information about how ambulation might be affected, but it cannot determine the effects that will be observed during chronic infusion and dose titration over several months.

Timing of Pump Insertion

Given the size of the pumps that are presently available, there are no longer any size or age limitations on pump insertion. The Medtronic SynchroMed 20 mL pump (Medtronic Inc., Minneapolis, Minnesota) is small enough to insert into an infant, although the umbilicus may need to be mobilized to obtain adequate space medially. Realistically, however, pumps are often not needed to treat spasticity in children younger than 4 years.

ITB is indicated whenever it is clear that nonsurgical management is inadequate, ideally before the development of significant contractures. There is some controversy about the timing of pump insertion in children with posttraumatic spasticity because of a previous recommendation that ITB be delayed for 1 year after the head injury. That recommendation is inappropriate, however. For children with severe posttraumatic spasticity, by 1 year (in fact, often by 6 weeks after injury) spasticity usually has resulted in contractures at several sites, and the children require multilevel orthopedic surgery. In my opinion and the opinion of others, spasticity that develops rapidly after traumatic brain injury should be treated with dantrolene, botulinum toxin injections, and ankle casting, but if definite improvement is not seen within 1 month, ITB should be used.[6] A child may improve over the first year after TBI and not require ITB indefinitely. If that is the case, the child at 1 year will have fewer contractures than would have developed otherwise, and the pump can be turned down or removed.

Surgical Techniques

Techniques for pump and catheter insertion were reviewed by Albright et al.[7] Pumps can be inserted either above or below the abdominal fascia. In young and thin patients, the subfascial position is preferable because it is associated with a considerably better cosmetic appearance and with less tension on the healing skin edges than if the pump is inserted above the fascia. Pumps with a 40 mL reservoir can usually be implanted in children weighing 40 lb or more; smaller children usually receive pumps with a 20 mL reservoir. Pumps with suture eyelets allow the pump to be secured to muscle or fascia more easily than the Dacron pouches that were previously used. Removal of Dacron pouches is difficult and results in the development of a substantial seroma at that site for days afterward.

There is controversy over the site where the intrathecal catheter tip should be positioned. For patients with spastic diplegia, there is uniform agreement that the tip should be positioned as it was in the earliest reports of ITB for spastic paraplegia of spinal cord origin: at the T10–T12 region, near the lumbar enlargement of the spinal cord, the site where baclofen will work in these patients. For patients with spastic quadriparesis, catheter tips are currently positioned in either the midthoracic region or the cervicothoracic junction. Grabb et al reported better reduction of spasticity in the upper extremities if the catheter was positioned in the midthoracic region rather than in the lower thoracic region, thinking that the higher catheter tip would result in a higher baclofen concentration in the cervicothoracic CSF.[8] I position the tip at C5–T2 for patients with spastic quadriparesis and have observed better upper extremity effects (e.g., decreased tone and increased range of motion) with no increase in side effects. Occasionally, a patient with a cervical catheter will demonstrate less effect in the lower extremities than desired.

If the child is fused or is expected to need a spine fusion, it is easier to tunnel the catheter to the cervical region and insert it into the thecal sac via a small laminectomy than to try to insert it by drilling through the lumbar fusion (**Fig. 19.1**).

When replacing an intrathecal catheter, there is debate about the management of the initial catheter. Surgical options include removing the catheter or tying it off and leaving it in place. In my experience, removal is often followed by CSF tracking along the catheter and accumulating around the new pump, sometimes with leakage through the incision. Because of that, it is probably safer to tie off the catheter and leave it in place.

Patient Management

After pump insertion, patients are typically kept at flat bed rest for 48 hours in an attempt to prevent CSF leaks around the intrathecal catheter. I know of no data showing that bed rest decreases that risk, but it seems intuitively to make sense. Some neurosurgeons, however, are implanting pumps in adults on an outpatient surgery basis, a policy that seems less appropriate for pediatric patients. Pumps are turned on on the day of surgery and programmed to infuse a priming bolus to fill the catheter, then to infuse

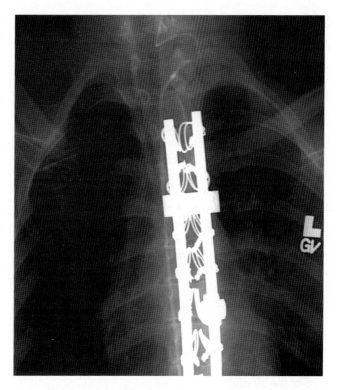

Fig. 19.1 Anteroposterior radiograph demonstrating a catheter tunneled subcutaneously cephalad and inserted into the cervical thecal sac via a small laminectomy.

baclofen, usually at a constant rate of 100 μg/day when treating spasticity. Doses are increased daily as needed. Because the half-life of intrathecal baclofen is ~4 to 5 hours, and 5 half-lives are needed to reach steady state, doses are increased only once a day. Increases of 10 to 20% per day are recommended, but larger doses may be indicated, depending on patient size, severity of spasticity, and response to the initial infusion. Baclofen is infused in a continuous mode in nearly all patients with spasticity, although additional boluses can be programmed to treat spasticity that is more severe at certain times of the day. Complex dosing can be used if there is inadequate response to higher doses (e.g., 600 μg/day), but there are no data to document better results than seen with continuous infusions.

There is controversy about the use of compounded baclofen solutions for ITB. Baclofen is supplied commercially in either 500 μg/mL or 2000 μg/mL solutions. Some pharmacists have compounded baclofen in higher concentrations (e.g., 4000 μg/mL) in an attempt to decrease the frequency of pump refills or to improve patient response. The solubility of baclofen at those concentrations is unreliable; precipitation may occur (within the pump), and high concentrations invalidate the pump warranty. Most patients who require high doses for spasticity (e.g., > 800 μg/day) either have a suboptimally functioning system or have associated dystonia that requires higher ITB doses.

Outcomes

Two studies have provided class I evidence of the effect of ITB on spasticity in bolus screening trials.[9,10] Numerous other studies, mostly providing Class II to IV evidence, have documented improved spasticity in the lower and upper extremities after chronic ITB administration.[3]

In 2003, we published the results of a prospective, open-label follow-up study of long-term ITB infusion in 68 patients, 54 with cerebral palsy.[11] Their mean age at pump implantation was 12.6 years, and the mean follow-up was 70 months (range 14.6–133.4 months). Spasticity was significantly decreased in both the upper and lower extremities ($p < .005$) and remained decreased for up to 10 years.

ITB has been associated with improved function. Krach et al evaluated Gross Motor Function Measure scores in 31 patients, ages 4 to 29 years, at baseline and 12 months after ITB therapy and found improved scores in all patients in all dimensions except running and walking.[12] Awaad et al performed the Pediatric Evaluation of Disability Index (PEDI) in 39 patients receiving ITB therapy, in a prospective, open-label 18-month study.[13] They observed improved self-case, improved social function, and less reliance on caregivers in 29 of the 39 subjects.

The effects of ITB on gait were reported by Gerszten et al, who graded ambulation in four functional levels (community, household, nonfunctional, and nonambulatory) in 24 patients who were partially ambulatory pre-ITB.[14] Ambulation improved by one level in 9, was unchanged in 12, and worsened in 3.

The relationship between ITB and seizures is controversial. Although increased seizure frequency has been reported after the administration of oral baclofen, there are few reports that ITB increases seizure frequency. In perhaps the largest series addressing that issue, Buonaguro et al evaluated the effects of ITB on seizures in 150 children.[15] Before ITB, 40% of the children had seizures; after ITB, their seizures decreased in 13% and increased in 2%. Of the 60% of children with no seizures before ITB, only one child developed seizures after ITB.

The effects of ITB on musculoskeletal deformities are less clear. In 1996, we reported that ITB appeared to reduce the need for subsequent orthopedic surgery in 40 subjects who were evaluated by an orthopedist before and after pump insertion, with a mean follow-up period of 53 months.[16] The effects of ITB on hip migration were evaluated by Krach et al in 33 patients whose ages ranged from 4 to 31 years. Postoperatively, the hip migration index was unchanged in 90% in the year after ITB.[17] The question about the relationship between ITB and scoliosis is controversial. Sansone et al observed rapid progression of scoliosis in four children after ITB, but in a substantially larger series of 80 patients with gross motor function classification system (GMFCS) level IV or V whose mean age was 11 years, no patient had rapid progression of scoliosis in the year after ITB therapy.[18,19]

Conclusion

LDR and ITB are excellent treatments for distinctly different clinical indications—in general, LDR for spastic diplegia and ITB for spastic quadriparesis. Relatively good data indicate that ITB decreases spasticity significantly in the upper and lower extremities. Moderately reliable data indicate that ITB improves function, quality of life, and caregiver burden. Controversy about the effect of ITB on scoliosis is related to the paucity of good data about the issue.

◆ Selective Dorsal Rhizotomy

Richard C. E. Anderson, Christopher E. Mandigo, and David W. Pincus

The treatment of childhood spasticity remains a difficult problem for both health care providers and patients.[20] Cerebral palsy is the most common cause of spasticity and physical disability in children. It defines a range of nonprogressive syndromes of posture and motor impairment that results from an insult to the developing central nervous system (CNS) either in utero or within the first 2 years of life.[21] The prevalence of cerebral palsy is not known, but it is estimated at ~2 per 1000 children, and its incidence may be increasing due to advances in neonatal intensive care units and improved survival of low birth weight infants.[22] Common features of cerebral palsy include movement disorders, muscle weakness, ataxia, rigidity, and spasticity.

Spasticity is defined as a velocity-dependent increased resistance to passive muscle stretch, or alternatively, as inappropriate involuntary muscle activity associated with upper motor neuron paralysis.[23,24] It is a hallmark of cerebral palsy, but it can occur with other genetic and metabolic diseases that cause dysfunction or damage to the developing CNS. Spasticity is demonstrated in children as increased muscle tone, hyperactive deep tendon reflexes, persistent primitive reflexes, and difficulty with normal motor skills. Spasticity inhibits effective use of motor control and strength and can lead to progressive musculoskeletal complications, such as joint and muscular contractures, bony deformation, and joint subluxation or dislocation.[25] Proper treatment for spasticity can halt progression of contractures or deformity and often can return some function to affected limbs. Both prospective and retrospective studies of children treated for spasticity have demonstrated improved ease of caregiving, decreased pain, and increased quality of life.[26]

Spasticity in children can result from any disease process that affects the upper motor neuron within the CNS. Injury to the upper motor neuron will decrease cortical input to the descending reticulospinal and corticospinal tracts, which causes weakness, loss of motor control, and reduction in the number of voluntarily active motor units. The reduction of these descending tracts removes the normal inhibition of the reflex arcs within the gray matter of the spinal cord, leading to a hyperactive reflex arc and spasticity. In addition to cerebral palsy, spasticity may result from any injury to the brain or spinal cord, including trauma, infection, immunological disorders, and neurodegenerative disease.

The diagnosis of spasticity requires a complete history and physical examination, with ancillary testing as needed. The history should inquire about possible gestational and perinatal events, as well as motor and cognitive development. The physical exam should focus on motor power, muscle tone, active and passive range of motion of joints, sensation, deep tendon reflexes, station (pelvis and leg alignment while standing), presence of limb deformity, spinal alignment, and extent of movement disorders. Ancillary testing usually includes imaging studies, particularly magnetic resonance imaging to evaluate for evidence of hemorrhage, hydrocephalus, or structural abnormalities of the CNS. Spasticity is most commonly quantified by the Ashworth spasticity scale (**Table 19.1**)[27,28]

Management of Spasticity

Spasticity treatment involves multiple modalities, including observation, physical and occupational therapy, orthotics, oral medicines, intramuscular injections, and both neurosurgical and orthopedic surgery. A combination of methods is typically employed to synergistically increase the beneficial effects of each strategy. A multidisciplinary team, including pediatricians, physical and occupational therapists, neurologists, orthotists, orthopedic surgeons, neurologic surgeons, and other health care professionals, is best suited to treat children with spasticity, and a specialized

spasticity clinic is ideal. Therapy should be guided by the clinical scenario and specifically targeted at treating pain, increased tone, muscle contractures, joint deformities, and abnormal motor control.

Spasticity should be addressed at an early age to prevent permanent contractures, joint subluxation, dislocation, and bony deformity. In general, young children generally respond well to physiotherapy, orthotics, intramuscular injections, and neurosurgical procedures. Older children will benefit from these therapies as well, but they may also need orthopedic surgery to address musculoskeletal deformity. An approach directed by the location and severity of the spasticity is used to identify the appropriate therapeutic intervention. Treatment should be directed toward achieving realistic goals determined in concert with caregivers and ideally should be monitored by the use of clearly defined outcome measures.[26]

Nonpharmacological Therapy

Physical and occupational therapy, orthotics, and casting are just a few of the nonpharmacological therapies employed to improve joint range of motion, strengthen muscles, inhibit spastic agonist muscles, and assist with motor development. There is a paucity of evidence-based information addressing these therapies for the treatment of spasticity, largely because outcome measures are commonly used that have not been validated or may not be functionally relevant.[29] However, decades of clinical experience support their use for maximizing the benefit of medical and surgical intervention.

Oral Medications

Oral medications are often used to reduce spasticity. The most common are baclofen, diazepam, dantrolene, and tizanidine (**Table 19.2**). These have different mechanisms of action, with the common goal of reducing spasticity. Additional agents under investigation include cannabinoids, gabapentin, and 4-aminopyridine. Although improvements in clinical measures of spasticity have been noted with several of these medications, few have demonstrated significant functional benefit. Frequently, negative side effects are reached before a clinically significant effect of the medication can be obtained. Antispasmodic medications are useful adjuncts to more invasive therapies and physiotherapy.[30]

Intramuscular Injections

Although not currently approved by the U.S. Food and Drug Administration for spasticity, botulinum toxin has been used clinically since 1988 to treat spasticity associated with cerebral palsy. When botulinum toxin is injected into spastic muscle tissue, it acts at the neuromuscular junction to inhibit the release of acetylcholine and balance muscle

Table 19.1 Ashworth Scale of Muscle Tone

1	No increase in tone
2	Slight increase in tone; "catch" when limb is moved
3	Marked increase in tone; passive movements difficult
4	Considerable increase in tone; passive movements difficult
5	Affected part rigid in flexion or extension

Table 19.2 Oral Medications Used in the Treatment of Spasticity

Medication	Mechanism of Action	Half-Life (Hrs)	Initial Dosage	Maintenance	Side Effects
Baclofen (Lioresal)	GABA-β agonist	3–4	2.5–10 mg/day	20–90 mg/day t.i.d.	Drowsiness, ataxia, confusion
Diazepam (Valium)	Benzodiazepine receptor agonist	36	0.1–0.2 mg/kg/day	0.1–0.8 mg/kg/day t.i.d.	Lethargy, tolerance
Dantrolene (Dantrium)	Impedes Ca²⁺ influx into muscle SR	3–9	0.5–1.0 mg/kg/day	12 mg/kg/day q.i.d.	Weakness, diarrhea, rash, liver problems
Tizanidine (Zanaflex)	Alpha-2 adrenergic agent; inhibits aspartate output	2–3	4–8 mg/day	8–24 mg/day q.i.d.	Sedation, dizziness, hypotension

Abbreviations: GABA, γ-aminobutyric acid; q.i.d., four times a day; SR, sarcoplasmic reticulum; t.i.d., three times a day.

forces across the joint.[31] It also acts locally, so it is not effective in reducing global spasticity. The general indications for botulinum toxin are temporary management of focal spasticity and evaluation of the effects of denervating a spastic muscle. Although specific timing varies, the effects of botulinum toxin generally begin after 1 to 3 days, peak around 21 days, and usually have little effect after 3 to 6 months. The dose varies according to the muscle size and formulation of the toxin, but in general, a dose of 2 to 6 U per kilogram of body weight is used.[32] Botulinum toxin can be injected into spastic muscles with or without the use of electromyogram (EMG) guidance. There are several randomized clinical trials that have demonstrated the efficacy and safety of botulinum toxin injections.[33–36] These trials have shown a significant reduction in spasticity and improved function in both lower and upper extremities. The drug has a very good safety profile and has infrequent side effects, mostly related to an allergic reaction to the medicine.[37] The efficacy of botulinum toxin injections often fades with successive injections, as antibodies can develop that limit the clinical impact.

Orthopedic Surgery

A wide variety of surgical options are available for the orthopedic surgeon to treat spasticity and its long-term consequences on the musculoskeletal system.[21] In general, orthopedic procedures have been used to improve the biomechanics of patients with spasticity. The goals of surgery include lengthening of contracted muscles and tendons, balancing of joint forces, reduction of joint subluxation, fusion of unstable joints, and diminishment of painful spasticity. The surgical techniques include tenotomy, arthrodesis, osteotomy, and tendon transfer or lengthening. The procedures used are tailored to the clinical situation and the age of the patient, as the natural course of specific musculoskeletal abnormalities is factored into the decision-making process.

Intrathecal Baclofen

Baclofen was first used for spasticity in the late 1960s. Baclofen is an agonist of γ-aminobutyric acid (GABA) at GABA-β receptors within the dorsal horn of the spinal cord. These inhibitory GABAergic cells reduce the excitatory input to the α motor neuron. The effectiveness of oral baclofen is often limited by dose-related side effects such as sedation, respiratory depression, confusion, and hallucinations. A profound response to the intrathecal administration of baclofen was first demonstrated in adult patients with spasticity from spinal cord injury or multiple sclerosis. A dramatic reduction of tone was achieved with dosages that were many orders of magnitude less than oral doses. Albright et al in 1991 reported the first experience with ITB therapy in children with cerebral palsy, demonstrating a significant reduction of spasticity and an acceptable complication rate.[38] Since then, many clinical studies have demonstrated the efficacy of intrathecal baclofen in reducing both upper and lower extremity tone, as well as improving function and ease of care in patients (**Fig. 19.2**).[39–42]

It is difficult in some circumstances to determine which patients are better suited for selective dorsal rhizotomy (SDR) and which are better for ITB therapy. Two main groups of children generally have a better outcome if treated with ITB therapy. First are those who have severe spastic quadriparesis, are functionally debilitated, and are completely dependent for care. These children often respond well to ITB because a global reduction in tone can lead to improvements in comfort, positioning, and daily care.[43] The second group of patients are those children with a spastic diparesis who use their increased tone for ambulation and functional mobility. If an SDR is performed in these children, it is possible that reduction in tone might unmask underlying weakness and impair function. ITB therapy can be effective because the intrathecal dosing can be titrated to balance tone reduction with functional improvement.

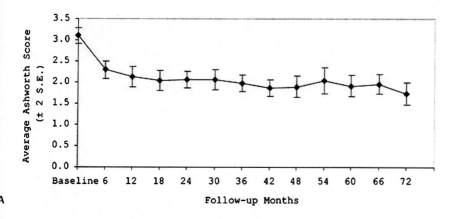

A

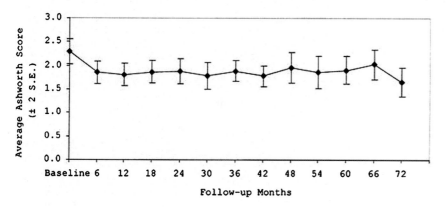

B

Fig. 19.2 (A) Graph demonstrating the mean Ashworth scores in the lower extremities at 6-month intervals after pump implantation. The scores were significantly decreased at 1 and 2 years following implantation ($p < .005$). **(B)** Graph demonstrating the mean Ashworth scores in the upper extremities at 6-month intervals after pump implantation. The scores were significantly decreased at 1 and 2 years following implantation ($p < .005$). S.E., standard error. (From Albright AL, Gilmartin R, Swift D, Krach LE, Ivanhoe CB, McLaughlin JF. Long-term intrathecal baclofen therapy for severe spasticity of cerebral origin. J Neurosurg 2003;98(2):291–295. Reprinted by permission.)

The main benefit of ITB therapy is the adjustable and nondestructive nature of the treatment. The amount of drug delivery can be adjusted to meet the needs of each specific child. Because no nervous tissue is destroyed, the effect of the therapy is also reversible. One disadvantage, however, is that complications are frequent. Baclofen overdose and withdrawal are potentially life-threatening complications of pump and catheter malfunction. Patients can be overdosed with baclofen with subsequent hypotonia and lethargy, which are usually managed with supportive care and adjustments of the pump rate. Catheter migration, disconnection, or fractures can occur, as well as other surgical problems, such as seromas, CSF leaks, and infections.[44] Gooch et al provided a retrospective analysis of complications seen with ITB therapy in the pediatric population.[45] At 1 year, 24 patients (24%) within a group of 100 experienced 48 total complications. The most common complications were catheter disconnection (9%), catheter dislodgement (8%), pump site infection (4%), and CSF infection (1%).[45] Lastly, baclofen withdrawal can occur, leading to rebound spasticity, high fevers, and mental status changes. After this study was conducted, smaller pumps that are more appropriate for pediatric patients became available. Although no new studies have been done, the combination of smaller pumps and subfascial placement of the pump is likely to

reduce the incidence of wound complications, especially in small children.

In addition to these common complications, other downsides to ITB are the cost and ongoing care and maintenance that are required. Device costs are high, and often compensation to the hospital may not cover the expense. Regular office visits are necessary for pump refills. In addition, average battery life is 6 to 7 years, thus necessitating additional surgery and hardware costs.

Surgical Rhizotomy

Surgical and chemical lesioning of peripheral nerves has been proven to be effective in treating spasticity. This can be accomplished through surgical exposure and transection of all or a portion of the nerve or through injection of ethanol or phenol around the nerve. Recently, ethanol and phenol injections have largely been abandoned due to the greater precision of surgical rhizotomy.

The objective of rhizotomy is to expose and isolate the nerve branches that supply the spastic muscle. A complete or partial division is then performed depending on both the particular muscle involved and a preoperative plan designed to balance spasticity with motor weakness. The technique involves intraoperative neurophysiologic monitoring and active stimulation of the nerves to better target lesioning.

History and Pathophysiology

SDR was derived from late-19th-century procedures for spasticity during which a complete nerve root transection was performed. These initial attempts effectively eliminated pathologic tone and spasticity but resulted in complete loss of motor, sensory, and proprioceptive function. After being abandoned until the 1960s, a modification of this approach has now been accepted as an effective treatment for spasticity. SDR was made possible after the exact anatomical localization of the Ia sensory input to the spinal cord at the dorsal root entry zone by Sindou et al in 1974.[46] It is believed that these sensory fibers help mediate the abnormal reflex arc in spasticity. Selective lesioning of these fibers should result in reduction of tone without loss of other sensory input or motor control at that spinal cord level. This finding was further supported by the development of techniques that help differentiate nerve rootlets responsible for spasticity from normal rootlets less involved in the pathologic process. This method, originally described by Fasano et al, uses electric stimulation of dorsal sensory rootlets with 30 to 50 Hz sustained impulses to activate the hyperactive reflex arc.[47,48] These stimulated motor responses are thought to occur in the abnormal nerve rootlets because of the loss of descending cortical inhibitory pathways.

The ability of SDR to reduce spasticity can be explained by the pathophysiology of spasticity. Motor control and tone of the muscle are ultimately controlled by the α motor neuron in the spinal cord. Interneurons within the spinal cord gray matter have a regulatory influence on the activity of the α motor neuron. These interneurons generally have an inhibitory effect on the α motor neuron and are activated by descending input from cortical upper motor neurons. However, interneurons are inhibited by the local spinal reflex arc, which is mediated by Ia sensory fibers. With damage to the brain or spinal cord, the balance of input is disrupted, and the reflex arc becomes hyperactive, leading to increased limb tone and spasticity. By selectively lesioning sensory nerve rootlets, SDR reduces the amount of Ia sensory input and helps restore a more normal balance to the α motor neuron (**Fig. 19.3**).

Surgical Technique

SDR is best suited for the treatment of children with primarily lower extremity spasticity, or spastic diplegia. Patients who benefit the most from SDR are those with pure spasticity involving the lower extremities, normal intelligence, good strength, minimal contractures, and postural stability. The ideal patient age is not known and is probably best determined by the individual clinical scenario. The typical

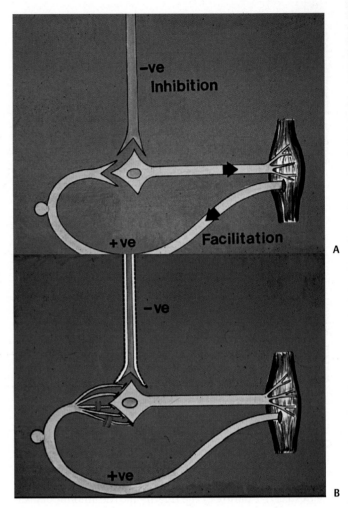

Fig. 19.3 Schematic drawings representing the excitatory and inhibitory influences on the spinal cord α motor neuron, which innervates the muscle fibers. **(A)** Normal physiology with a balance of inhibitory influence from descending neurons and excitatory influence from the sensory spinal reflex arc. **(B)** In children with spasticity, injury to the upper motor neuron results in a decrease in the descending inhibitory influence, leaving a hyperactive spinal cord reflex arc. By cutting some of the dorsal rootlets, selective dorsal rhizotomy can help restore balance to the α motor neuron by reducing the amount of excitatory influence on the neuron. (Courtesy of Jack Walker, professor of neurosurgery at the University of Utah, Primary Children's Medical Center, Salt Lake City, Utah.)

age ranges from 3 to 8 years, but teenagers may benefit as well.

General anesthesia is administered, but long-acting muscle relaxants and propofol are avoided to prevent any effects on neurophysiologic monitoring. Patients are positioned prone on a suitable frame or bolsters. EMG needles are then placed in the major lower extremity muscle groups (hip adductors, quadriceps, tibialis anterior, hamstring, and gastrocnemius) and sphincter muscles. The procedure as described by Peacock et al[49] involves a 5- to 6-inch skin incision. A five-level laminoplasty is elevated with the high-speed drill. L2 through S2 nerve roots are identified anatomically and electrophysiologically. The dorsal roots are carefully separated from the ventral roots and divided into multiple fascicles. Dorsal rootlets are then stimulated with two hook electrodes. The reflex threshold is determined by increasing the stimulus intensity of 0.1 msec square wave pulses at 0.5 Hz until muscle contraction is achieved. A 1-second 50 Hz train of tetanic stimulation is then applied to each fascicle. Sensory rootlets that result in spastic responses when stimulated are divided until a rhizotomy of between 40 and 60% of the nerve is achieved. The process is repeated bilaterally from L2 to S2. A simple grading system of abnormal responses has been described by Phillips and Park.[50] Grade 0 is a normal unsustained response. Grade 1 is a prolonged response within the root's normal distribution. Grade 2 involves response not only with the nerve's normal distribution but in the adjacent root's territories as well. The most abnormal grades, 3 and 4, demonstrate spread to distant ipsilateral muscles and to contralateral muscles, respectively.

Peacock et al's technique is easy to perform and provides clear identification of root levels, as each nerve can be traced until it exits its foramen. However, it requires a long incision and extensive bone removal. Even with replacement of the lamina, there is increased potential for postlaminotomy deformity[51,52] and spinal stenosis.[53] In response to concerns of deformity, pain, blood loss, and lengthy postoperative recovery, Park and colleagues developed a limited access approach for SDR.[54] This method employs a single-level laminectomy directly over the distal conus. Fluoroscopy or a plain radiograph is initially used to identify the L1 spinous process, and an ~1.5-inch incision is made exposing the T12–L1 interspace. After ligament removal, the intraoperative ultrasound is used to localize the conus, and a single-level laminectomy is performed.[55] Intraoperative ultrasound is again used to confirm that adequate exposure just caudal to the conus is available, and the dura is opened to expose the conus and nerve roots (**Fig. 19.4**). Under the operating microscope, the natural planes are then developed that separate both the dorsal from ventral roots just below the conus and the left- and right-sided nerve roots. The L3–S1 sensory roots on one side are wrapped with a Silastic sheet to separate them from the other roots. The L2 root is identified as it exits its corresponding neural foramen. The root is separated into its ventral and dorsal components, then stimulated individually to establish both motor and sensory thresholds. The sensory root is divided into four to eight smaller rootlets and selectively lesioned. The remaining sensory roots from L3 to S1 can then be tentatively identified moving from a lateral to medial fashion, with S1 typically being the largest root. Confirmatory additional information is obtained with stimulation of the roots and recording EMGs from the innervated muscles, as well as manual palpation of the lower extremity muscles by a physical therapist, physiatrist,

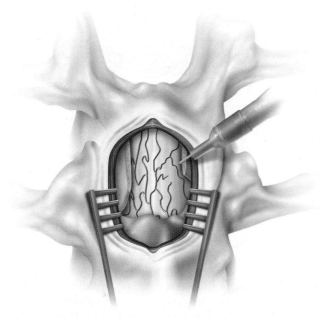

A

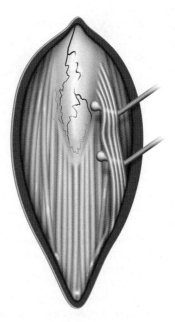

B

Fig. 19.4 **(A)** After the conus is clearly identified, a single laminectomy is done entirely with a Midas Rex craniotome. At least 5 mm of the caudal conus should be exposed. The laminectomy extends laterally close to the facet joint. **(B)** After the dural incision, an operating microscope is brought into the field. The L1 and L2 spinal roots are identified at the corresponding intervertebral foramina, and the filum terminale in the midline is found. *(Continued on page 236)*

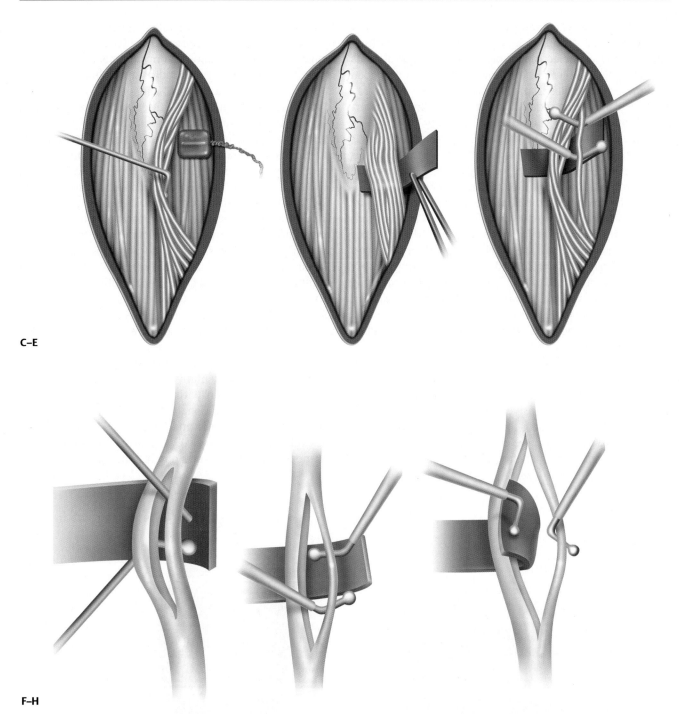

C–E

F–H

Fig. 19.4 (*Continued*) **(C)** The L2 dorsal root and the dorsal roots medial to the L2 root are retracted medially to separate the L2–S2 dorsal roots from the ventral roots. The thin S3–5 spinal roots exiting from the conus are identified. A cotton patty is placed over the ventral roots and lower sacral roots. **(D)** A 5 mm Silastic sheet is placed under the L2–S2 dorsal roots, after which the sugeon again inspects the L2 dorsal root at the foraminal exit, the lateral surface of the conus between the dorsal and ventral roots, and the lower sacral roots near the filum terminale. The inspection ensures placement of only the L2–S2 dorsal roots on top of the Silastic sheet. **(E)** The L2 dorsal root is easily identified. In an attempt to identify the L3–S2 dorsal roots, all the dorsal roots are spread over the Silastic sheet and grouped into presumed individual dorsal roots. Then the innervation pattern of each dorsal root is examined with electromyographic (EMG) responses to electrical stimulation with a threshold voltage. **(F)** With a Scheer needle, each dorsal root is subdivided into three to five rootlet fascicles, which are subjected to EMG testing. **(G)** Stimulation of an L2 rootlet fascicle elicits an unsustained discharge to a train of titanic stimuli. **(H)** The rootlet is thus spared from sectioning and placed behind the Silastic sheet.

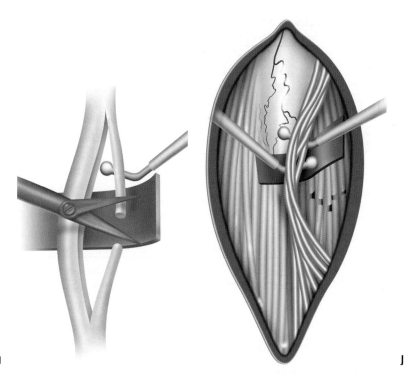

I   J

Fig. 19.4 *(Continued)* **(I)** Stimulation of a rootlet is thus sectioned. **(J)** The rootlets spared from sectioning are under the Silastic sheet, and the roots to be tested are on top of the Silastic sheet. Note the EMG testing and sectioning of the dorsal roots are performed caudal to the conus. (From Goodrich, J. Neurosurgical Operative Atlas: Pediatric Neurosurgery, Second Edition. New York: Thieme Publishers: 2008.) (From Park TS, Gaffney PE, Kaufman BA, Molleston MC. Selective lumbosacral dorsal rhizotomy immediately caudal to the conus medullaris for cerebral palsy spasticity. Neurosurgery 1993;33(5):929–933, discussion 933–934. Reprinted by permission.)

or neurologist. Selective lesioning is performed in a similar fashion on the contralateral side.

Recovery from surgery typically takes 2 to 3 days, followed by discharge to home with intensive outpatient rehabilitation or to acute inpatient rehabilitation. Long-term physical and occupational therapy is employed to ensure optimal outcomes.

Outcomes

There have been several excellent long-term outcome studies for SDR. The outcome measures examined include muscle tone, flexibility, gait pattern, functional positioning, and the ability of the child to deal with his or her environment. Nearly all studies investigating SDR have demonstrated a significant and persistent decrease in spasticity without a return of hypertonicity over time. Improved function and ambulation are commonly seen regardless of the preoperative abilities.[56–61] Despite the impressive decrease in spasticity after the procedure, some patients will still suffer from loss of joint mobility and require subsequent orthopedic surgery for tendon lengthening or transfer. Long-term outcome data for children with spastic diplegia who underwent SDR in Capetown, South Africa, demonstrated that significant improvements in both range of motion and quality of gait

(cadence and step length) persisted over a 20-year period.[57] Importantly, in this prospective cohort study, SDR did not abolish the need for subsequent orthopedic surgery, as approximately half of these children still required lengthening of the rectus femoris, hamstrings, and/or Achilles tendon.

McLaughlin et al reported a comparative analysis and meta-analysis of three randomized clinical trials.[62] Eighty-two children with spastic diplegia received either SDR and physiotherapy or physiotherapy alone. Outcome measures were used for spasticity (Ashworth scale) and function (Gross Motor Function Measure) and applied at a 12-month follow-up visit. As shown in **Fig. 19.5**, selective dorsal rhizotomy with physical therapy was more effective than physical therapy alone in reducing spasticity and improving overall function in children with spastic diplegia. Interestingly, multivariate analysis in the SDR group also revealed a direct relationship between the percentage of dorsal root tissue transected and functional improvement.

Although many studies have documented the efficacy of SDR and ITB therapy on the treatment of spasticity, only recently has information comparing these treatments directly become available. Kan and colleagues reported a consecutive series of 71 children who underwent SDR for spasticity and compared them with another group of 71 children who underwent ITB therapy

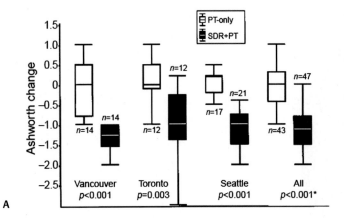

A

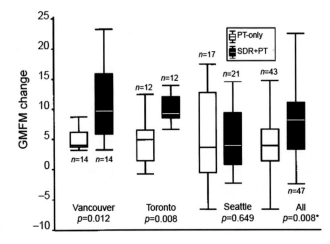

B

Fig. 19.5 Summary of meta-analysis data after selective dorsal rhizotomy. **(A)** Ashworth change score and **(B)** Gross Motor Function Measure (GMFM) change score; physical therapy (PT) only and selective dorsal rhizotomy (SDR) + PT group data for individual studies and pooled meta-analysis. Interval is from baseline to 12 months after beginning treatment (9 months for Vancouver). Boxes represent the 25th, 50th, and 75th percentiles. Whiskers represent minimum and maximum values excluding outliers beyond 1.5 times the interquartile range. Probability values are based on Wilcoxon's tests, with blocking on site for combined test. (From McLaughlin J, Bjornson K, Temkin N, et al. Selective dorsal rhizotomy: meta-analysis of three randomized controlled trials. Dev Med Child Neurol 2002;44(1):17–25. Reprinted by permission.)

matched by age and preoperative score on the GMFCS.[63] At 1 year postoperatively, both SDR and ITB therapy decreased tone, increased passive range of motion (PROM), and improved function. Compared with ITB therapy, however, SDR provided a significantly larger magnitude of improvement in tone, PROM, and gross motor function. In addition, fewer patients in the SDR group required subsequent orthopedic procedures (19.1% vs 40.8%). Overall review of the literature supports the findings summarized in **Table 19.3**.

Table 19.3 Summary of Some of the Reported Outcomes after Selective Dorsal Rhizotomy

Class I	• Decrease in lower limb spasticity (Ashworth): up to 12 years
	• Increase in lower extremity range of motion: up to 5 years
	• Improvement in motor function (GMFM)
Class II	• Improvement in disability (PEDI) and ADL performance
	• Improvement in gait, including increased stride length and velocity
	• Improvement in suprasegmental effects, including upper limb function and cognition
Class III	• Reduction in the need for future orthopedic procedures

Abbreviations: ADL, activities of daily living; GMFM, Gross Motor Function Measure; PEDI, Pediatric Evaluation of Disability Index.

Complications

Complications can occasionally be seen following SDR, the most common being pain or transient neurologic dysfunction, including weakness, sensory loss, and bladder dysfunction. The majority of these are temporary, with permanent dysfunction occurring in < 5% of patients.[64] Retrospective studies have drawn attention to the possibility of an increased incidence of scoliosis and hip subluxation after SDR.[51,52] Because these conditions are a common finding in children with spasticity who do not have SDR, it is unclear what role SDR plays in the development of scoliosis or hip subluxation.[65–67] It remains to be seen if minimally invasive SDR through a single-level rather than a multilevel laminectomy reduces the incidence of these conditions.

Conclusion

The management of childhood spasticity requires a multidisciplinary effort. With input from pediatricians, pediatric physiatrists, physical and occupational therapists, neurologists, orthotists, orthopedic surgeons, neurologic surgeons, and other health care personnel, effective treatment for spasticity can be initiated and maintained that can lead to meaningful improvement in the quality of life for a vast number of children. Neurosurgical treatment of spasticity will continue to evolve and be refined as procedures and techniques are appropriately evaluated with reliable and validated outcome measures. SDR remains an important treatment, particularly for spastic diplegia in children. For children with moderate to severe spasticity, SDR may be more effective than ITB therapy in reducing the degree of spasticity and improving function.

♦ Lessons Learned

There is nothing much to be added to the exceptional clarity of the contribution by Leland Albright. We learn the indications for ITB and some clear insights into a long and experienced practice. For instance, the discontinuation of test infusions is something that many will find a new thing. But it certainly makes a lot of sense.

Many of us will find new impetus in using ITB for tetraparetic patients quite early, as early as 1 month after injury, when the source of spasticity is severe traumatic brain injury.

Anderson and colleagues' contribution on selective dorsal rhizotomy describes the indications and surgical technique. This procedure is best suited for the treatment of children with primarily lower extremity spasticity, as the children who benefit the most are those with pure spasticity, normal intelligence, good strength, and minimal contractures. The ideal patient age is still not known, but the typical age in the literature ranges from 3 to 8 years. This technique is more invasive than intrathecal baclofen but has very good long-term favorable outcomes relative to the cost of the procedure. This must be considered for certain children as the procedure of choice as compared with the baclofen pump. There also have been significant advances in the surgical technique by performing the procedure in a one- or two-level laminotomy rather than an extensive operative exposure.

References

1. Dan B, Bouillot E, Bengoetxea A, Cheron G. Effect of intrathecal baclofen on gait control in human hereditary spastic paraparesis. Neurosci Lett 2000;280(3):175–178
2. Albright AL, Barron WB, Fasick MP, Polinko P, Janosky J. Continuous intrathecal baclofen infusion for spasticity of cerebral origin. JAMA 1993;270(20):2475–2477
3. Butler C, Campbell S; AACPDM Treatment Outcomes Committee Review Panel. Evidence of the effects of intrathecal baclofen for spastic and dystonic cerebral palsy. Dev Med Child Neurol 2000;42(9):634–645
4. Albright AL, Barry MJ, Fasick MP, Janosky J. Effects of continuous intrathecal baclofen infusion and selective posterior rhizotomy on upper extremity spasticity. Pediatr Neurosurg 1995;23(2):82–85
5. Albright AL, Barry MJ, Shafton DH, Ferson SS. Intrathecal baclofen for generalized dystonia. Dev Med Child Neurol 2001;43(10):652–657
6. François B, Vacher P, Roustan J, et al. Intrathecal baclofen after traumatic brain injury: early treatment using a new technique to prevent spasticity. J Trauma 2001;50(1):158–161
7. Albright AL, Turner M, Pattisapu JV. Best-practice surgical techniques for intrathecal baclofen therapy. J Neurosurg 2006;104(4, Suppl):233–239
8. Grabb PA, Guin-Renfroe S, Meythaler JM. Midthoracic catheter tip placement for intrathecal baclofen administration in children with quadriparetic spasticity. Neurosurgery 1999;45(4):833–836, discussion 836–837
9. Albright AL, Cervi A, Singletary J. Intrathecal baclofen for spasticity in cerebral palsy. JAMA 1991;265(11):1418–1422
10. Van Schaeybroeck P, Nuttin B, Lagae L, Schrijvers E, Borghgraef C, Feys P. Intrathecal baclofen for intractable cerebral spasticity: a prospective placebo-controlled, double-blind study. Neurosurgery 2000;46(3):603–609, discussion 609–612
11. Albright AL, Gilmartin R, Swift D, Krach LE, Ivanhoe CB, McLaughlin JF. Long-term intrathecal baclofen therapy for severe spasticity of cerebral origin. J Neurosurg 2003;98(2):291–295
12. Krach LE, Kriel RL, Gilmartin RC, et al. GMFM 1 year after continuous intrathecal baclofen infusion. Pediatr Rehabil 2005;8(3): 207–213
13. Awaad Y, Tayem H, Munoz S, Ham S, Michon AM, Awaad R. Functional assessment following intrathecal baclofen therapy in children with spastic cerebral palsy. J Child Neurol 2003;18(1):26–34

14. Gerszten PC, Albright AL, Johnstone GF. Intrathecal baclofen infusion and subsequent orthopedic surgery in patients with spastic cerebral palsy. J Neurosurg 1998;88(6):1009–1013
15. Buonaguro V, Scelsa B, Curci D, Monforte S, Iuorno T, Motta F. Epilepsy and intrathecal baclofen therapy in children with cerebral palsy. Pediatr Neurol 2005;33(2):110–113
16. Gerszten PC, Albright AL, Johnstone GF. Intrathecal baclofen infusion and subsequent orthopedic surgery in patients with spastic cerebral palsy. J Neurosurg 1998;88(6):1009–1013
17. Krach LE, Kriel RL, Gilmartin RC, et al. Hip status in cerebral palsy after one year of continuous intrathecal baclofen infusion. Pediatr Neurol 2004;30(3):163–168
18. Sansone JM, Mann D, Noonan K, Mcleish D, Ward M, Iskandar BJ. Rapid progression of scoliosis following insertion of intrathecal baclofen pump. J Pediatr Orthop 2006;26(1):125–128
19. Gooch JL, Oberg WA, Grams B, Ward LA, Walker ML. Care provider assessment of intrathecal baclofen in children. Dev Med Child Neurol 2004;46(8):548–552
20. Mandigo CE, Anderson RC. Management of childhood spasticity: a neurosurgical perspective. Pediatr Ann 2006;35(5):354–362
21. Koman LA, Smith BP, Shilt JS. Cerebral palsy. Lancet 2004;363(9421):1619–1631
22. O'Shea TM, Preisser JS, Klinepeter KL, Dillard RG. Trends in mortality and cerebral palsy in a geographically based cohort of very low birth weight neonates born between 1982 to 1994. Pediatrics 1998;101(4 Pt 1):642–647
23. Goldstein EM. Spasticity management: an overview. J Child Neurol 2001;16(1):16–23
24. Sanger TD, Delgado MR, Gaebler-Spira D, Hallett M, Mink JW; Task Force on Childhood Motor Disorders. Classification and definition of disorders causing hypertonia in childhood. Pediatrics 2003;111(1):e89–e97
25. Flett PJ. Rehabilitation of spasticity and related problems in childhood cerebral palsy. J Paediatr Child Health 2003;39(1):6–14
26. Gooch JL, Oberg WA, Grams B, Ward LA, Walker ML. Care provider assessment of intrathecal baclofen in children. Dev Med Child Neurol 2004;46(8):548–552
27. Ashworth B. Preliminary trial of carisoprodol in multiple sclerosis. Practitioner 1964;192:540–542

28. Bohannon RW, Smith MB. Interrater reliability of a modified Ashworth scale of muscle spasticity. Phys Ther 1987;67(2):206–207

29. Watanabe T. The role of therapy in spasticity management. Am J Phys Med Rehabil 2004;83(10, Suppl):S45–S49

30. Zafonte R, Lombard L, Elovic E. Antispasticity medications: uses and limitations of enteral therapy. Am J Phys Med Rehabil 2004;83(10, Suppl):S50–S58

31. Koman LA, Mooney JF III, Smith B, Goodman A, Mulvaney T. Management of cerebral palsy with botulinum-A toxin: preliminary investigation. J Pediatr Orthop 1993;13(4):489–495

32. Gormley ME, Gaebler-Spira D, Delgado MR. Use of botulinum toxin type A in pediatric patients with cerebral palsy: a three-center retrospective chart review. J Child Neurol 2001;16(2):113–118

33. Baker R, Jasinski M, Maciag-Tymecka I, et al. Botulinum toxin treatment of spasticity in diplegic cerebral palsy: a randomized, double-blind, placebo-controlled, dose-ranging study. Dev Med Child Neurol 2002;44(10):666–675

34. Corry IS, Cosgrove AP, Walsh EG, McClean D, Graham HK. Botulinum toxin A in the hemiplegic upper limb: a double-blind trial. Dev Med Child Neurol 1997;39(3):185–193

35. Koman LA, Mooney JF III, Smith BP, Walker F, Leon JM; BOTOX Study Group. Botulinum toxin type A neuromuscular blockade in the treatment of lower extremity spasticity in cerebral palsy: a randomized, double-blind, placebo-controlled trial. J Pediatr Orthop 2000;20(1):108–115

36. Sutherland DH, Kaufman KR, Wyatt MP, Chambers HG, Mubarak SJ. Double-blind study of botulinum A toxin injections into the gastrocnemius muscle in patients with cerebral palsy. Gait Posture 1999;10(1):1–9

37. Francisco GE. Botulinum toxin: dosing and dilution. Am J Phys Med Rehabil 2004;83(10, Suppl):S30–S37

38. Albright AL, Cervi A, Singletary J. Intrathecal baclofen for spasticity in cerebral palsy. JAMA 1991;265(11):1418–1422

39. Albright AL, Gilmartin R, Swift D, Krach LE, Ivanhoe CB, McLaughlin JF. Long-term intrathecal baclofen therapy for severe spasticity of cerebral origin. J Neurosurg 2003;98(2):291–295

40. Armstrong RW, Steinbok P, Cochrane DD, Kube SD, Fife SE, Farrell K. Intrathecally administered baclofen for treatment of children with spasticity of cerebral origin. J Neurosurg 1997;87(3):409–414

41. Plassat R, Perrouin Verbe B, Menei P, Menegalli D, Mathé JF, Richard I. Treatment of spasticity with intrathecal baclofen administration: long-term follow-up, review of 40 patients. Spinal Cord 2004;42(12):686–693

42. Rawicki B. Treatment of cerebral origin spasticity with continuous intrathecal baclofen delivered via an implantable pump: long-term follow-up review of 18 patients. J Neurosurg 1999;91(5):733–736

43. Middel B, Kuipers-Upmeijer H, Bouma J, et al. Effect of intrathecal baclofen delivered by an implanted programmable pump on health related quality of life in patients with severe spasticity. J Neurol Neurosurg Psychiatry 1997;63(2):204–209

44. Albright AL, Awaad Y, Muhonen M, et al. Performance and complications associated with the synchromed 10-ml infusion pump for intrathecal baclofen administration in children. J Neurosurg 2004;101(1, Suppl):64–68

45. Gooch JL, Oberg WA, Grams B, Ward LA, Walker ML. Complications of intrathecal baclofen pumps in children. Pediatr Neurosurg 2003;39(1):1–6

46. Sindou M, Quoex C, Baleydier C. Fiber organization at the posterior spinal cord-rootlet junction in man. J Comp Neurol 1974;153(1):15–26

47. Newberg NL, Gooch JL, Walker ML. Intraoperative monitoring in selective dorsal rhizotomy. Pediatr Neurosurg 1991–1992;17(3):124–127

48. Fasano VA, Broggi G, Zeme S, Lo Russo G, Sguazzi A. Long-term results of posterior functional rhizotomy. Acta Neurochir Suppl (Wien) 1980;30:435–439

49. Peacock WJ, Arens LJ. Selective posterior rhizotomy for the relief of spasticity in cerebral palsy. S Afr Med J 1982;62(4):119–124

50. Phillips LH, Park TS. Electrophysiologic mapping of the segmental anatomy of the muscles of the lower extremity. Musle Nerve 1991;14:1213–1218

51. Peter JC, Hoffman EB, Arens LJ, Peacock WJ. Incidence of spinal deformity in children after multiple level laminectomy for selective posterior rhizotomy. Childs Nerv Syst 1990;6(1):30–32

52. Turi M, Kalen V. The risk of spinal deformity after selective dorsal rhizotomy. J Pediatr Orthop 2000;20(1):104–107

53. Gooch JL, Walker ML. Spinal stenosis after total lumbar laminectomy for selective dorsal rhizotomy. Pediatr Neurosurg 1996;25(1):28–30

54. Park TS, Gaffney PE, Kaufman BA, Molleston MC. Selective lumbosacral dorsal rhizotomy immediately caudal to the conus medullaris for cerebral palsy spasticity. Neurosurgery 1993;33(5):929–933, discussion 933–934

55. Park TS, Owen JH. Surgical management of spastic diplegia in cerebral palsy. N Engl J Med 1992;326(11):745–749

56. Engsberg JR, Olree KS, Ross SA, Park TS. Spasticity and strength changes as a function of selective dorsal rhizotomy. J Neurosurg 1998;88(6):1020–1026

57. Langerak NG, Lamberts RP, Fieggen AG, et al. A prospective gait analysis study in patients with diplegic cerebral palsy 20 years after selective dorsal rhizotomy. J Neurosurg Pediatr 2008;1(3):180–186

58. McLaughlin J, Bjornson K, Temkin N, et al. Selective dorsal rhizotomy: meta-analysis of three randomized controlled trials. Dev Med Child Neurol 2002;44(1):17–25

59. Mittal S, Farmer JP, Al-Atassi B, et al. Long-term functional outcome after selective posterior rhizotomy. J Neurosurg 2002;97(2):315–325

60. Mittal S, Farmer JP, Al-Atassi B, et al. Functional performance following selective posterior rhizotomy: long-term results determined using a validated evaluative measure. J Neurosurg 2002;97(3):510–518

61. Subramanian N, Vaughan CL, Peter JC, Arens LJ. Gait before and 10 years after rhizotomy in children with cerebral palsy spasticity. J Neurosurg 1998;88(6):1014–1019

62. McLaughlin JF, Bjornson KF, Astley SJ, et al. Selective dorsal rhizotomy: efficacy and safety in an investigator-masked randomized clinical trial. Dev Med Child Neurol 1998;40(4):220–232

63. Kan P, Gooch J, Amini A, et al. Surgical treatment of spasticity in children: comparison of selective dorsal rhizotomy and intrathecal baclofen pump implantation. Childs Nerv Syst 2008;24(2):239–243

64. Steinbok P, Schrag C. Complications after selective posterior rhizotomy for spasticity in children with cerebral palsy. Pediatr Neurosurg 1998;28(6):300–313

65. Chicoine MR, Park TS, Kaufman BA. Selective dorsal rhizotomy and rates of orthopedic surgery in children with spastic cerebral palsy. J Neurosurg 1997;86(1):34–39

66. Greene WB, Dietz FR, Goldberg MJ, Gross RH, Miller F, Sussman MD. Rapid progression of hip subluxation in cerebral palsy after selective posterior rhizotomy. J Pediatr Orthop 1991;11(4):494–497

67. Mooney JF III, Millis MB. Spinal deformity after selective dorsal rhizotomy in patients with cerebral palsy. Clin Orthop Relat Res 1999; (364):48–52

20 Syringomyelia

◆ Syringosubarachnoid Shunts

Sudesh J. Ebenezer and Richard G. Ellenbogen

Syringomyelia is a disorder of the spinal cord characterized by a fluid-filled cavity within the cord substance. When the cavity is a dilated central canal of the spinal cord, the term *hydromyelia* has been applied, reserving the term *syringomyelia* for cavities in the cord extending lateral to or independent of the central canal.[1] The term *communicating syringomyelia* also refers to an enlargement of the central canal, whereas *noncommunicating syringomyelia* refers to a cyst not in communication with the central canal, but rather arising from the cord substance. The term *syringohydromyelia* reflects the difficulties in classification and terminology.[2] Others have used the terms *syringomyelia* and *syrinx* in a general manner to represent any spinal cord cyst, and we shall also use these terms in the same general sense in this discussion.[3]

Epidemiology

There is a prevalence of 8.4 cases per 100,000 population of syringomyelia related to nontrauma, according to Heiss and Oldfield.[4] In patients with Chiari I malformation, the incidence and prevalence of syringomyelia vary depending on the series quoted. For example, between 3 and 75% will have a syrinx seen on magnetic resonance imaging (MRI).[5–9] In a study by the senior author (RE), 80.5% of pediatric patients with Chiari I malformation had associated syringomyelia.[10] Twenty to 95% of those with Chiari II malformations will have a syrinx on neuroimaging.[11] In a study by Rossier et al, 3.2% of 951 patients with spinal cord injuries followed for 11 years developed syringomyelia.[12] Heiss and Oldfield found that 4% of intramedullary spinal cord tumors have associated syringomyelia.[4]

Pathophysiology

Syringomyelia develops due to an alteration of cerebrospinal fluid (CSF) circulation at the foramen magnum or around the spinal cord.[13] Important theories of syringomyelia formation include the water-hammer theory of Gardner,[14–17] the craniospinal dissociation theory of Williams,[18,19] Ball and Dayan's theory involving Virchow-Robin spaces,[20] and Oldfield et al's theory of the cerebellar tonsils moving down with systolic pulses, producing a systolic pressure wave in the spinal CSF that acts on the spinal cord surface.[21] Ellenbogen et al found that in patients having Chiari I malformation with and without syringomyelia, aberrant CSF flow profiles were observed at the craniocervical junction.[10] A syringosubarachnoid shunt provides an outflow route for CSF during external cord compression, which occurs during cardiac systole.[22]

Communicating syringomyelia is usually observed with pathology involving the foramen magnum. Examples of this are Chiari I malformation and basilar arachnoiditis. Occult spinal dysraphism can also cause communicating syringomyelia. Noncommunicating syringomyelia can be caused by trauma, neoplasm, intradural arachnoid cysts, arteriovenous malformations, and arachnoiditis. The causes for syringomyelia are very diverse. Yet all of the conditions share a common feature: an alteration in the normal CSF dynamics in the spinal subarachnoid space.[23]

Clinical Presentation

The classic description of the "syringomyelia syndrome" consists of a dissociative sensory loss (loss of pain and temperature sensation with relative sparing of light touch and perception) in a cape-like distribution with upper extremity weakness of a lower motoneuron type and lower extremity weakness of an upper motoneuron type.[24] The clinical presentation can vary greatly and may include weakness, sensory loss, pain, gait abnormality, scoliosis, and changes in bladder or bowel function.[25] Physical findings can include an ascending sensory level, increased motor deficits, depressed tendon reflexes, atrophy, increased spasticity, hyperhidrosis, autonomic dysreflexia, and myelopathy.

Indications

First, one must determine if the syrinx is causing significant or progressive neurologic symptoms or deficits. If it is felt that the syrinx is responsible for the progressive symptoms or signs, one must always first attempt to discover and treat the underlying etiology of syringomyelia in the individual patient. There is no medical or pharmacological treatment for syringomyelia. Primary treatment of syringomyelia can include posterior fossa decompression in the setting of Chiari I malformation. Many surgeons argue that decompression of the posterior fossa to enlarge the volume of the posterior fossa at the craniovertebral junction and establish normal CSF flow patterns should be the primary goal of surgical intervention in patients with Chiari I malformation and syringomyelia. In patients who have undergone posterior fossa decompression and a symptomatic syrinx persists, reexploration can be considered after appropriate radiologic evaluation to look for an etiology such as a pseudomeningocele or obstruction to normal CSF flow. Shunting of the syrinx should be used only if the patient fails treatment of the underlying cause of the syringomyelia. A shunt cannot correct the initial pathophysiology of syringomyelia formation, and for this reason it is always best to aim treatment initially at the causative mechanism. It is also possible that a patient has a syrinx without an obvious cause. If no cause of a significant syrinx is found, consideration for exploration of the craniocervical junction may be considered in selected patients.[26,27] Primary syringosubarachnoid shunting can also be useful for this population.

Contraindications

Shunting procedures of the syrinx as the initial mode of treatment for Chiari I malformation have a relative contraindication because of concern that further herniation by spinal cord collapse and compromise of the brainstem will be precipitated by such a procedure.[28–30] Van den Bergh found that in patients with Chiari I malformation, if only a syringosubarachnoid shunt is inserted, the headache attacks may become more severe, because the shunt makes the craniospinal pressure difference even greater.[31] There also can be a danger of cerebellar coning with apnea. These observations do not uniformly hold for children with Chiari II malformations.

A syringosubarachnoid shunt should not be chosen as a first-line treatment for syringomyelia. Its use should be considered only after failed attempts to treat the underlying pathophysiology of the syrinx. Use of the syringosubarachnoid shunt also is dependent on a normal flow of CSF in the subarachnoid space. Hence, patients with a history of arachnoiditis may not be candidates. A person with a history of chemical or tuberculous meningitis can have diffuse arachnoiditis and is thus not an ideal patient for syringosubarachnoid

shunting. Arachnoid flow can be significantly altered in post-trauma patients; thus, this population may be less responsive to syringosubarachnoid shunting. In patients with prior arachnoiditis and trauma, it is possible that the distal shunt should be positioned in the peritoneum or pleural space, rather than in the subarachnoid space.

Recognition of septa within the syrinx on MRI may hinder drainage through a shunt.[28] This therefore can also be considered a contraindication to shunting procedures. However, free communication within the syrinx can exist despite septation seen on MRI.[32]

Operative Procedure

Intraoperative neurophysiologic monitoring is set up after the patient is anesthetized. This includes motor evoked potentials and somatosensory evoked potentials (SSEPs). The patient is positioned prone on bolsters on the operating room table. Towel, foam, or gel rolls are used to serve as bolsters in the adolescent patient. The arms are positioned up at 90-degree angles if operating on the thoracic or lumbar region. The arms are placed at the patient's side if the syrinx is located at the cervical region. All pressure points are adequately padded. A single prophylactic dose of antibiotics is administered by the anesthesiologist 30 to 45 minutes before skin incision. A laminotomy is planned at the levels with the largest cord expansion caused by the syrinx. Intraoperative fluoroscopy is first used to mark the relevant levels of the spinous processes, to plan the extent of the initial skin incision. Subperiosteal dissection is then continued to complete the exposure of spinous processes and lamina. A Leksell rongeur, Kerrison punch, and/or high-speed drill is used to perform the laminotomy. Conservative bone removal is employed to avoid iatrogenically induced instability. Intraoperative ultrasound may be used to confirm the underlying syrinx and define its borders. The microscope is brought into the field at this point to open the dura. Special care is taken not to violate the arachnoid layer. The dura is tacked laterally using 4–0 Nurolon sutures. A beaver or arachnoid microblade is used to vertically cut the arachnoid and pia in the midline or at the dorsal root entry zone (DREZ). Often, the surgeon chooses the region with the thinnest and most transparent trajectory to the syrinx-filled cord. Care should be taken to maintain the subarachnoid space. Hemostasis is important so blood does not track in the subarachnoid space. The blade is then carefully used to perform a 2 mm midline or DREZ myelotomy and then enter the syrinx. Once the syrinx is entered, fluid rushes out, decompressing the syrinx. We use a K-shaped syringosubarachnoid shunt made of nonreactive Silastic of the Pudenz type (Medtronic PS Medical, Goleta, California). This has multiple fenestrations at the ends. One end of the K is tunneled into the syrinx rostrally. Another end is placed caudally in the syrinx. The distal end of the K tube is placed

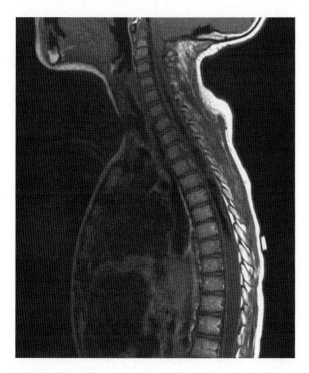

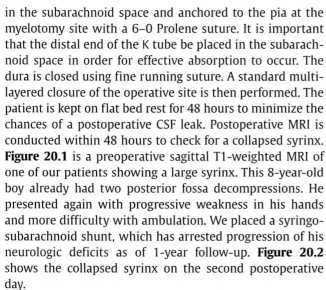

Fig. 20.1 Preoperative sagittal T1-weighted magnetic resonance imaging (MRI).

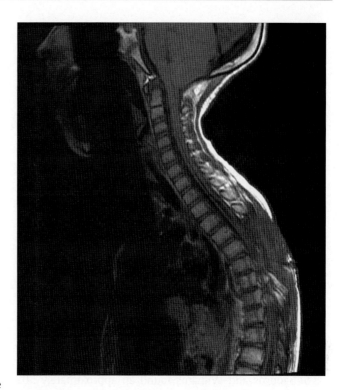

Fig. 20.2 Postoperative sagittal T1-weighted MRI.

in the subarachnoid space and anchored to the pia at the myelotomy site with a 6–0 Prolene suture. It is important that the distal end of the K tube be placed in the subarachnoid space in order for effective absorption to occur. The dura is closed using fine running suture. A standard multi-layered closure of the operative site is then performed. The patient is kept on flat bed rest for 48 hours to minimize the chances of a postoperative CSF leak. Postoperative MRI is conducted within 48 hours to check for a collapsed syrinx. **Figure 20.1** is a preoperative sagittal T1-weighted MRI of one of our patients showing a large syrinx. This 8-year-old boy already had two posterior fossa decompressions. He presented again with progressive weakness in his hands and more difficulty with ambulation. We placed a syringo-subarachnoid shunt, which has arrested progression of his neurologic deficits as of 1-year follow-up. **Figure 20.2** shows the collapsed syrinx on the second postoperative day.

Rhoton advocated that the myelotomy and placement of a cavity to subarachnoid shunt should be made in the DREZ because this is the thinnest portion of the spinal cord when cavitation takes place.[33] Theoretically, this prevents loss of bladder control and prevents neurologic deficit.[6] We agree with Menezes, who noted a paucity of neurologic deficits with midline myelotomy when this has been the thinnest portion of the spinal cord in a distended hydromyelic sac.[6]

Results

We present, in chronological order, the highlights of several studies that discuss the use of syringosubarachnoid shunts in pediatric patients.

1. Vaquero et al described a 14-year-old male patient with syringomyelia who had a 1-year history of dissociated sensory loss and light spasticity in the legs. A syringosubarachnoid shunt was placed, and at the 2-year follow-up he had subjectively improved.[34]
2. Dauser et al reported on five pediatric patients who underwent syringosubarachnoid shunt placement.[35] One patient had a syringosubarachnoid shunt placed at age 3 that improved his symptoms (a myelogram had showed low cerebellar tonsils and a wide cord from C2 to T2). Five years later, he had rapid acceleration in scoliosis, and 3 years subsequently, he developed upper extremity weakness. The child, then 11 years old, had posterior fossa decompression. This stopped the neurologic progression, and the child remained stable 2 years later. In the four other pediatric patients, ages 4 to 11 years, posterior fossa decompression and syringosubarachnoid shunting were performed. The authors reported good outcomes in these four cases. Pain resolved, and there was no scoliosis progression. Follow-up on these patients ranged from 16 months to 2.5 years.

3. Phillips et al reviewed four children ages 3, 5, 15, and 15 with scoliosis and syringomyelia, three of whom were followed to skeletal maturity.[36] Each patient had the syrinx drained by a syringosubarachnoid shunt. The average follow-up was 8 years. Three of the four patients' neurology improved after drainage. The other patient was stabilized. The older two patients had spinal fusions after the drainage operations. Fusions were felt to be less risky after syringosubarachnoid shunt placement. One child had kyphosis at the laminectomy site in follow-up. Progression of scoliosis was arrested only temporarily by syrinx drainage in the 3- and 5-year-olds. The authors concluded that long-term follow-up shows progression of scoliosis even with drainage of the syrinx plus management with orthotics.

4. Nagib described one pediatric patient with a Chiari I malformation and syrinx that were treated by a suboccipital craniectomy but later required syringosubarachnoid shunting, due to the generous nature of the syringomyelic cavity.[37] Resolution of the cavity was noted. Details of the case were not described.

5. Sgouros and Williams found an approximately 50% rate of longevity for 73 patients who had a syrinx shunt procedure.[38] A 15.7% complication rate was noted, as well. In the study, 56 had syringopleural shunts and 14 had syringosubarachnoid shunts. The mean age was 37.5, with a range of 11–77 years of age. Seven of the 14 syringosubarachnoid shunt patients had a good long term result. The experience and outcomes of the syringopleural and syringosubarachnoid shunt was similar in this study.

6. In a study of children with syringomyelia and scoliosis, Farley et al included 17 patients ages 1 to 14 years in whom syringosubarachnoid shunts were placed.[39] With respect to neurologic function postoperatively, four improved, eight showed no change, four worsened, and one was not followed. The authors felt that the drainage of the syrinx was not predictive of curve progression.

7. Chapman and Frim performed syringosubarachnoid shunting in three children with symptomatic syringomyelia that arose following retethering of lipomeningomyelocele.[40] Syringosubarachnoid shunting arrested the progression of deficits but only partially reversed them.

8. Vernet et al included 13 pediatric cases of syringosubarachnoid shunting.[41] They included four cases of Chiari I and two of Chiari II malformations, four cases of shunted hydrocephalus, two cases of spina bifida aperta, and five cases of spina bifida occulta. Six patients had prior posterior fossa decompression. Eight had new onset weakness or a progressive deterioration of a preexisting motor handicap. A urologic

difficulty was the presenting feature in five patients. Scoliosis was seen in five of the cases. Holocord syrinx was found in three, a cervicothoracic syrinx was seen in two, a thoracic syrinx was present in five, and a lumbar syrinx was seen in three patients. After syringosubarachnoid shunt placement, one patient improved, eight stabilized, three worsened neurologically, and one was lost to follow-up. The three patients with poor postoperative outcome exhibited a rapid clinical and radiologic deterioration, occurring a few weeks after syringosubarachnoid shunt placement. One of these patients had the syringosubarachnoid shunt removed and a syringopleural shunt placed 5 months later due to clinical and radiologic deterioration. A second had repeat syringosubarachnoid shunting done and remained stable for 3 years. The last patient who deteriorated refused further surgery. Radiologically, one cavity was collapsed, six were significantly reduced, two were unchanged, and three had enlarged. The follow-up period ranged from 1 to 10 years.

9. Koyanagi et al described four pediatric patients in which syringosubarachnoid shunts were placed (two patients having syringomyelia with occult spinal dysraphism and two with a history of myelomeningocele).[13] Details of the cases were not provided. Collapse of the syrinx was achieved in all. Neurologically, one patient showed improved muscle power of the upper limbs after surgery. The authors concluded that a large syrinx in the case of spinal dysraphism should be surgically treated.

10. Caldarelli et al reported two syringosubarachnoid cases in pediatric patients. The patients presented with progressive neurologic deterioration.[42] MRI showed mainly unilocular, severely dilated, and extended hydromyelic cavities. The patients showed reduction of the cavity on MRI. One patient remained clinically stable, and the other had partial clinical improvement.

11. Weinberg et al described one 2-year-old patient who presented with vertex headaches and syncope.[43] Tonsillar descent was noted to C1 along with a large C4–T6 syrinx. The patient underwent posterior fossa decompression with obex plugging, as well as placement of a syringosubarachnoid shunt. The patient was neurologically intact postoperatively. The short- and long-term outcomes were described as excellent. The authors reported the patient to be asymptomatic along with no progression of symptoms and no new complaints. Complete collapse of the syrinx was noted on postoperative MRI.

12. Hida et al reviewed 16 patients ages 3 to 15 years with syringomyelia and Chiari I malformation.[44] Syringosubarachnoid shunting was performed initially

in nine patients due to large syrinxes. The authors reported the result of surgery as "successful" with no major operative complications. Follow-up ranged from 6 to 128 months. One patient required repeat surgery. In this patient, the shunt tube was loosened and pulled out. It was felt that scoliosis in affected patients was improved or stabilized.

13. Iwasaki et al reported on 24 patients in whom partial hemilaminectomy and syringosubarachnoid shunting had been performed.[45] Twenty of these patients were ages 9 to 16 years. They were patients who had syringomyelia with Chiari malformation, spinal cord trauma, and spinal arachnoiditis. Syringosubarachnoid shunting was chosen due to the large size of the syrinx on MRI and the main symptoms associated with the syrinx, such as dissociated sensory disturbance, motor weakness of extremities, and local pain. Syringosubarachnoid shunting was chosen also for new neurologic deficits thought to be related to the syrinx. There were no operative complications. Postoperative follow-up was from 6 months to 5 years. Collapse of the cavity was shown in all cases by MRI an average of 11.8 days after surgery. No patient developed spinal deformity or relapse of the syrinx. In the Chiari malformation group, neurologic improvement was seen in 84%. In the posttrauma and postmeningitis groups, improvement of new or delayed symptoms was seen in 90% and 75%, respectively.

14. In Ellenbogen et al's study, two pediatric patients had undergone syringosubarachnoid shunting previously.[10] This ultimately resulted in a new syrinx formation and a recurrence of symptoms. One of these children presented with quadriparesis and apnea caused by the development of a new cervicomedullary syrinx that developed after prior placement of a syringosubarachnoid shunt caused a cervicothoracic syrinx to collapse. On a cine MRI, significant dorsal obstruction to CSF flow was seen, along with borderline tonsillar ectopia. This finding directed a posterior fossa decompression rather than another syringosubarachnoid shunt. Collapse of the syrinx and resolution of apnea and weakness occurred within 6 weeks of surgery.

15. Sade et al placed syringosubarachnoid shunts in two pediatric patients.[46] These children had occult spina bifida associated with a terminal syrinx at the time of initial presentation. After the primary releasing procedure, they developed enlargement of the syrinx. A 9-year-old patient had a syringosubarachnoid shunt placed due to new orthopedic symptomatology with the progression of syrinx. Despite the collapse of the syrinx, the clinical status did not improve with syringosubarachnoid shunting, and a new untethering procedure was done. The other 2-year-old patient had no neurologic deficit in the pre- and postoperative periods relating to her primary untethering operation and was operated on to preserve the neurologic status when the syrinx progression was detected.

16. Emmez et al described a 5-day-old girl with a spinal dermal sinus, type II split cord malformation, tethered cord, and a small terminal syrinx.[47] At 5 months of age, the cord was untethered. Her neurologic deficits resolved completely. Four years later, she was admitted with weakness of the foot. A syringosubarachnoid shunt was placed after MRI showed a holocord syrinx from C1 to L5 and no Chiari malformation. Adhesive arachnoiditis was not observed during the operation. Significant relief of neurologic deficits was detected postoperatively.

Complications

Complications of syringosubarachnoid shunting can include obstruction (proximal and distal), dislocation, tethering of the spinal cord by the shunt, and shunt-related infection.[38] Complications can also involve development of a new syrinx[10] and myelotomy-associated neurologic deficits.[48] Fortunately, deficits associated with myelotomy are usually minor and transient.

Based on the pediatric studies highlighted here and other studies involving children and adults, up to 100% of patients seem to have eventual clinical deterioration and shunt failure when followed over time.[38,49,50]

Discussion

A meaningful scientific discussion of the use of syringosubarachnoid shunts in the pediatric population is complicated due to the heterogeneity of etiologies. Patient numbers are small, and studies are usually retrospective.

Surgical techniques are not standardized and also are not fully described in all studies. This involves but is not limited to length of the catheter; type of tubing; amount of bone removed versus laminoplasty; level of drainage; entering the syrinx via the midline versus DREZ; distal insertion of the tube into the dorsal, dorsolateral, or anterior subarachnoid space; type of suture used; and suturing the tube to the pia versus the arachnoid versus no suturing of the tube. Moreover, different surgical techniques and even different shunts (syringosubarachnoid, syringopleural, and syringoperitoneal) are sometimes discussed together in the same study.

Patients have had varied indications for insertion of a syringosubarachnoid shunt, as well as varied pathogenesis causing their syringomyelia. Age ranges in studies are wide. The patients who undergo syringosubarachnoid shunting also often have had a varied surgical history prior to insertion: some patients undergo syringosubarachnoid shunting as a primary operation, other patients have had syringosubarachnoid shunting at the same time of posterior fossa decompression, whereas other patients have undergone syringosubarachnoid shunting only if posterior fossa decompression fails.

Even the technique of diagnosis of syringomyelia is not always uniform within the same study, diagnosis being made by plain myelography, computed tomography–myelography, or MRI. The size and location of the syrinx have not always been reported. We are not always told if the syrinx is loculated or not. The criteria for evaluation of results have differed greatly, especially with respect to objective versus subjective neurologic improvement. Follow-up times quoted in the literature are also highly variable.

An advantage of shunt placement includes immediate cyst drainage with reduction in cyst size.[48] In addition, the procedure is technically easy. However, drainage of septated cysts can be difficult. Drainage of a syrinx below adherent arachnoid scar may place traction on the spinal cord. Syringosubarachnoid shunting may be less likely to cause tethering compared with shunts draining to peritoneal or pleural cavities. However, it assumes the distal subarachnoid space is open and able to absorb CSF, which may not be possible in those with diffuse scarring. Drainage into the subarachnoid space following syringostomy is not always free. Absorption of fluid from the cavity may be imperfect, and reflux from the subarachnoid space to the syrinx can occur.[51] Vernet et al felt that their failures may include the absence of a significant pressure gradient between the syringomyelic cavity and the subarachnoid space, the fact that arachnoiditis affects perimedullary CSF circulation, and with arachnoiditis it may be hard to establish whether the distal tube is in the subarachnoid space.[41] Iwasaki et al asserted that by placing the syringosubarachnoid shunt via the DREZ into the anterior subarachnoid space in front of the dentate ligaments, they decreased the incidence of neuronal and spinal complications and avoided subarachnoid adhesions around the shunt tube.[45] The spinal subarachnoid space shows different anatomical features in the anterior and posterior aspects.[52,53] It is known that the arachnoid septum exists in the posterior subarachnoid space but not anteriorly. Hida et al felt the syringosubarachnoid shunt would be patent for a longer term by inserting the catheter tip into the anterior subarachnoid space because of less chance of adhesions.[54] They also felt that the minimal exposure of the spinal subarachnoid space via a hemilaminectomy may also decrease the chance of postoperative subarachnoid adhesions.[54] In their study, adhesions in the anterior subarachnoid space were not encountered, and there was no shunt malfunction during the time of follow-up.[54] Hida et al also recommended that when treating posttraumatic syringomyelia with a syringosubarachnoid shunt, it was best to choose a site as far from the initial injury as possible.[54] This may avoid arachnoiditis at the injury site.[55]

Intraoperative monitoring and pre- and postoperative assessment with SSEP have shown measurable improvement in the neurophysiologic properties of the spinal cord around

a syrinx after placement of a shunt.[56] This may be due to the relieved mechanical stretching of the axons.[57]

There are no accepted imaging parameters on which to base the decision of whether to place a shunt.[58] The issue of whether a syringosubarachnoid shunt is necessary regardless of the syrinx size is also not resolved. In a patient with Chiari I malformation, Alzate et al asserted that an associated syringomyelia can be treated with a syringosubarachnoid shunt if the syrinx is of significant size and causes symptoms.[58] Vaquero et al recommended syringosubarachnoid shunting for patients with syringomyelia without significant descent of the tonsils or in those cases where posterior fossa operations have failed to obtain good results and the patients show a progressive neurologic picture.[34] Hida et al and Iwasaki et al favored the shunt in cases of rapid neurologic deterioration because they claim it facilitates and accelerates neurologic recovery.[50,59] Koyanagi et al stated that if a patient has a large syrinx and shows signs and symptoms mainly caused by the syrinx, such as progressive motor weakness or pain in the upper limbs, syringosubarachnoid shunting would be their primary method of surgical treatment.[13] Syringosubarachnoid shunt placement also seems to be an effective treatment in symptomatic cases of terminal syringomyelia.[13,40,42,46]

Conclusion

Placement of a syringosubarachnoid shunt should not be considered a first-line treatment for syringomyelia. Based on history and cine MRI, an attempt should be made to determine the cause of the syringomyelia. If the patient is symptomatic from the syringomyelia, surgical treatment should be directed at the underlying presumed etiology. In cases where a patient presents with rapid progressive neurologic deterioration, and prior surgery aimed at the causative mechanism of syringomyelia formation has failed, syringosubarachnoid shunting can be useful at stabilizing the progressive neurologic deterioration. However, over long-term follow-up of 10 years, it can be expected that ~50% of syringosubarachnoid shunts will eventually fail.[38] The failure of shunting with long-term follow-up is particularly important when a pediatric age group is considered, given the expected long-term survival of these patients.[60] This is especially important when we know that a syringosubarachnoid shunt does not address the pathophysiologic mechanism of syrinx formation or if the subarachnoid space is not patent and cannot absorb the syrinx fluid.

Shunting of a syrinx will never reinstitute normal physiologic conditions or provide causative treatment. Because the mechanism of syrinx development is left undisturbed, shunting will be susceptible to failure. The realistic goal of surgical treatment is stabilization of the patient's neurologic status.[61]

We believe, along with Klekamp et al, that optimal results are obtained if the cause of the syrinx is treated rather than the syrinx shunted.[61] Klekamp and colleagues go as far as saying that idiopathic syringomyelia does not exist, insisting there is always a cause for a syrinx.[61] Every effort should be made to identify areas of CSF flow obstruction. In cases of failed foramen magnum procedures in patients with Chiari I malformation, the senior author (RE) agrees with Klekamp et al that it may be necessary to reinvestigate the foramen magnum area for evidence of CSF flow obstruction due to arachnoid scarring. As the senior author has shown, cine MRI can be used to direct a reoperation of the posterior fossa.[10] A second operation at the foramen magnum to establish a free CSF pathway can give far better results than syrinx shunts.[62]

There is no prospective study discussing syringosubarachnoid shunts in the pediatric population with follow-up information over 5 to 10 years. Such a study would be nearly impossible at a single center, given the low patient numbers involved. Despite controversy, syringosubarachnoid shunting certainly has its role in the stabilization and possible neurologic improvement of a patient with syringomyelia, where previous surgery at the underlying cause has failed, and the patient presents with rapid progressive neurologic deterioration.

Acknowledgment The authors thank Dr. Jacob Zauberman for assistance in formatting the MR images.

♦ Lessons Learned

Ebenezer and Ellenbogen illustrate the prevalence of syringomyelia that is idiopathic or associated with other conditions, such as Chiari malformations and spinal cord tumors. The authors highlight the treatment options for these syrinxes. The most important questions to be answered before any surgical procedure are to determine the etiology of the syrinx and determine if the syrinx is symptomatic. The surgeon should not rush to treat a syrinx until he or she ensures that the cervicomedullary decompression is adequately performed, the spinal cord tumor removed, or spinal dysraphism corrected. The authors stress that shunting or stenting of the syrinx should be performed only after treatment of the underlying condition. The other key pearl is that there is communication of the syringes even when septations or haustra are seen on MRI scans. The authors review the literature concerning the surgical technique for syringosubarachnoid stents and the overall results, which are very promising. This is an excellent source for all who care for children with syringomyelia.

References

1. Larroche JC. Malformations of the nervous system: syringomyelia and syringobulbia. In: Adams JH, Corsellis J, Duchin EW, eds. Greenfield's Neuropathology. 4th ed. New York: Wiley and Sons
2. Harwood-Nash DC, Fitz CR. Myelography and syringohydromyelia in infancy and childhood. Radiology 1974;113(3):661–669
3. Peerless SJ, Durward QJ. Management of syringomyelia: a pathophysiological approach. Clin Neurosurg 1983;30:531–576
4. Heiss JD, Oldfield EH. Pathophysiology and treatment of syringomyelia. Contemp Neurosurg 2003;25(3):1–8
5. Oakes WJ, Tubbs RS. Chiari malformations. In: Winn HR, ed. Youmans Neurological Surgery: A Comprehensive Guide to the Diagnosis and Management of Neurosurgical Problems. 5th ed. Philadelphia: WB Saunders; 1993
6. Menezes AH. Chiari I malformations and hydromyelia—complications. Pediatr Neurosurg 1991–1992;17(3):146–154
7. Batzdorf U. Chiari I malformation with syringomyelia: evaluation of surgical therapy by magnetic resonance imaging. J Neurosurg 1988;68(5):726–730
8. Cahan LD, Bentson JR. Considerations in the diagnosis and treatment of syringomyelia and the Chiari malformation. J Neurosurg 1982;57(1):24–31
9. Carmel PW, Markesbery WR. Early descriptions of the Arnold-Chiari malformation: the contribution of John Cleland. J Neurosurg 1972;37(5):543–547
10. Ellenbogen RG, Armonda RA, Shaw DW, Winn HR. Toward a rational treatment of Chiari I malformation and syringomyelia. Neurosurg Focus 2000;8(3):E6
11. Iskandar B, Oakes W. Chiari malformation and syringomyelia. In: Albright L, Pollack I, Adelson P, eds. Principles and Practice of Pediatric Neurosurgery. New York: Thieme Medical Publishers; 1999:165–187
12. Rossier AB, Foo D, Shillito J, Dyro FM. Posttraumatic cervical syringomyelia: incidence, clinical presentation, electrophysiological studies, syrinx protein and results of conservative and operative treatment. Brain 1985;108(Pt 2):439–461
13. Koyanagi I, Iwasaki Y, Hida K, Abe H, Isu T, Akino M. Surgical treatment of syringomyelia associated with spinal dysraphism. Childs Nerv Syst 1997;13(4):194–200
14. Gardner WJ, Angel J. The cause of syringomyelia and its surgical treatment. Cleve Clin Q 1958;25(1):4–8
15. Gardner WJ, Angel J. The mechanism of syringomyelia and its surgical corrections. Clin Neurosurg 1959;6:131–140
16. Gardner WJ, Goodall RJ. The surgical treatment of Arnold-Chiari malformation in adults: an explanation of its mechanism and importance of encephalography in diagnosis. J Neurosurg 1950;7(3):199–206
17. Gardner WJ. Hydrodynamic mechanism of syringomyelia: its relationship to myelocele. J Neurol Neurosurg Psychiatry 1965;28:247–259
18. Williams B. The distending force in the production of "communicating syringomyelia." Lancet 1969;2(7613):189–193

19. Williams B. Pathogenesis of syringomyelia. Acta Neurochir (Wien) 1993;123(3–4):159–165

20. Ball MJ, Dayan AD. Pathogenesis of syringomyelia. Lancet 1972; 2(7781):799–801

21. Oldfield EH, Muraszko K, Shawker TH, Patronas NJ. Pathophysiology of syringomyelia associated with Chiari I malformation of the cerebellar tonsils. Implications for diagnosis and treatment. J Neurosurg 1994;80(1):3–15

22. Heiss JD, Patronas N, DeVroom HL, et al. Elucidating the pathophysiology of syringomyelia. J Neurosurg 1999;91(4):553–562

23. Holly LT, Batzdorf U. Syringomyelia associated with intradural arachnoid cysts. J Neurosurg Spine 2006;5(2):111–116

24. Adams RD, Victor M. Principles of Neurology. 4th ed. New York: McGraw-Hill; 1989

25. La Marca F, Herman M, Grant JA, McLone DG. Presentation and management of hydromyelia in children with Chiari type II malformation. Pediatr Neurosurg 1997;26(2):57–67

26. Iskandar BJ, Hedlund GL, Grabb PA, Oakes WJ. The resolution of syringohydromyelia without hindbrain herniation after posterior fossa decompression. J Neurosurg 1998;89(2):212–216

27. Tubbs RS, Elton S, Grabb P, Dockery SE, Bartolucci AA, Oakes WJ. Analysis of the posterior fossa in children with the Chiari 0 malformation. Neurosurgery 2001;48(5):1050–1054, discussion 1054–1055

28. Vaquero J, Martínez R, Arias A. Syringomyelia-Chiari complex: magnetic resonance imaging and clinical evaluation of surgical treatment. J Neurosurg 1990;73(1):64–68

29. Wisoff JH, Epstein F. Management of hydromyelia. Neurosurgery 1989;25(4):562–571

30. Ergün R, Akdemir G, Gezici AR, et al. Surgical management of syringomyelia-Chiari complex. Eur Spine J 2000;9(6):553–557

31. Van den Bergh R. Headache caused by craniospinal pressure dissociation in the Arnold-Chiari-syringomyelia syndrome. J Neurol 1992;239(5):263–266

32. Lederhaus SC, Pritz MB, Pribram HFW. Septation in syringomyelia and its possible clinical significance. Neurosurgery 1988;22(6 Pt 1): 1064–1067

33. Rhoton AL Jr. Microsurgery of Arnold-Chiari malformation in adults with and without hydromyelia. J Neurosurg 1976;45(5):473–483

34. Vaquero J, Martínez R, Salazar J, Santos H. Syringosubarachnoid shunt for treatment of syringomyelia. Acta Neurochir (Wien) 1987; 84(3–4):105–109

35. Dauser RC, DiPietro MA, Venes JL. Symptomatic Chiari I malformation in childhood: a report of 7 cases. Pediatr Neurosci 1988;14(4):184–190

36. Phillips WA, Hensinger RN, Kling TF Jr. Management of scoliosis due to syringomyelia in childhood and adolescence. J Pediatr Orthop 1990;10(3):351–354

37. Nagib MG. An approach to symptomatic children (ages 4–14 years) with Chiari type I malformation. Pediatr Neurosurg 1994;21(1): 31–35

38. Sgouros S, Williams B. A critical appraisal of drainage in syringomyelia. J Neurosurg 1995;82(1):1–10

39. Farley FA, Song KM, Birch JG, Browne R. Syringomyelia and scoliosis in children. J Pediatr Orthop 1995;15(2):187–192

40. Chapman PH, Frim DM. Symptomatic syringomyelia following surgery to treat retethering of lipomyelomeningoceles. J Neurosurg 1995;82(5):752–755

41. Vernet O, Farmer JP, Montes JL. Comparison of syringopleural and syringosubarachnoid shunting in the treatment of syringomyelia in children. J Neurosurg 1996;84(4):624–628

42. Caldarelli M, Di Rocco C, La Marca F. Treatment of hydromyelia in spina bifida. Surg Neurol 1998;50(5):411–420

43. Weinberg JS, Freed DL, Sadock J, Handler M, Wisoff JH, Epstein FJ. Headache and Chiari I malformation in the pediatric population. Pediatr Neurosurg 1998;29(1):14–18

44. Hida K, Iwasaki Y, Koyanagi I, Abe H. Pediatric syringomyelia with Chiari malformation: its clinical characteristics and surgical outcomes. Surg Neurol 1999;51(4):383–390, discussion 390–391

45. Iwasaki Y, Koyanagi I, Hida K, Abe H. Syringo-subarachnoid shunt for syringomyelia using partial hemilaminectomy. Br J Neurosurg 1999;13(1):41–45

46. Sade B, Beni-Adani L, Ben-Sira L, Constantini S. Progression of terminal syrinx in occult spina bifida after untethering. Childs Nerv Syst 2003;19(2):106–108

47. Emmez H, Güven C, Kurt G, Kardes O, Dogulu F, Baykaner K. Terminal syringomyelia: is it as innocent as it seems? Case report. Neurol Med Chir (Tokyo) 2004;44(10):558–561

48. Batzdorf U. Primary spinal syringomyelia: a personal perspective. Neurosurg Focus 2000;8(3):E7

49. Klekamp J, Batzdorf U, Samii M, Bothe HW. The surgical treatment of Chiari I malformation. Acta Neurochir (Wien) 1996;138(7):788–801

50. Hida K, Iwasaki Y, Koyanagi I, Sawamura Y, Abe H. Surgical indication and results of foramen magnum decompression versus syringosubarachnoid shunting for syringomyelia associated with Chiari I malformation. Neurosurgery 1995;37(4):673–678, discussion 678–679

51. Suzuki M, Davis C, Symon L, Gentili F. Syringoperitoneal shunt for treatment of cord cavitation. J Neurol Neurosurg Psychiatry 1985;48(7):620–627

52. Nauta HJW, Dolan E, Yasargil MG. Microsurgical anatomy of spinal subarachnoid space. Surg Neurol 1983;19(5):431–437

53. Tator CH, Koyanagi I. Vascular mechanisms in the pathophysiology of human spinal cord injury. J Neurosurg 1997;86(3):483–492

54. Hida K, Iwasaki Y, Imamura H, Abe H. Posttraumatic syringomyelia: its characteristic magnetic resonance imaging findings and surgical management. Neurosurgery 1994;35(5):886–891, discussion 891

55. Tator CH. Comments. Neurosurgery 1994;35(5):886–891

56. Wagner W, Perneczky A, Mäurer JC, Hüwel N. Intraoperative monitoring of median nerve somatosensory evoked potentials in cervical syringomyelia: analysis of 28 cases. Minim Invasive Neurosurg 1995;38(1):27–31

57. Milhorat TH, Kotzen RM, Capocelli AL Jr, Bolognese P, Bendo AA, Cottrell JE. Intraoperative improvement of somatosensory evoked potentials and local spinal cord blood flow in patients with syringomyelia. J Neurosurg Anesthesiol 1996;8(3):208–215

58. Alzate JC, Kothbauer KF, Jallo GI, Epstein FJ. Treatment of Chiari I malformation in patients with and without syringomyelia: a consecutive series of 66 cases. Neurosurg Focus 2001;11(1):E3

59. Iwasaki Y, Hida K, Koyanagi I, Abe H. Reevaluation of syringosubarachnoid shunt for syringomyelia with Chiari malformation. Neurosurgery 2000;46(2):407–412, discussion 412–413

60. Krieger MD, McComb JG, Levy ML. Toward a simpler surgical management of Chiari I malformation in a pediatric population. Pediatr Neurosurg 1999;30(3):113–121

61. Klekamp J, Batzdorf U, Samii M, Bothe HW. Treatment of syringomyelia associated with arachnoid scarring caused by arachnoiditis or trauma. J Neurosurg 1997;86(2):233–240

62. Goel A, Desai K. Surgery for syringomyelia: an analysis based on 163 surgical cases. Acta Neurochir (Wien) 2000;142(3):293–301, discussion 301–302

Index

Note: Page numbers followed by *f* and *t* indicate figures and tables, respectively.